The Cardiovascular System:
Key Concepts

The Cardiovascular System: Key Concepts

Edited by **Janice Hunter**

FOSTER
ACADEMICS

New Jersey

Published by Foster Academics,
61 Van Reypen Street,
Jersey City, NJ 07306, USA
www.fosteracademics.com

The Cardiovascular System: Key Concepts
Edited by Janice Hunter

International Standard Book Number: 978-1-63242-388-7 (Hardback)

Printed in the United States of America.

Contents

Permissions

List of Contributors

Preface

This book presents a detailed analysis of the key concepts in cardiovascular system. The cardiovascular system consists of the heart located centrally in the thorax and the vessels of the body which transport blood. The cardiovascular (or circulatory) system supplies oxygen from the air that we inspire, via the lungs to the tissues around the body. It is also responsible for the removal of carbon dioxide via the air that we expire from the lungs. It also supplies the nutrients like amino acids, electrolytes, enzymes, hormones that are important for cellular respiration, immunity and metabolism. The book contains selected information contributed by veterans in this field which describes the latest developments in general and clinical sciences. It covers topics under Clinical Impact of Cardiovascular Physiology and Pathophysiology.

Significant researches are present in this book. Intensive efforts have been employed by authors to make this book an outstanding discourse. This book contains the enlightening chapters which have been written on the basis of significant researches done by the experts.

Finally, I would also like to thank all the members involved in this book for being a team and meeting all the deadlines for the submission of their respective works. I would also like to thank my friends and family for being supportive in my efforts.

Editor

Clinical Impact of Cardiovascular Physiology and Pathophysiology

Physical Activity and Cardiovascular Health

Raul A. Martins
University of Coimbra,
Faculty of Sport Science and Physical Education,
Portugal

1. Introduction

The approach of this chapter makes the assumption that relationships between levels of physical activity and cardiovascular health are complex. The theoretical framework considers that physical activity can influence cardiovascular health by itself but can also influence health-related fitness, which in turn may be able to influence cardiovascular health and the level of habitual physical activity. To add more complexity, all these relationships are thought to occur in a reciprocal manner.

Cardiovascular disease corresponds to a group of disorders occurring in the heart and in the blood vessels. The various manifestations of the disease include sudden death, myocardial infarction, angina pectoris, stroke (ischemic or hemorrhagic), or peripheral vascular disease. The risk factors for the cardiovascular diseases are classified usually considering the positive or negative association with the disease and the modifiable or non-modifiable nature. On the other hand, the definition of criterions to some risk factors could be dependent of the context of prevention – primordial, primary, secondary, tertiary or even quaternary. Additionally, it is necessary the plausibility theoretic and biological, and the reversibility of the effect by the reduction or suspension of the risk factor. Modifiable risk factors like dyslipidemia, hypertension, diabetes, excess of adipose tissue, pro-coagulant state, pro-inflammatory state, ignorance, sedentariness or low fitness play alone or, more frequently, in conjunction with each others, augmenting exponentially the risk of disease.

White Paper on Sport (CEC, 2007) was released by the European Union (EU) to give strategic orientation on the role of sport in Europe. The document use the definition of "sport" established by the Council of Europe: "all forms of physical activity which, through casual or organized participation, aim at expressing or improving physical fitness and mental well-being, forming social relationships or obtaining results in competition at all levels." With the ratification of the Lisbon Treaty in late 2009, sport was assumed as contributing to the EU strategic objectives of solidarity and prosperity. This follows the Olympic ideal, born in Europe, of developing sport to promote peace and understanding among nations and cultures as well as the education of young people. Member States are encouraged to implement evidence-based policies in order to improve their provision of sporting facilities and opportunities. This means that for the first time the EU is actively aiming to promote sport and physical activity at the policy level – not only with a view to improving physical wellbeing and health across the EU, which is the main focus of this chapter, but also to enhance the role of sport in boosting social cohesion and its educational value. This chapter will explore the relationship of cardiovascular health with sport, as the European understanding, or physical activity in the North American understanding. Physical activity concept, physical activity epidemiology and cardiovascular health, physical activity guidelines, prevalence of sedentariness in Europe and USA, physical activity and life expectancy, and pro-inflammatory state and physical activity are topics explored in this chapter.

2. Physical activity

Physical activity comprises any body movement produced by the skeletal muscles that results in a substantial increase over the resting energy expenditure (Bouchard & Shephard, 1994). Included in this large umbrella is considered the leisure-time physical activity (LTPA), daily physical activities, intentionally practiced exercise (frequency, intensity, type, time) and sport, or occupational work, together with other physical expressions that modify the total energy expenditure. Within the concept of physical activity, physical exercise is a narrow concept, usually defined as planned and repeated movements intending to maintain or to improve one or more components of the health-related fitness or of the performance-related fitness. Physical activity has been understood as a behavior that could also change health-related or performance-related fitness. However, it is also taken in account as a determinant behavior to health and functionality. When one is talking about the potential benefits on health, obviously, all determinants of human energy expenditure should be under careful consideration. Contrarily, sedentariness refers that people remain sitting much of the labor and leisure times.

There are a lot of methods to characterize and measure the behavior *physical activity* including calorimetry (direct and indirect), physiologic markers (heart rate or maximal oxygen uptake) mechanical and electronic devices (pedometers and accelerometers), the observation of behaviors, or the caloric intake (Welk, 2002). Independently of the selected method, the investigator should consider the complex nature of the behavior physical activity and the errors derived from the method usually used with largest number of participants – the self-reported questionnaires. The use of questionnaires imply low costs but sometimes introduces considerable error because, for instance, could exist social tendency to associate physical activity to sport participation. It means that it is desirable to use direct methods as pedometers or accelerometers. Pedometers count the number of steps but are not able to distinguish different levels of activity. This limitation is overcome by the accelerometry, and the last National Health and Nutrition Examination Survey (NHANES) realized in 2003-2004 evaluated physical activity of around 4867 American citizens with accelerometry (Troiano et al., 2008).

3. Prevalence of sedentariness

A national representative study of Portuguese people has measured directly physical activity by accelerometry (Baptista et al., 2011). Volunteered to participate 5231 adolescents (10-17 years-old; 1456 males; 1755 females), adults (18-64 years-old; 441 males; 803 females), and older adults (65+ years-old; 303 males; 473 females). All participants were measured during four days (two week days and two weekend days). The cut-off points for moderate intensity were 3-5,9 METs (adults and older adults) and 4-6,9 METs (adolescents), and for vigorous intensity were 6+ METs (adults and older adults) and 7+ METs (adolescents). Adolescents with less than 60 minutes/day of moderate/vigorous physical activity on 5 days/week, and adults or older adults with less than 30 minutes/day on 5 days/week were classified as 'insufficiently active'.

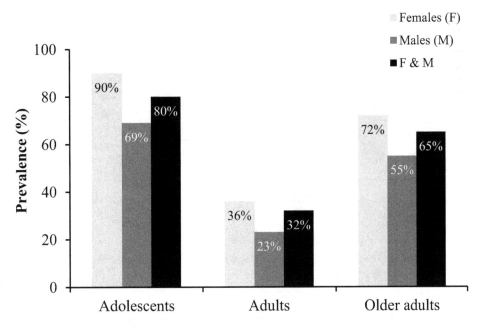

Source: Baptista et al., 2011.

Fig. 1. Prevalence of 'insufficiently active' Portuguese people measured by accelerometry.

As illustrated by Figure 1, the prevalence of insufficiently active people was particularly high in the adolescents (80%) but also in the older adults (65%). The adult people (18-64 years old) attained only 32%, which represents the group with higher volume of moderate/vigorous weekly physical activity. The prevalence of insufficiently active in all the people evaluated was 67%. Males are more active than females, in each one of the three groups, with higher difference (21%) among adolescents and lower difference among adults (13%). One can speculate that the indirect methods like self-reported questionnaires tend to overestimate physical activity when compared with a direct measure (accelerometry), as seems to result when one compares these overall data (67%) with data provided from Eurobarometer 2003 (30%) and Eurobarometer 2010 (52%) on Figure 2. However, the high prevalence of insufficiently active, particularly in adolescents and older adults, claim for the adoption of specific strategies to change these sedentary behaviors.

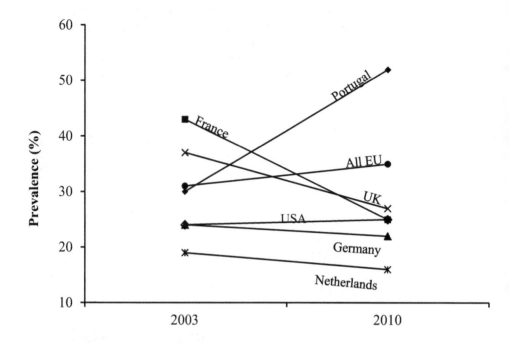

USA data is No Leisure-Time Physical Activity in 2003, and 2008.

http://www.cdc.gov/nccdphp/dnpa/physical/stats/leisure_time.htm. Extracted on 24/Oct/2011.

Fig. 2. Prevalence of the sedentariness in some EU Member States measured by self-reported questionnaires.

Data from the 2003 Eurobarometer (EC, 2003) are presented in Figure 2. Sedentary people are those not meeting the threshold for low activity. Cut-off points for low physical activity participation were 30 minutes of walking or moderate-intensity activity on at least 5 days/week, or 20 minutes of vigorous-intensity activity on at least 3 days/week. Participated people from each one of the EU Member States with 15+ years-old (N=16230), randomly sampling with probability proportional to population size (for a total coverage of the country) and to population density (metropolitan, urban, and rural areas). It was used the International Physical Activity Questionnaire (IPAQ) to characterize physical activity in a face-to-face interview in people's home and in the appropriate national language. Frequency of 5+ days/week of moderate intensity physical activity was not achieved by 72% of EU Member States citizens (equal for women and men) while 74% did not achieve 3+ days/week of vigorous intensity physical activity (81% on women, and 68% on men). Prevalence of people who do not practiced 3+ days/week of vigorous intensity increases with age from 66% (15-25 years) to 69% (26-44 years), to 76% (45-64 years), and to 89% (65+ years). Prevalence of people not engaged on 5+ days/week of moderate intensity also increases with age: 70% (15-25 years), 70% (26-44 years), 72% (45-64 years), and 79% (65+ years).

The 2010 Eurobarometer (EC, 2010) analyzed people with 15+ years-old of 27 EU Member States (N=26788), with a different self-reported questionnaire than IPAQ, and revealed a prevalence of 27% for people saying they engage in physical activity regularly at least 5 times/week, while 38% answered that exercising with some regularity (1-4 times/week) (Figure 2). The other 35% EU citizens never engage in any physical activity or engage below the desirable level (1-3 times/month). By analyzing data from some EU Member States it is possible to observe clear discrepancies in the values from 2003 to 2010. These discrepancies maybe is reflecting partially the utilization of different instruments with different self-reported answers. Sedentariness was considered in Eurobarometer 2010 to the people that engage only 1-2 times/month or even less in physical activities. With these cut-off points, sedentariness was respectively in 2003 and 2010: Portugal - 30% and 52%; France - 43% and 25%; Germany – 24% and 22%; UK – 37% and 27%; Netherlands – 19% and 16%; All EU – 31% and 35%.

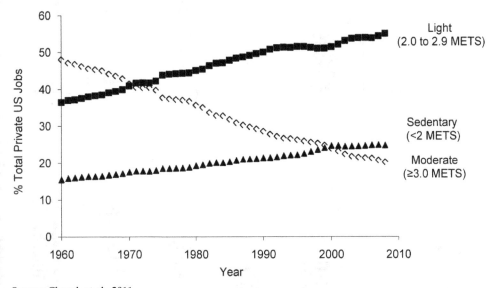

Source: Church et al., 2011.

Fig. 3. Trends in the prevalence of sedentary, light and moderate intensity occupations from 1960 to 2008.

Troiano and colleagues (2008) have described physical activity levels of children (6-11 years old), adolescents (12-19 years old), and adults (20+ years old), using objective data obtained with accelerometers from a representative sample of the U.S. population. The results were attained from the 2003-2004 National Health and Nutritional Examination Survey (NHANES), a cross-sectional study of a complex, multistage probability sample of the civilian, noninstitutionalized population. Data are described from 6329 participants who provided at least 1 day of accelerometer data and from 4867 participants who provided 4+ days of accelerometer data. Males were more physically active than females. Authors observed that physical activity declines dramatically across age groups between childhood (42% obtained the recommended 60 minutes/day) and adolescence (8% achieve 60 minutes/day) and continues to decline in adults (less than 5% attained 30 minutes/day). Objective and subjective measures of physical activity gave qualitatively similar results regarding gender and age patterns of activity. However, adherence to physical activity recommendations according to accelerometer-measured activity is substantially lower than according to self-reported questionnaire. Occupational work is also an important expression of physical activity contributing to energy expenditure and to the energy balance.

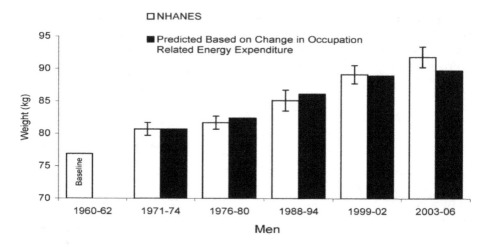

Men

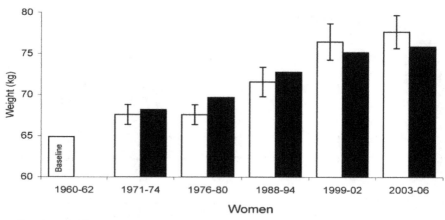

Women

Source: Church et al., 2011.

Fig. 4. Predicted mean U.S. body weight based on change in occupation related daily energy expenditure since 1960 compared to mean U.S. weight gain based on the NHANES examination periods for 40–50 year old.

Trends in occupational physical activity during the past 5 decades (Figure 3), and the concurrent changes in body weight in the U.S. were explored by Church and colleagues (2011). Authors observed that in 1960 almost half the jobs (48%) in private industry in the

U.S. required at least moderate intensity physical activity whereas in 2008 less than 20% demand this level of energy expenditure. While there has been a steady increase in the prevalence of sedentary and light intensity physical activity occupations since 1960, the prevalence of moderate intensity physical activity occupations has decreased. At the same period (1960-2008) there was a drop in occupation-related daily energy expenditure of about 142 calories for men and 124 calories for women. Authors estimate that the decrease of 142 calories in men would result in an increase in mean weight from 76.9 kg (1960-62) to 89.7 kg (2003-06), with the results having similar pattern for women (Figure 4).

Over the last 50 years the prevalence of Americans in the labor force has increased approximately 40% to 50%, with women assuming a growing prevalence in the work force from 43% in 1970 to 60% in 2007. This fact helps to explain the decrease in the pattern of occupation-related energy expenditure (Lee & Mather, 2008). Given this, it is unlikely a return to occupations demanding moderate levels of physical activity, which addresses further strong evidence of the public health importance of promoting physically active lifestyles outside of the work day. The reduction of 124 (women) and 142 calories (men) per day in occupation-related energy expenditure over the last 50 years would have been adequately compensated for by meeting the 2008 Physical Activity Guidelines of 150 minutes/week of moderate intensity activity or 75 minutes/week of vigorous intensity activity (USDHHS, 2011). While it is often noted that the prevalence of Americans who achieve this recommendation has been constant over recent decades, the fact remains that based on self-report data only 25% adults achieve this level (CDC, 2008), but when physical activity is assessed with accelerometers the number of adult people achieving the recommendations drops dramatically to less than 5% (Troiano et al., 2008). Therefore, since energy expenditure of the labor activities has largely been removed, the relative importance of LTPA has increased and should be considered as a major focus of public health interventions and research.

Brownson and colleagues (2005) developed a revision to describe current patterns and long-term trends (up to 50 years when possible) related to (i) physical activity, (ii) employment and occupation, (iii) travel behavior, (iv) land use, and (v) related behaviors (e.g., television watching). Available data allows the following trends: relatively stable or slightly increasing levels of LTPA, declining work-related activity, declining transportation activity, declining activity in the home, and increasing sedentary activity. These reflect an overall trend of declining total physical activity, with large differences noted in the rates of walking for transportation across metropolitan areas, and a strong linear increase in vehicle miles traveled per person, coupled with a strong and consistent trend toward people living in suburbs. Authors concluded that although difficult to quantify, it appears that a combination of changes to the built environment and increases in the proportion of the population engaging in sedentary activities put the majority of the population at high risk of physical inactivity.

4. Physical activity guidelines

Vigorous activity was centrally considered to health promotion until 1995 when recommendations of the Center for Disease Control (CDC) and the American College of Sports Medicine (ACSM) pointed out for adults to accumulate at least 30 minutes of moderate-intensity physical activity on most days of the week (Pate et al., 1995). These recommendations were described in the 1996 U.S. Surgeon General's Report on Physical Activity and Health (USDHHS, 1996), and served as cornerstone for the Healthy People 2010 (HP 2010) goals on physical activity (USDHHS, 2000), inspiring public policies and programs over the next years. The HP 2010 objectives stated that adults should engage in vigorous LTPA (60-84%VO_{2Res} or %HR_{Res}; 77-93%HR_{max}; >60%VO_{2max}; >6 METs) for at least 20 minutes, at least 3 times/week, or moderate LTPA (40-59%VO_{2Res} or %HR_{Res}; 64-76%HR_{max}; 40-60%VO_{2max}; 3-6 METs) for at least 30 minutes, at least 5 times/week.

For the purposes of HP 2010, lesser amounts of vigorous and moderate activities could not be combined. In 2007, the CDC/ACSM recommendations published in 1995 were updated and clarified, emphasizing the potential health benefits of combinations of moderate and vigorous-intensity activities and of strengthening activities (Haskell et al., 2007). Meantime, the Healthy People 2020 (HP 2020) goals on physical activity were released (USDHHS, 2010) introducing some modifications, and establishing and encouraging to increase the prevalence of "sufficiently active" adults engaging in moderate-intensity aerobic physical activity of at least 150 minutes/week or vigorous-intensity aerobic activity of at least 75 minutes/week or an equivalent combination. The HP 2020 also pursue to increase the prevalence of "highly active" adults engaging in aerobic physical activity of at least moderate intensity for more than 300 minutes/week or more than 150 minutes/week of vigorous intensity or an equivalent combination. And, finally, to increase the prevalence of adults who perform muscle-strengthening activities on 2 or more days/week of 7 large muscle groups.

5. Physical activity and life expectancy

Mortality differentials by level and intensity of physical activity have been documented, with Lollgen and colleagues (2009) obtaining significant association of lower all-cause mortality for active individuals comparing with sedentary persons. Highly active men had a 22% lower risk of all-cause mortality (RR=0.78; 95% CI: 0.72 to 0.84), and women had 31% (RR=0.69; 95% CI: 0.53 to 0.90) comparing to mildly active men and women, respectively. The authors also found a similar and significant association of activity to all-cause mortality in older participants.

Schoenborn and Stommel (2011) studying the benefits of accomplish the 2008 Physical Activity Guidelines for Adults (USDHHS, 2011), which are similar to the HP 2020 goals, achieved 27% lower risk of all-cause mortality among people without existing chronic comorbidities, and by almost half among people with chronic comorbidities (such as heart disease, stroke, diabetes, cancer, respiratory conditions, or any functional limitation), regardless of age and obesity levels. Assuming several limitations present on causal interpretations, when examining for interactions of physical activity with smoking and alcohol consumption, data suggest that relative survival benefits associated with physical activity are largest among current smokers and light-moderate drinkers.

Figure 5 shows the survival curves associated with four types of adherence to the 2008 Guidelines for all adults: meeting both the aerobic and muscle-strengthening guidelines, the aerobic only, the muscle-strengthening only, and neither of the minimum recommendations. This figure suggests that meeting the 2008 Guidelines is associated with survival benefits, with stronger benefits for both the aerobic and muscle-strengthening exercises; also suggests that aerobic activity alone promotes stronger benefits than muscle strengthening alone.

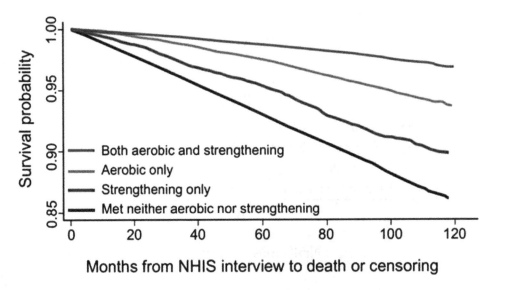

Months from NHIS interview to death or censoring

Note: U.S. adults aged ≥ 18 years (weighted); respondents not linked to death records were considered "censored", meaning they were presumed to be alive as of December 31, 2006. NHIS, National Health Interviews Survey, 1997-2004.

Adapted from Schoenborn and Stommel (2011)

Fig. 5. Survival probabilities by levels of adherence to 2008 Physical Activity Guidelines.

Figure 6 illustrates that higher volumes of aerobic exercise are associated with higher increase in survival probabilities. Those who engage in none aerobic leisure-time activity attained lower survival probability while people that engaged in more than 300 minutes/week have the higher survival probability. In other words, it means that additional survival benefits can be achieved with higher levels of aerobic leisure-time activity.

6. Epidemiology of physical activity and cardiovascular health

Epidemiology has been defined as "the study of the distribution and determinants of health-related states or events in specified populations, and the application of this study to the prevention and control of health problems" (Last, 2001). When this definition considers 'health-related states or events' instead of the former 'disease frequency' is having in account the contemporary definition of health that considers positive health states, as a good quality of life, or well succeeded aging, and not only the absence of disease. The word 'epidemiology' is derived from the Greek words: *epi* "upon", *demos* "people", and *logos* "study". In fact, epidemiology origin based on Hippocrates observation, made more than 2000 years ago, that environmental factors could be determinant for the occurrence of a disease. However, it was only in second half of the XIX century when the first truly epidemiologic investigations appeared (Bonita et al., 2006).

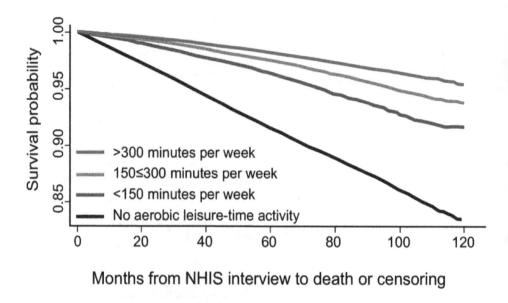

Months from NHIS interview to death or censoring

Note: U.S. adults aged ≥ 18 years (weighted); respondents not linked to death records were considered "censored", meaning they were presumed to be alive as of December 31, 2006. NHIS, National Health Interviews Survey, 1997-2004.

Adapted from Schoenborn and Stommel (2011).

Fig. 6. Survival probabilities by levels of adherence to 2008 aerobic physical activity guidelines.

Physical activity and the relationship with cardiovascular health was firstly studied in an epidemiologic basis by Morris and colleagues (1953a,b). Works were conducted to understand how both vocational and LTPA relate to fitness and risk of coronary heart disease (CHD). Authors studied London transit workers, and other occupations as postal service employees and civil servants. Initially they found bus conductors on London's double-decker omnibuses to be at lower risk than bus drivers; what disease the conductors did develop was less severe, and they were more likely to survive an attack. The conductors, who walked up and down stairs in a daily basis, often for decades, experienced roughly half the number of heart attacks and sudden death as the drivers. After that, Morris and colleagues (1990) studied a random sample of 3591 British civil servants during a follow-up of 8-year period ending in 1977, during which time 268 men died. Subjects were classified as having engaged in vigorous activities (>6 METs), or not. Of the subjects 22% reported some kind of vigorous exercise and their death rate was 4,2%. The remaining 78% reported no vigorous exercise and their mortality rate was 8,2%, i.e., twice as high. This differential in death rates persisted when controlling for age, smoking, obesity and successive intervals of follow up.

Several other populations have been studied for physical activity and physiological fitness in relation to health and specifically cardiovascular health (USDHHS, 1996). One of the most remarkable studies was conducted with 17549 men who entered Harvard College between

1916 and 1950 (Paffenbarger et al., 1978), and when aged 55–84 years responded to a questionnaire on their personal characteristics, health status and lifestyle habits like current and former physical activity, as participation in student sport whilst at university. These patterns have been related to cardiovascular disease mortality over a 16-year follow-up period (1962 to 1978), during which 1413 men died (Paffenbarger et al., 1986a,b).

Among Harvard alumni there were strong significant inverse associations between death rates and levels of each of the following physical activity: walking, stair climbing, sports play and combinations of these activities, measured in kJ/week. Gradients of benefit from more active lifestyles were consistent throughout, and maintained after controlling for age, smoking, hypertension and obesity. As compared with the one-third of least active men, the middle third experienced a 23 % reduction in death rate during follow-up and the one-third of most active men, a 32 % reduction. Light activities (<4METs), moderate activities (4–5METs), and vigorous activities (>6METs) each predicted lower death rates. Physical activity related inversely to total mortality, primarily to death due to cardiovascular or respiratory causes. Death rates declined steadily as energy expended on such activities increased from less than 500kcal/week to 3500kcal/week, beyond which rates increased slightly. This relationship was independent of the presence or absence of hypertension, cigarette smoking, extremes or gains in body weight, or early parental death (Figure 7).

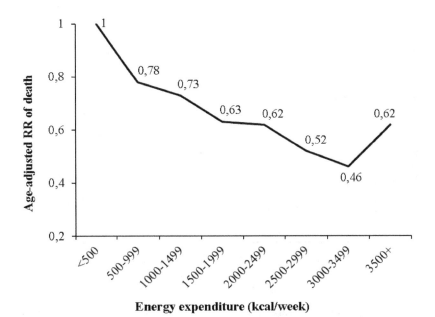

Source: Paffenbarger et al., 1986a.

Notes: Participated 16936 men. A total of 1413 alumni died during 12 to 16 years of follow-up (1962-1978). Exercise reported as walking, stair climbing, sports play, and combinations of these activities.

Fig. 7. Inverse association between weekly energy expenditure and RR of all-cause mortality.

Those men were studied for the effect on all-cause mortality from changing physical activity habits. Men who had increased or decreased their activity by less than 250kcal/week between the 1960s and 1977 were considered in an 'unchanged' category. Compared with their death rates, gradient reductions in mortality were observed with increased levels of physical activity, and gradient increases in mortality with decreased levels of activity. At the extremes of this gradient, men who had increased their energy expenditure by 1250kcal/week had a 20% lower risk of death than men in the unchanged category; men who decreased their activity by 1250kcal/week had a 26% higher risk (Paffenbarger et al., 1993, 1994).

Vigorous activity should be encouraged. Not only because in today's world, where time is a precious commodity, a short period of vigorous exercise expends as much energy as does moderate activity carried out for two or three times as long (Figures 8 and 9), but also because the kind of stimulation over tissues and systems could be more benefic to compensate lost, asymptomatic in an initial stage, that tends to occur with aging.

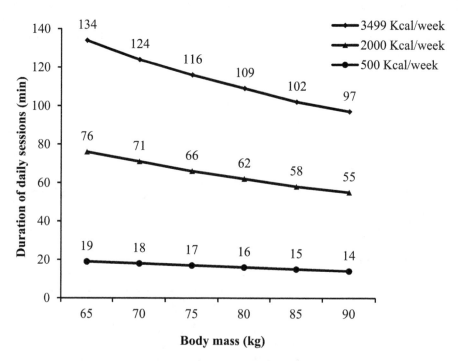

Fig. 8. Duration (min) of daily walking sessions, with moderate intensity (velocity of 80m/min; 3,3METs), for people with different body masses, to gain cardiovascular health (500kcal/week: RR=1,00; 2000kcal/week: RR≈0,62; 3499kcal/week: RR≈0,46).

Figure 8 illustrates time spent with walking at moderate intensity (velocity of 80m/min, or 4,8km/h) by people of different body masses, within the range 500-3499kcal/week (Paffenbarger et al., 1986a). A person weighting 75kg will needs to walk 116 minutes per each one of the 7 days of the week to maximize the potential benefits of physical activity on cardiovascular health, i.e. to spend 3499kcal/week (RR=0,46). In other words, and taking in account the work of Paffenbarger and colleagues (1986a) illustrated by the Figure 1, a person of 75kg will obtain progressive cardiovascular gain from 17 minutes of horizontal walking (RR=1,0) to 116 minutes of daily horizontal walking (RR=0,46). However, if that same person of 75kg of body mass decides to exercise at vigorous intensity (Figure 9), 40 minutes of horizontal running at 150m/min (9km/h) will be enough to maximize the potential gains on cardiovascular health.

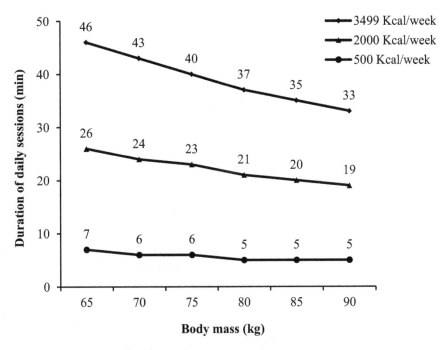

Fig. 9. Duration (min) of daily running sessions, with vigorous intensity (velocity of 150m/min; 9,6METs), for people with different body masses, to gain cardiovascular health (500kcal/week: RR=1,00; 2000kcal/week: RR≈0,62; 3499kcal/week: RR≈0,46).

7. Pro-inflammatory state and physical activity

Inflammation has emerged some years ago as a key pathophysiological event in vascular diseases and the consequent cardiovascular and cerebral injury. Inflammation is a complex process involving multiple cellular and molecular components, and is triggered by different pro-inflammatory mediators generated directly and indirectly by microbial invasion, endotoxins, immune complexes, and cytokines. Vascular endothelium is subjected to pro-inflammatory insults but fortunately is awarded with strong anti-inflammatory molecules that confer resistance to damage by transient pro-inflammatory attacks.

Inflammation is a natural response to infection or damage that intends to destroy or to inactivate the foreign agents permitting tissues repairing. Inflammation could be a local or systemic response, and the key mediators are the cells that act as phagocytes, with the most important being neutrophils, macrophages, and macrophages-like cells. The sequence of local events in a typical nonspecific inflammatory response includes: (i) vasodilatation of the microcirculation in the infected area, leading to increased blood flow; (ii) large increase in protein permeability of the capillaries and venules in the infected area, with resulting diffusion of protein and filtration of fluid into the interstitial fluid; (iii) chemotaxis: movement of leukocytes from the venules into the interstitial fluid of the infected area; (iv) destruction of bacteria in the tissue either through phagocytosis or by other mechanisms; (v) tissue repair (Widmaier et al., 2011). The events of inflammation, such as vasodilation, are induced and regulated by several chemical mediators including kinins, complement, products of blood clotting, histamine, eicosanoids, platelet-activating factors, cytokines, nitric oxide, C-reactive protein (CRP). CRP is an acute phase protein produced by the liver, always found at some concentration in the plasma, and act to minimize the extent of local tissue damage. CRP can bind nonspecifically to carbohydrates or lipids in the cell wall of microbes and facilitate opsonization to enhance phagocytosis.

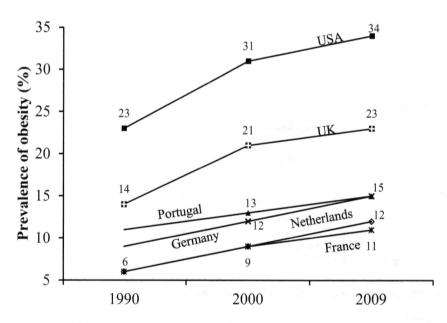

Source: OECD Health Data 2011. Extracted on 25 Oct 2011 from:

http://stats.oecd.org/Index.aspx?DataSetCode=HEALTH_LVNG

Notes: Data of Portugal are self-reported, in 1999 and 2006; data of France are self-reported, in 1990, 2000 and 2008; data of Germany are self-reported, in 1999 and 2009; data of UK are measured in 1991, 2000 and 2009; data of Netherlands are self-reported, in 1990, 2000 and 2009; data of USA are measured in 1991, 2000 and 2008.

Fig. 10. Decennial evolution of obesity (BMI ≥ 30kg/m²) in % of total population.

There is scientific evidence indicating to atherosclerosis as an inflammatory disease (De Haro et al., 2008; Hamer & Stamatakis, 2008; Virani et al., 2008). In fact, some of the most prevalent risk factors for cardiovascular diseases have been shown to have a pro-inflammatory action including hypertension (Imatoh et al., 2007; Hamer & Stamatakis, 2008), diabetes (Porrini et al., 2007; Hwang et al., 2008), dyslipidemia (Kim et al., 2007), and overweight or obesity (Hamer & Stamatakis, 2008; Piestrzeniewicz et al., 2008). As high-sensitivity C-reactive protein (hs-CRP) is a sensitive marker of inflammation, it has been pointed as the golden marker of inflammation, with Berk and colleagues (1990) establishing for the first time a positive association between hs-CRP and angina pectoris. Other authors have also found positive association of the hs-CRP with risk of vascular disease (Koenig et al., 1999; Kuller et al., 1996; Ridker et al., 1998a; Ridker et al., 2002; Ridker et al., 2003). Since then, various investigations have concentrated on the effects of physical activity on hs-CRP (Church et al., 2002; Martins et al., 2010a; Martins et al., 2010b; Mora et al., 2006; Wannamethee et al., 2002).

Figure 10 illustrates decennial evolution of obesity, self-reported or measured, in different countries of Europe and North America. United States of America and United Kingdom attained higher values of obesity (BMI $\geq$ 30kg/m^2) prevalence, according to the Organization for Economic Co-Operation and Development (OECD) 2011 health data, with 34% and 23% in 2009, respectively. The importance of this risk factor in this context is related with pro-inflammation action, as referred above. One would yet speculate that self-reported data by people in Portugal, France, Germany, and Netherlands are below to the real prevalence, which addresses for a rise of prevalence of obesity in these countries to values close to the measured ones in the USA and UK.

	Before	After
Body weight (kg)	73 (11)	72 (11)*
Waist circumference (cm)	94 (10)	91 (10)**
Body mass index (kg/m^2)	30.6 (5.0)	30.3 (4.9)*
Blood pressure (mm Hg)		
Systolic	149 (21)	150 (19)
Diastolic	77 (10)	74 (9)*
Triglycerides (mmol/l)	1.35 (0.58)	1.20 (0.54)*
Total cholesterol (mmol/l)	5.64 (0.86)	5.29 (1.03)*
HDL-cholesterol (mmol/l)	1.31 (0.25)	1.37 (0.32)*
LDL-cholesterol (mmol/l)	2.36 (0.77)	2.05 (0.86)**
Total Cholesterol/HDL-cholesterol	4.40 (0.92)	4.02 (0.81)**
hs-CRP (mg/l)	5.4 (3.9)	4.0 (2.0)*
6-minute walk distance (m)	387 (76)	437 (83)**

Values are mean (SD). *p<0.05, **p<0.01 compared with before.

Source: Martins RA et al., (2010b).

Table 1. Exercising group.

Measurement of cholesterol by itself do not allow the recognition of about of the individuals who will present later with myocardial infarctions (Rifai & Ridker, 2001), and a number of studies (Ridker et al., 1998b; Ridker et al., 2001; Ridker et al., 2002; Onat et al., 2001; Torres & Ridker, 2003) reinforce the idea that introducing markers of inflammation in the models of diagnosis, beyond the lipid profile, result in more accuracy to predict atherogenic events, comparing with lipid-based models only. High serum levels of CRP have also been found not only in patients with elevated blood pressure but also in those with congestive heart failure (Barbieri et al., 2003; Torre-Amione, 2005), type 2 diabetes, metabolic syndrome and obesity (Das, 2001; Pradham et al., 2001; Ridker et al., 2003). Therefore, factors that may impact negatively hs-CRP levels, like physical activity, should be further studied, particularly in populations at increased risk of the above diseases.

	Before	After
Body weight (kg)	71 (12)	70 (13)
Waist circumference (cm)	93 (10)	91 (10)**
Body mass index (kg/m²)	29.0 (4.4)	28.8 (4.7)
Blood pressure (mm Hg)		
Systolic	146 (20)	142 (24)
Diastolic	76 (9)	75 (13)
Triglycerides (mmol/l)	1.10 (0.35)	1.15 (0.35)
Total cholesterol (mmol/l)	5.14 (0.94)	5.27 (1.02)
HDL-cholesterol (mmol/l)	1.33 (0.28)	1.32 (0.29)
LDL-cholesterol (mmol/l)	2.39 (0.86)	2.27 (0.61)
Total Cholesterol/HDL-cholesterol	3.99 (0.98)	4.07 (0.83)
hs-CRP (mg/l)	5.5 (3.5)	5.1 (2.3)
6-minute walk distance (m)	342 (126)	343 (170)

Values are mean (SD). *$p<0.05$, **$p<0.01$ compared with before.

Source: Martins RA et al., (2010b).

Table 2. Control group.

Inflammatory processes have been positively associated with aging (Pedersen et al., 2003), with studies suggesting that physical activity would benefit atherosclerotic disease, at least partially, by reducing the inflammatory level (Wannamethee et al., 2002; Reuben et al., 2003). Serum CRP levels has been negatively associated with physical activity or physical fitness, but also with BMI and other adiposity measures (Church et al., 2002; Wannamethee et al., 2002; Mora et al., 2006; Martins et al., 2010b). These studies suggest that regular physical exercise might lower CRP levels, acting as an anti-inflammatory agent, by the effects over adipose tissue and/or by the effects on the muscle mass.

Martins and colleagues (2010b) present results (Table 1) showing beneficial effects of two exercising programs (i.e., aerobic and strength-based) in older adults with significant differences on body weight (-1%), waist circumference (-3%), BMI (-1%), diastolic blood pressure (-4%), triglycerides (-11%), total cholesterol (-6%), HDL-cholesterol (5%), LDL-cholesterol (-13%), total cholesterol/HDL-cholesterol relationship (-9%), hs-CRP (-26%), and 6-minute walk distance (13%), while the control group (Table 2) only had significant differences on waist circumference (-2%). At baseline, BMI correlated with total cholesterol ($r=0.35$, $p=0.007$), triglycerides ($r=0.38$, $p=0.004$), and hs-CRP ($r=0.46$, $p=0.001$). Waist circumference correlated with total cholesterol ($r=0.30$, $p=0.022$), triglycerides ($r=0.35$, $p=0.010$), hs-CRP ($r=0.38$, $p=0.010$), and total cholesterol/HDL-cholesterol ($r=0.38$, $p=0.005$). Finally, body weight also correlated with total cholesterol ($r=0.33$, $p=0.011$), triglycerides ($r=0.27$, $p=0.044$), hs-CRP ($r=0.40$, $p=0.006$), and total cholesterol/HDL-cholesterol ($r=0.33$, $p=0.016$).

Studies examining the effects on cardiovascular health by endurance and strength training have generally found either positive changes in lipid profile or no changes at all. More pronounced dyslipidemia at baseline has been pointed has having more favorable changes after training (Laaksonen et al., 2000), mediated by the reduction of body fat (Leon & Sanchez, 2001). On the other hand, older people are known to be under the effects of sarcopenia, which is characterized by loss of skeletal muscle mass and strength weakness. Sarcopenia has been associated not only with functional fitness impairment (Reid et al., 2008) but also with systemic inflammation (Visser et al., 2002). Resistance training (Marini et al., 2008) has been suggested to be an effective way to prevent the adverse outcomes of sarcopenia whereas the effects of aerobic training are not as clear.

The mechanisms underlying the positive effects of the physical activity on inflammation remain under discussion, being considered the hypothesis of reduction of body fat, and/or the increase of muscle mass. Some have hypothesized about changes in circulating inflammatory cytokine levels alter hs-CRP hepatic production. Reductions of serum IL-18, IL-6 and CRP have been reported after 10 months of aerobic exercise but not after flexibility/resistance exercise (Kohut et al., 2006). However, others failed to obtain exercise-induced effects in plasmatic inflammatory cytokines, including IL-6, TNF-α and IL-1β after 12 weeks of combined aerobic/resistance and flexibility training (Stewart et al., 2007). Additionally, TNF-α may contribute directly to sarcopenia once can disrupt the differentiation process in cultured muscle cells and promotes catabolism in mature muscle cells. Muscle mass is a primary site for glucose and triglyceride disposal (Dinneen et al., 1992) and the major determinant of metabolic rate (Zurlo et al., 1994). Age-related muscle loss may contribute to insulin resistance, dyslipidemia and increased adiposity. IL-6 protein is expressed in contracting muscle fibers and released from skeletal muscle during exercise whereas this is not the case for TNF-α (Steensberg et al., 2002). IL-6 is able to inhibit TNF-α, and IL-1 production stimulates the production of IL-1ra and IL-10 and the release of soluble TNF-receptors (Steensberg et al., 2003). In synthesis, a chronic training-induced reduction on hs-CRP concentrations in older adults is supported by various studies having as key factors increase in muscular mass and reduction in body fat.

8. Summary

Exercise and physical activity, or a wide concept of sport as defined by the Council of Europe, are cornerstones to act at different levels of prevention for cardiovascular health. Physical activity comprises any voluntary movement that substantially increases oxygen uptake above the resting level. Prevalence of sedentariness should be considered as a key point for public health initiatives across all ages, with particular emphasis in older adults because not only they have the higher prevalence of inactivity, but also the higher costs of health services. On the other side, energy expenditure related with occupational work has been diminishing, which addresses more importance to the leisure-time physical activity to the energy balance. Physical activity and cardiovascular fitness, i.e. oxygen uptake capacity, are both risk factors for cardiovascular health. Sometimes, questions arise about the most appropriate kind of exercise to burn energy and enhance oxygen uptake. However, the question seems to be easily answered since all fuel used in the body is ultimately processed by the aerobic energy pathways. This means that we can use the amount of oxygen consumed during the activity to calculate caloric burn. The impact of physical activity on fat mass is a sensitive point, and the question about the most appropriate intensity to burn fat also arises occasionally. Again, the answer seems to be very easy. Each individual should practice with the higher possible intensity, according to their risk stratification. The time necessary to reach the same level of energy expenditure is about one third when comparing vigorous intensity with moderate intensity, addressing for the lack of importance to discuss about the right zone to burn fat. Moreover, it is very well known that after about 2 minutes of exercising at high intensity the aerobic pathway (using fat free acids as fuel) becomes predominant over glycolytic pathway. Recent risk factors, as inflammation, have been considered. Again, exercise seems to be very promising in reducing the inflammatory processes, with the actual discussion centered on the acute and chronic effects of different modes of exercise, and on the underlying mechanisms.

9. References

Baptista F, Silva AM, Santos, DA, Mota J, Santos R, Vale S, Ferreira JP, Raimundo A, Moreira H (2011) Livro Verde da Actividade Física. Instituto do Desporto de Portugal, I.P. Lisboa

Barbieri M, Ferruci L, Corsi AM, Macchi C, Laurentani F, Bonafe M, Olivieri F, Giovagnetti S, Franceschi C, Paolisso G (2003) Is chronic inflammation a determinant of blood pressure in the elderly? American Journal of Hypertension 16:537-543

Berk BC, Weintraub WS, Alexander RW (1990) Elevation of C-reactive protein in "active" coronary artery disease. American Journal of Cardiology 65:168-172

Bonita R, Beaglehole R, Kjellstrom T (2006). Basic Epidemiology, 2nd edn. World Health Organization, Geneva

Bouchard C, Shephard RJ (1994) Physical activity, fitness, and health: the model and key concepts. In: Bouchard C, Shephard RJ, Stephens T (eds) Physical Activity, Fitness, and Health: International Proceedings and Consensus Statement. Human Kinetics Champaign, IL pp 77-88

Brownson RC, Boehmer TK, Luke DA (2005) Declining rates of physical activity in the United States: what are the contributors? Annual Review of Public Health 26:421-443

Center for Disease Control and Prevention (2008) U.S. Physical Activity Statistics: 1998–2007 No Leisure-Time Physical Activity Trend Chart, http://www.cdc.gov/nccdphp/dnpa/physical/stats/leisure_time.htm

Church TS, Barlow CE, Earnest CP, Kamper JB, Priest EL, Blair SN (2002) Associations between cardiorespiratory fitness and C-reactive protein in men. Arteriosclerosis, Thrombosis and Vascular Biology 22:1869-1876

Church TS, Thomas DM, Tudor-Locke C, Katzmarzyk PT, Earnest CP, Rodarte RQ, Martin CK, Blair SN, Bouchard C (2011) Trends over 5 Decades in U.S. Occupation-Related Physical Activity and Their Associations with Obesity. PLoS ONE 6:e19657. doi:10.1371/journal.pone.0019657

Commission of the European Communities (2007) White Paper on Sport. Commission of the European Communities, Brussels

Das UN (2001) Is obesity an inflammatory condition? Nutrition 17:953-966

De Haro J, Acin F, Lopez-Quintana A, Medina FJ, Martinez-Aguilar E, Florez A, March JR (2008) Direct association between C-reactive protein serum levels and endothelial dysfunction in patients with claudication. European Journal of Vascular Endovascular Surgery 35:480-486

Dinneen S, Gerich J, Rizza R (1992) Carbohydrate metabolism in non-insulin-dependent diabetes mellitus. New England Journal of Medicine 327:707-713

EC (2003) Special Eurobarometer 183-6 on Physical Activity / Wave 58.2. European Opinion Research Group EEIG, European Comission, Brussels

EC (2010) Special Eurobarometer 334 on Sport and Physical Activity / Wave 72.3. TNS Opinion & Social, European Comission, Brussels

Hamer M, Stamatakis E (2008) The accumulative effects of modifiable risk factors on inflammation and haemostasis. Brain, Behaviour and Immunity 22:1041-1043

Haskell WL, Lee IM, Pate RR, Powell KE, Blair SN, Franklin BA, Macera CA, Heath GW, Thompson PD, Bauman A (2007) Physical activity and public health: updated recommendation for adults from the American College of Sports Medicine and the American Heart Association. Medicine and Science in Sports and Exercise 39:1423-1434

Hwang JS, Wu TL, Chou SC, Ho C, Chang PY, Tsao KC, Huang JY, Sun CF, Wu JT (2008) Development of multiple complications in type 2 diabetes is associated with the increase of multiple markers of chronic inflammation. Journal of Clinical Laboratory Analysis 22:6-13

Imatoh T, Miyazaki M, Une H (2007) Does elevated high-sensitivity serum C-reactive protein associate with hypertension in non-obese Japanese males? Clinical Experimental Hypertension 29:395-401

Kim ES, Im JA, Kim KC, Park JH, Suh SH, Kang ES, Kim SH, Jekal Y, Lee CW, Yoon YJ, Lee HC, Jeon JY (2007) Improved insulin sensitivity and adiponectin level after exercise training in obese Korean youth. Obesity 15:3023-3030

Koenig W, Sund M, Fröhlich M, Fischer HG, Löwel H, Döring A, Hutchinson WL, Pepys MB (1999) C-Reactive protein, a sensitive marker of inflammation, predicts future risk of coronary heart disease in initially healthy middle-aged men: results from the MONICA (Monitoring Trends and Determinants in Cardiovascular Disease) Augsburg Cohort Study, 1984 to 1992. Circulation 99:237-242

Kohut ML, McCann DA, Russell DW, Konopka DN, Cunnick JE, Franke WD, Castillo MC, Reighard AE, Vanderah E (2006) Aerobic exercise, but not flexibility/resistance exercise, reduces serum IL-18, CRP, and IL-6 independent of b-blockers, BMI, and psychosocial factors in older adults. Brain Behaviour and Immunity 20:201-209

Kuller LH, Tracy RP, Shaten J, Meilahn EN (1996) Relation of C-reactive protein and coronary heart disease in the MRFIT nested case-control study. Multiple Risk Factor Intervention Trial. American Journal of Epidemiology 144:537-547

Laaksonen DE, Atalay M, Niskanen LK, Mustonen J, Sen CK, Lakka TA, Uusitupa MI (2000) Aerobic exercise and the lipid profile in type 1 diabetic men: a randomized controlled trial. Medicine and Science in Sports and Exercise 32:1541-1548

Last JM (2001) A Dictionary of Epidemiology, 4th edn. Oxford University Press, Oxford

Lee MA, Mather M (2008) Population Bulletin: U.S. Labor Force Trends. www.prb.org

Leon AS, Sanchez OA (2001) Response of blood lipids to exercise training alone or combined with dietary intervention. Medicine and Science in Sports and Exercise 33:S502-S515, discussion S528-S529

Lollgen H, Bockenhoff A, Knapp G (2009) Physical activity and all-cause mortality: an updated meta-analysis with different intensity categories. International Journal of Sports Medicine 30:213–224

Marini M, Sarchielli E, Brogi L, Lazzeri R, Salerno R, Sgambati E, Monaci M (2008) Role of adapted physical activity to prevent the adverse effects of the sarcopenia. A pilot study. Italian Journal of Anatomy and Embryology 113:217-225

Martins RA, Neves AP, Coelho-Silva MJ, Veríssimo MT & Teixeira AM (2010a) High-sensitivity C-reactive protein, body fat and physical exercise in older people. European Journal of Applied Physiology 110:161-169

Martins RA, Veríssimo MT Coelho-Silva MJ, Cumming SP & Teixeira AM (2010b) Effects of aerobic and strength-based training on metabolic health indicators in older adults. Lipids in Health and Disease, 9:76

Mora S, Lee IM, Buring JE, Ridker PM (2006) Association of physical activity and body mass index with novel and traditional cardiovascular biomarkers in women. JAMA 295:1412–1419

Morris JN, Clayton DG, Everitt MG, Semmence AM, Burgess EH (1990) Exercise in leisure time: coronary attack and death rates. British Heart Journal, 63:325-334

Morris JN, Heady JA, Raffle PAB, Roberts CG, Parks JN (1953a) Coronary heart disease and physical activity of work. Lancet 2:1053–1057

Morris JN, Heady JA, Raffle PAB, Roberts CG, Parks JN (1953b) Coronary heart disease and physical activity of work. Lancet 2:1111–1120

Onat A, Sansoy V, Yildirim B, Keles I, Uysal O, Hergenc G (2001) C-reactive protein and coronary heart disease in western Turkey. American Journal of Cardiology 88:601-607

Paffenbarger RS, Wing AL & Hyde RT (1978) Physical activity as an index of heart attack risk in college alumni. American Journal of Epidemiology 108:161-175

Paffenbarger RS Jr, Hyde RT, Wing AL & Hsieh C-c (1986a) Chronic disease in former college students: XXX. Physical activity, all-cause mortality, and longevity of college alumni. New England Journal of Medicine 314:605-613

Paffenbarger RS Jr, Hyde RT, Wing AL, Hsieh C-c (1986b) Chronic disease in former college students: XXX. Physical activity, all-cause mortality, and longevity of college alumni. New England Journal of Medicine 315:399-401

Paffenbarger RS Jr, Hyde RT, Wing AL, Lee I-M, Jung DL, Kampert JB (1993) Chronic disease in former college students: XXXVII. The association of changes in physical activity level and other lifestyle characteristics with mortality among men. New England Journal of Medicine 328:538-545

Paffenbarger RS Jr, Kampert JB, Lee I-M, Hyde RT, Leung RW, Wing AL (1994) Chronic disease in former college students: LII. Changes in physical activity and other lifeway patterns influencing longevity. Medicine and Science in Sports and Exercise 26:857–865

Pate RR, Pratt M, Blair SN, Haskell WL, Macera CA, Bouchard C, Buchner D, Ettinger W, Heath GW, King AC, Kriska A, Leon AS, Marcus BH, Morris J, Paffenbarger RS, Patrick K, Pollock ML, Rippe JM, Sallis J, Wilmore JH (1995) Physical activity and public health. A recommendation from the CDC and the American College of Sports Medicine. JAMA 273:402-407

Pedersen M, Bruunsgaard H, Weis N, Hendel HW, Andreassen BU, Eldrup E, Dela F, Pedersen BK (2003) Circulating levels of TNF-alpha and IL-6-relation to truncal fat mass and muscle mass in healthy elderly individuals and in patients with type-2 diabetes. Mechanisms of Ageing and Development 124:495-502

Piestrzeniewicz K, Łuczak K, Komorowski J, Maciejewski M, Jankiewicz-Wika J, Goch JH (2008) Resistin increases with obesity and atherosclerotic risk factors in patients with myocardial infarction. Metabolism: Clinical and Experimental 57:488-493

Porrini E, Gomez MD, Alvarez A, Cobo M, Gonzalez-Posada JM, Perez L, Hortal L, García JJ, Dolores-Checa M, Morales A, Hernández D, Torres A (2007) Glycated haemoglobin levels are related to chronic subclinical inflammation in renal transplant recipients without pre-existing or new onset diabetes. Nephrology and Dialysis Transplantation 22:1994-1999

Pradhan AD, Manson JE, Rifai N, Buring JE, Ridker PM (2001) C-reactive protein, interleukin-6 and risk of developing type 2 diabetes mellitus. JAMA 286:327-334

Reid KF, Naumova EN, Carabello RJ, Phillips EM, Fielding RA (2008) Lower extremity muscle mass predicts functional performance in mobility-limited elders. Journal of Nutrition, Health and Aging 12:493-498

Reuben DB, Judd-Hamilton L, Harris TB, Seeman TE (2003) The associations between physical activity and inflammatory markers in high-functioning older persons: MacArthur Studies of Successful Aging. Journal of the American Geriatrics Society 51:1125-1130

Ridker PM, Buring JE, Cook NR, Rifai N (2003) C-reactive protein, the metabolic syndrome, and risk of incident cardiovascular events: an 8-year follow-up of 14719 initially healthy American women. Circulation 107:391-397

Ridker PM, Buring JE, Shih J, Matias M, Hennekens CH (1998a) Prospective study of C-reactive protein and the risk of future cardiovascular events among apparently healthy women. Circulation 25:731-733

Ridker PM, Glynn RJ, Hennekens CH (1998b) C-reactive protein adds to the predictive value of total and HDL cholesterol in determining risk of first myocardial infarction. Circulation 97:2007-2011

Ridker PM, Rifai N, Rose L, Buring JE, Cook NR (2002) Comparison of C-reactive protein and low-density lipoprotein cholesterol levels in the prediction of first cardiovascular events. New England Journal of Medicine 347:1557-1565

Ridker PM, Stampfer MJ, Rifai N (2001) Novel risk factors for systemic atherosclerosis: a comparison of C-reactive protein, fibrinogen, homocysteine, lipoprotein(a), and standard cholesterol screening as predictors of peripheral arterial disease. Journal of the American Medical Association 285:2481-2485

Rifai N, Ridker PM (2001) High-sensitivity C-reactive protein: a novel and promising marker of coronary heart disease. Clinical Chemistry 47:403-411

Schoenborn CA, Stommel M (2011) Adherence to the 2008 adult physical activity guidelines and mortality risk. American Journal of Preventive Medicine 40:514-521

Steensberg A, Keller C, Starkie RL, Osada T, Febbraio MA, Pedersen BK (2002) IL-6 and TNF-alpha expression in, and release from, contracting human skeletal muscle. American Journal of Physiology, Endocrinology and Metabolism 283:E1272-E1278

Steensberg A, Fischer CP, Keller C, Moller K, Pedersen BK (2003) IL-6 enhances plasma IL-1ra, IL-10, and cortisol in humans. American Journal of Physiology, Endocrinology and Metabolism 285:E433-E437

Stewart LK, Flynn MG, Campbell WW, Craig BA, Robinson JP, Timmerman KL, McFarlin BK, Coen PM, Talbert E, (2007) The influence of exercise training on inflammatory cytokines and C-reactive protein. Medicine and Science in Sports and Exercise 39:1714-1719

Torre-Amione G (2005) Immune activation in chronic heart failure. American Journal of Cardiology 95:3C-8C

Torres JL, Ridker PM (2003) Clinical use of high sensitivity C-reactive protein for the prediction of adverse cardiovascular events. Current Opinion in Cardiology 18:471-478

Troiano RP, Berrigan D, Dodd KW, Masse LC, Tilert T, McDowell M (2008) Physical activity in the United States measured by accelerometer. Medicine and Science in Sports Exercise 40:181-188

USDHHS (1996) Physical Activity and Health. A Report of the Surgeon General. USDHHS, CDC, National Center for Chronic Disease Prevention and Health Promotion, Atlanta GA

USDHHS (2000) Healthy People 2010: Understanding and Improving Health. 2nd ed. US Government Printing Office, Washington, DC

USDHHS (2010) Healthy People 2020. US Government Printing Office, Washington, DC

USDHHS (2011) Physical activity guidelines for Americans. USDHHS. Washington DC. www.health.gov/paguidelines/, accessed on October 19th

Virani SS, Polsani VR, Nambi V (2008) Novel markers of inflammation in atherosclerosis. Current Atherosclerosis Reports 10:164-170

Visser M, Pahor M, Taaffe DR, Goodpaster BH, Simonsick EM, Newman AB, Nevitt M, Harris TB (2002) Relationship of interleukin-6 and tumor necrosis factor-alpha with muscle mass and muscle strength in elderly men and women: the Health ABC Study. The Journals of Gerontology. Series A, Biological Sciences and Medical Sciences 57:M326-M332

Wannamethee SG, Lowe GD, Whincup PH, Rumley A, Walker M, Lennon L (2002) Physical activity and haemostatic and inflammatory variables in elderly men. Circulation 105:1785-1790

Welk GJ (2002) Physical Activity Assessments for Health-Related Research. Human Kinetics, Champaign, IL

Widmaier EP, Raff H, Strang KT, Vander AJ (2011) Vander's human physiology: the mechanisms of body function, 12th edn. McGraw-Hill Higher Education, New York

Zurlo F, Nemeth PM, Choksi RM, Sesodia S, Ravussin E (1994) Whole-body energy metabolism and skeletal muscle biochemical characteristics. Metabolism 43:481-486

2

Cardiovascular and Cerebrovascular Problems in the Development of Cognitive Impairment: For Medical Professionals Involved in the Treatment of Atherosclerosis

Michihiro Suwa
Department of Cardiology,
Hokusetsu General Hospital, Takatsuki, Osaka,
Japan

1. Introduction

When cognitive function declines at a rate greater than that expected based on the actual age, life circumstances and educational level, we define it as cognitive impairment (Blennow et al., 2006; Gauthier et al 2006). In the older generation, the neurodegenerative process is considered to occur several years before the development of clinically detectable cognitive impairment. Although aging is the most clear factor in the development of this disease process, several epidemiological studies have elucidated that cardiovascular risk factors, i.e., hyperlipidemia, hypertension, smoking and diabetes, are also associated with cerebrovascular disease processes that may deteriorate cognitive function and advance dementia (Casserly & Topol, 2004; Nash & Fillit, 2006; Whitmer et al., 2005). In this chapter, I would like to introduce the current positioning of cognitive impairment as a consequence of cardiovascular diseases as well as a form of cerebrovascular disease, to neurologists or psychiatrists as well as to general physicians or cardiologists.

2. Cognitive impairment

Currently, Alzheimer's disease is the most common form of dementia or cognitive impairment, but less than 20% of dementia patients exhibit the isolated form of Alzheimer's disease and around 50% of such patients exhibit a combination of Alzheimer's disease and intracerebral vascular disease. By contrast, the isolated vascular type only contributes 20% (Meguro et al., 2002). Therefore, various problems related to metabolic syndrome, i.e., hypertension, hyperlipidemia, diabetes, and smoking habit, contribute to the development or deterioration of cognitive impairment.

3. Cardiovascular problems in cognitive impairment

Furthermore, recent investigations have suggested that the incidence of cognitive impairment is higher in patients with congestive heart failure and that treatment for left ventricular (LV) systolic dysfunction may prevent or delay the development of dementia in elderly patients (Zuccala et al., 2003, 2005). An Italian investigation indicated that the incidence of congestive heart failure was markedly higher in subjects with Mini-Mental State Examination (MMSE) scores <24 (20.2%), compared with those with scores ≥24 (4.6%) (Zuccala et al., 2003). Also, the presence of cognitive impairment has been associated with increased in-hospital mortality in older patients with heart failure (Zuccala et al., 2005). These data may indicate that low cardiac output due to heart failure is related to the deterioration of cognitive function, although there have been no reports regarding the pathophysiology or etiology of heart failure in relation to cognitive impairment. Another investigation indicated an independent relation between the levels of b-type natriuretic peptide (BNP) and the degree of cognitive impairment in older subjects (>55years of age) with cardiovascular disease; despite the fact that the mechanism was unclear (Gunstad et al., 2006).

In patients with heart failure, more than half of them, especially in females, showed normal or preserved LV ejection fraction (EF), i.e., exhibited heart failure resulting from LV diastolic dysfunction (Hogg et al. ,2004). Also, in heart failure patients with cardiovascular risk factors, i.e., hyperlipidemia, hypertension, smoking and diabetes, heart failure with preserved EF is also common. Therefore, we evaluated the relationship between LV diastolic dysfunction and cognitive impairment in Japanese patients with cardiovascular diseases (Suwa & Ito, 2009).

In our study, patients were divided into 2 groups; those patients with normal cognitive function or mild cognitive impairment (MMSE>=24; n=68: group N) and those with depressed cognitive function (MMSE<24, n=13). Diastolic function was evaluated based upon the ratio of the early diastolic mitral flow velocity (E) by pulse-wave Doppler echocardiography to the early diastolic mitral annular myocardial velocity (e') by tissue Doppler echocardiography (Diastolic Doppler index: E/e'). BNP was also evaluated as an index of heart failure. Consequently, in depressed cognitive function, diastolic Doppler index, E/e', was deteriorated (6.1 ± 1.3 vs. N: 4.6 ± 1.3, p<0.0003) and BNP was higher (137 ± 142 pg/ml vs. N: 60 ± 49 pg/ml, p<0.007), compared with those with normal cognitive function. Furthermore, the number of patients with diabetes was also higher in depressed cognitive function than in normal cognitive function (46% vs. N: 18%). From these studies evaluating the relation between cardiac and cognitive function, heart failure due to LV systolic and diastolic dysfunction can affect the development and the deterioration of cognitive impairment.

Poor cerebral circulation:	Left ventricular systolic dysfunction
	Left ventricular diastolic dysfunction
Stroke:	Atrial fibrillation, Atherosclerotic vascular diseases including of carotid artery stenosis
Deep white matter hyperintensity in brain MRI:	Atherosclerotic abnormalities, due to hypertension, diabetes, hyperlipidemia, and smoking
Hippocampal atrophy in brain:	Senile process

MRI: magnetic resonance imaging

Table 1. Relationship between cardiovascular abnormalities and cerebrovascular diseases affecting the decline of cognitive function

The occurrence of atrial fibrillation (AF) is a risk of stroke, and stroke increases the risk of cognitive decline and dementia. Therefore, AF has been reported to be associated with cognitive decline and dementia (Jozwiak et al., 2006). Recently, even in stroke-free patients it has been shown that AF is a risk for cognitive impairment and hippocampal atrophy (Knecht et al., 2008). For these reasons, it was considered that AF was associated with abnormalities of hemostasis, endothelial damage, platelet dysfunction, and low cardiac output.

As another measurable index in the vascular system, the ankle to brachial index is also related to incidence of total dementia, vascular dementia and Alzheimer's disease, especially in carriers of the apolipoprotein E gene abnormality (Laurin et al. 2007).

4. Common interest between cardiovascular and cerebrovascular diseases

Brain magnetic resonance imaging is conducted to screen for cerebrovascular disease as well as cerebral disease, and hyperintensities in the deep white matter on T2-weighted images can be incidentally detected in 10-20% in adults aged 64 to 94% at age 82 in the general population (Fig.1 and Fig.2). At present, these white matter lesions are related to chronic hypoperfusion and disruption of the blood brain barrier due to small vessel disease in the lesion area (Debette & Markus, 2010). Also, white matter hyperintensities are more common in patients with cerebrovascular disease as well as cardiovascular disease, with risk factors affecting atherosclerosis, inclusive of hypertension (Hajjar et al., 2011). Furthermore, meta-analysis reveals that the white matter lesions predict an increased risk of stroke, dementia, and death. Although data that treatment for these risk factors reduces the progression of white matter hyperintensities are limited, it is also reported that antihypertensive therapy reduced the progression in patients with stroke (Saxby et al., 2008). Therefore, white matter hyperintensities may be important markers to not only detect the risk of stroke and dementia but also diagnose the atherosclerosis in cerebro-cervical vascular system. The progression of white matter lesions is independently related to baseline cerebral lesion, higher age, hypertension, and current smoking. Also, atherosclerotic processes in the carotid artery, connecting to the cerebral artery, are associated with the cerebral small vessel disease (Romero et al., 2009).

Modified Mini-Mental State Examination scale falls more according to the worsening of white matter grade (prominently in grade Two +). (Fig.3. Longstreth et al. 2005) (with permission, License No.2776831264727)

To date, some angiotensin receptor blockers have been reported to significantly reduce the incidence and progression of Alzheimer's disease and dementia, compared with the use of angiotensin converting enzyme inhibitors or other cardiovascular drugs, in a predominant male population (Saxby et al., 2008). Therefore, when prescribing antihypertensive drugs we may have to consider the contribution of such medicines.

At present, the CHADS2 score is widely used to validate the risk for stroke in patients with AF. A newer clinical study has shown that the CHADS2 score is useful to predict ischemic stroke in patients with stable coronary artery disease, even in those without baseline atrial fibrillation (Welles et al., 2011)

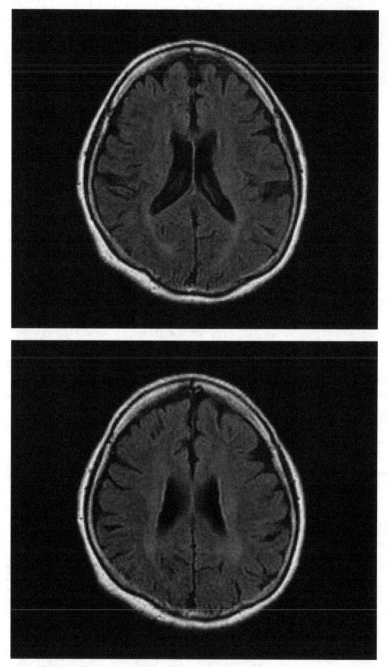

Fig. 1. Brain magnetic resonance imaging on T2 weighted images obtained from a 77 year old female without cognitive impairment and being under medication for hypertension. These images show somewhat brain atrophy but no white matter hyperintensities.

Cardiovascular and Cerebrovascular Problems in the Development of Cognitive Impairment: For Medical
Professionals Involved in the Treatment of Atherosclerosis

29

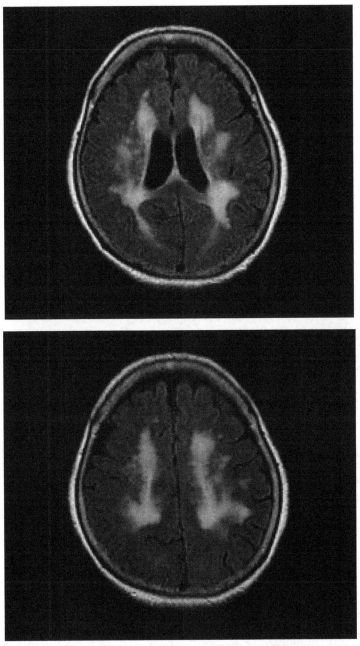

Fig. 2. White matter hyperintensities on brain magnetic resonance imaging from a 73 year
old female with advanced cognitive impairment (score 18 on MMSE). Extensive
hyperintensities can be seen in deep white matter, especially in periventricular region. She is
under medication for hypertension and hyperlipidemia

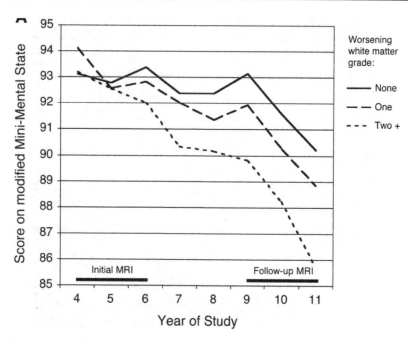

Fig. 3. Scores on modified Mini-Mental State Examination (vertical axis) for each year of study from initial to follow-up brain MRI scans (horizontal axis) by groups of participants (people aged 65 years and older) defined by worsening grade of white matter hyperintensity (three grade: None, grade One, and grade Two+).

Left ventricular systolic dysfunction:	Low left ventricular ejection fraction
Left ventricular diastolic dysfunction:	Reduced e′, Increased E/e′ ratio
B-type natriuretic peptide (BNP):	Increased BNP or N-terminal pro-BNP
Rhythm disturbance:	Development of atrial fibrillation
Ankle-brachial index (ABI):	Low ABI
Carotid ultrasonography	Internal carotid artery stenosis

e′: early diastolic mitral annular myocardial velocity by tissue Doppler echocardiography

E: early diastolic mitral flow velocity by pulse-wave Doppler echocardiography

Table 2. Cardiovascular indexes possibly to detect cognitive impairment

5. Relationship between echocardiographic parameters and age

Currently, LV diastolic function is evaluated based upon the following indices. Using pulse-wave Doppler echocardiography, the ratio of E velocity and the late diastolic transmitral flow velocity (A): (E/A ratio), and early diastolic flow deceleration time are measured. By tissue Doppler echocardiography of mitral annular motion, e′ myocardial velocity can be evaluated. Also, diastolic function was evaluated by the diastolic Doppler index (E/e′), and this index is also useful to evaluate LV end-diastolic pressure or left atrial pressure in patients with heart failure with depressed or normal LV EF (Ommen et.al., 2000).

Among the healthy subjects, the previous reports have evaluated the changes with age in various parameters. LV systolic function, obtained from LV EF by standard echocardiography or LV myocardial performance index using Doppler echocardiography, have shown minimum increments with age. However, LV diastolic function declined with age on echocardiographic parameters, i.e., E/A ratio and e' velocity decreased, and E/e' ratio increased (Munagala et al., 2003). Furthermore, LV wall thickness and LV mass increased gradually with age, and suggested depression of LV myocardial compliance (Daimon et al., 2008).

In some reports discussing the relationship between cognitive impairment and cardiovascular dysfunction, LV diastolic function was depressed with the deterioration of cognitive function, which may be more progressive than that with aging alone (Hogg et al. ,2004). Furthermore, in patients with heart failure, cognitive function is depressed, but there is no clear data as to whether LV systolic function is depressed with the decline of cognitive function and its decline is improved with the correction of systolic dysfunction.

6. Conclusion

While age is the most significant contributing factor to the development of cognitive impairment, several epidemiological studies have elucidated that cardiovascular risk factors, i.e., hyperlipidemia, hypertension, smoking and diabetes contribute to the deterioration of cognitive function. Furthermore, LV systolic and diastolic dysfunction, have been reported to cause cognitive impairment, likely as a result of the development of poor cerebral perfusion. Brain white matter hyperintensitiy and thromboembolic stroke due to atherosclerotic factors and atrial fibrillation are also related to producing cognitive impairment. Therefore, doctors and medical professionals, who are involved with medical treatment for cerebrovascular and cardiovascular diseases must keep in mind that atherosclerotic disease processes are also related to the development of cognitive impairment and progression of dementia.

7. References

Blennow, K et al (2006). Alzheimer's disease. Lancet, Vol.368, No.9533, pp. 387-403.

Casserly, I. & Topol, E. (2004) . Convergence of atherosclerosis and Alzheimer's disease: inflammation, cholesterol, and misfolded proteins. Lancet, Vol. 363, No.9514, pp. 1139-46.

Daimon M et al. (2008). Normal values of echocardiographic parameters in relation to age in a healthy Japanese population: The JAMP Study. CIrc J Vol.72, No.11, pp. 1859-1866.

Debette S & Markus HS. (2010). The clinical importance of white matter hyperintensities on brain magnetic resonance imaging: Systemic review and meta-analysis. BMJ Vol.341, pp c3666 (on-line)

Gauthier, S et al (2006). Mild cognitive impairment. Lancet, Vol. 367: No. No.9518, pp.1262-70.

Gunstad J et al. (2006). Relation of brain natriuretic peptide levels to cognitive dysfunction in adults > 55 years of age with cardiovascular disease. Am J Cardiol Vol.98, No.4, pp. 538-40.

Hajjar I et al. (2011). Hypertension, white matter hyperintensities, and concurrent impairments in mobility, cognition, and mood: The cardiovascular health study. Circulation Vol. 123, No.8, pp. 858-865.

Hogg K et al. (2004). Heart failure with preserved left ventricular systolic function: Epidemiology, clinical characteristics, and prognosis. J Am Coll Cardiol Vol 43, No 3, pp.317-327

Jozwiak A et al. (2006) Association of atrial fibrillation and focal neurologic deficits with impaired cognitive function in hospitalized patients ≥65 years of age. Am J Cardiol Vol. 98, No.9, pp.1238-41.

Knecht S et al. (2008). Atrial fibrillation in stroke-free patients is associated with memory impairment and hippocampal atrophy. Eur Heart J Vol. 29, No.17, pp. 2125-2132.

Laurin D et al. (2007) Ankle-to-brachial index and dementia. Honolulu-Asia aging study. Circulation Vol. 116, No.20, pp. 2269-2274.

Longstreth WT Jr. et al. (2005). Incidence, manifestation, and predictors of worsening white matter on serial cranial magnetic resonance imaging in the elderly. The cardiovascular health study. Stroke 36, No. 1, pp56-61

Meguro K et al. (2002). Prevalence of dementia and dementing diseases in Japan: the Tajiri project. Arch Neurol. Vol. 59, No. 7, pp. 1109-1114

Munagala VK et al. (2003). Association of newer diastolic function parameters with age in healthy subjects: A population-based study. J Am Soc Echocardiogr Vol. 16, No.10, pp. 1049-56

Nash DT & Fillit H. (2006). Cardiovascular disease risk factors and cognitive impairment. Am J Cariol, Vol. 97, No.8, pp.1262-65.

Ommen SR et.al (2000). Clinical utility of Doppler echocardiography and tissue Doppler imaging in the estimation of left ventricular filling pressures. A comparative simultaneous Doppler-catheterization study. Circulation Vol. 102, No.15, pp. 1788 – 94.

Romero JR et al. (2009). Carotid artery atherosclerosis, MRI indices of brain ischemia, aging, and cognitive impairment. The Framingham study. Stroke Vol. 40, No.5, pp.1590-1596

Saxby BK et al. (2008). Candesartan and cognitive decline in older patients with hypertension. Neurology Vol. 70, No.19 pt2, pp.1858-1866.

Suwa M & Ito T (2009). Correlation between cognitive impairment and left ventricular diastolic dysfunction in patients with cardiovascular diseases. Int J Cardiol, Vol. 136, No. 3, pp. 351-354.

Welles CC et al. (2011). The CHADS2 score predicts ischemic stroke in the absence of atrial fibrillation among patients with coronary heart disease: Data from the Heart and Soul Study. ACC. 2011, J Am Coll Cardiol Vol.57, No.14, suppl S, E607.

Whitmer RA et al (2005). Midlife cardiovascular risk factors and risk of dementia in late life. Neurology, Vol.64, No.2, pp. 277-81.

Zuccala G et al. (2003). The effects of cognitive impairment on mortality among hospitalized patients with heart failure. Am J Med Vol. 115, No.2, pp. 98-103.

Zuccala G et al. (2005). Correlates of cognitive impairment among patients with heart failure: Results of a multicenter survey. Am J Med. Vol.118, No.5, pp. 496-502

3

Cardiovascular Disease Risk Factors

Reza Amani and Nasrin Sharifi
Ahvaz Jondishapour University of Medical Sciences,
Iran

1. Introduction

Cardiovascular disease (CVD) is the leading cause of death not only in industrialized and developed countries but also in developing societies (WHO, 2008a). Changes in lifestyle of the population living in developing countries, which is due to the socioeconomic and cultural transition, are important reasons for increasing the rate of CVD. This observation has led to extensive research on prevention. Diagnosis the risk factors and predictors of CVD can help us detect high risk patients and prevent the disease, effectively.

Nowadays with a rapid progress in medical technology and diagnostic tools, more predictors are being added to the previous list of CVD risk factors. Therefore, we need to design updated risk assessment methods to screen high risk individuals early in their life span.

This chapter defines cardiovascular risk factors, classifies them, briefly describes how they interact, and discusses what strategies Should be implemented to prevent CVD progression.

2. Definitions

2.1 Coronary Heart Disease (CHD)

Coronary heart disease (CHD) is a condition in which the walls of arteries supplying blood to the heart muscle (coronary arteries) become thickened. This thickening, caused by development of lesions in the arterial wall, is called atherosclerosis; the lesions are called plaques. It can restrict the supply of blood to the heart muscle (the myocardium) and may manifest to the patient as chest pain on exertion (angina) or breathlessness on exertion. (Frayn 2005).

2.2 Cerebrovascular disease

Cerebrovascular disease involves interruption of the blood supply to part of the brain and may result in a stroke or a transient ischemic attack. The loss of blood supply to part of the brain may lead to irreversible damage to brain tissue. The blockage most commonly arises from the process of thromboembolism, in which a blood clot formed somewhere else (*e.g.* in the heart or in the carotid artery) becomes dislodged and then occludes an artery within the brain (cerebral arteries). Narrowing of the intracerebral arteries with atherosclerotic plaque may increase the risk, and may also lead to local formation of a blood clot. The etiology is similar to that of CHD (Frayn 2005).

2.3 Peripheral Vascular Disease (PVD)

Peripheral vascular disease (PVD) involves atherosclerotic plaques narrowing the arteries supplying other regions apart from the myocardium and brain. A common form involves narrowing of the arteries supplying blood to the legs. The result may be pain on exercise. In more severe cases, impaired blood supply leads to death of leg tissues, which requires amputation (Frayn 2005).

3. Epidemiology

3.1 Global and regional trends in CVD burden

In recent years, the dominance of chronic diseases as major contributors to total global mortality has emerged (WHO, 2008a). By 2005, the total number of cardiovascular disease (CVD) deaths (mainly coronary heart disease, stroke, and rheumatic heart disease) had increased globally to 17.5 million from 14.4 million in 1990(WHO, 2009a).

The World Health Organization (WHO) estimates there will be about 20 million CVD deaths in 2015, accounting for 30 percent of all deaths worldwide (WHO, 2005). Thus, CVD is today the largest single contributor to global mortality and will continue to dominate mortality trends in the future (WHO, 2009a).

Globally, there is an uneven distribution of age-adjusted CVD mortality that is mapped in Figure 1. The lowest age-adjusted mortality rates are in the advanced industrialized countries and parts of Latin America, whereas the highest rates today are found in Eastern Europe and a number of low and middle income countries(WHO, 2008a). The broad causes for the rise and, in some countries, the decline in CVD over time are well described. The key contributors to the rise across countries at all stages of development include tobacco use and abnormal blood lipid levels, along with unhealthy dietary changes (especially related to fats and oils, salt, and increased calories) and reduced physical activity(Hu, 2008;). Key contributors to the decline in some countries include declines in tobacco use and exposure, healthful dietary shifts, population-wide prevention efforts, and treatment interventions (Shafey et al, 2009; Davies et al, 2007).

4. Pathophysiology

Cardiovascular diseases, whether affecting the coronary, cerebral or peripheral arteries, share a common pathophysiology involving atherosclerosis and thrombosis (or clotting).

4.1 Atherosclerosis

Atherosclerosis is the most common cause of CVD and related mortality. The first observable event in the process of atherosclerosis is the accumulation of plaque (cholesterol from low-density lipoproteins [LDLs], calcium, and fibrin) in large and medium arteries.

This plaque can grow and produce ischemia either by insufficient blood flow if there is a high oxygen demand or by rupturing, forming a thrombus and occluding the lumen (Rudd et al., 2005). Only high-risk or vulnerable plaque forms thrombi. Characteristics of vulnerable

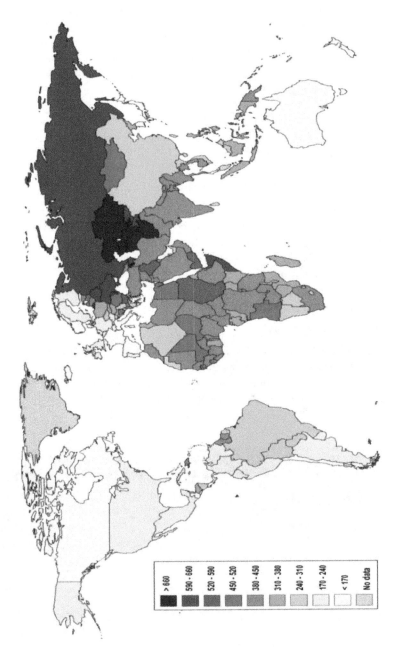

NOTE: Rates are age-standardized to WHO's world standard population.
SOURCES: WHO, 2009a

Fig. 1. Age-standardized deaths due to cardiovascular disease (rate per 100,000), 2004.

plaque are lesions with a thin fibrous cap, few smooth muscle cells, many macrophages (inflammatory cells),and a large lipid core(Figure 2) (Rudd et al., 2005). The site of plaque formation or atherogenesis is the endothelium in the artery wall. Normally the endothelium promotes dilation of the blood vessel ,less smooth muscle cell growth, and prevention of an anti-inflammatory response (Davignon and Ganz, 2004). In atherosclerosis the endothelium becomes dysfunctional before an atheroma or plaque, a more serious lesion, develops. This endothelial dysfunction results in the production of less nitric oxide, a key vasodilator, and the blood vessel becomes more constricted .It also becomes more permeable and allows LDL cholesterol to be taken up by macrophages, which then accumulate and form foam cells and eventually an early lesion known as a fatty streak.

5. Risk factors for cardiovascular disease

This section described the major risk factors for CVD in more detail. The section begins with lipid and inflammation-related factors, behavioral risk factors, including tobacco use, dietary factors, alcohol, and physical activity. This is followed by the major biological risk factors that mediate the role of these behaviors leading to CVD, including obesity, blood pressure, blood lipids, and diabetes.

5.1 Modifiable cardiovascular risk factors

5.1.1 Lipid-related factors

Lipid-related cardiovascular risk factors have attracted enormous attention over the past years, and consensus documents have been produced to implement treatment and preventive strategies. Essentially, this applies to the conventional risk factors such as high plasma total and low-density lipoprotein (LDL) cholesterol, low plasma high density lipoprotein (HDL) cholesterol and elevated plasma triglycerides.

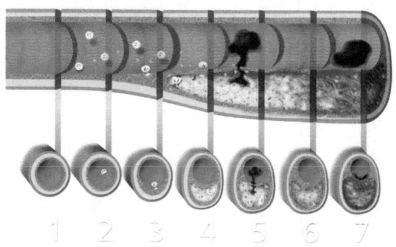

Fig. 2. Natural Progression of atherosclerosis

5.1.1.1 Atherogenic lipoproteins

A number of factors determine whether a cholesterol-containing lipoprotein particle resident in plasma has atherogenic properties. The size of the particle determines the ease by which the endothelium can be penetrated; small particles are more likely to be deposited in the arterial wall than large particles. The binding to the subendothelial matrix is also dependent on size, in which the smaller particles bind more avidly to proteoglycans (Anber *et al.*, 1997). The apoB protein, present as one molecule per lipoprotein particle, seems to be crucial. Firstly, lipoprotein particles without apoB are not atherogenic; secondly, apoB has multiple proteoglycan binding domains which enhance the retention of the particle in the subendothelial matrix (Skalen *et al.*, 2002). Finally, physicochemical and compositional characteristics, such as resistance factors against oxidative stress, are likely to be important in reducing the modification of lipoprotein particles.

5.1.1.2 Small, dense Low-Density Lipoprotein (LDL)

The formation of small, dense LDL particles is complex and can be seen as a genetic trait, but the major gene(s) responsible remain unknown. Environmental factors also play a major role, in that dietary factors can influence triglyceride as a major determinant. *In vitro* studies have shown that small, dense LDL particles are formed by sequential exchange of lipids between LDL and triglyceride-rich lipoproteins. The cholesteryl esters contained in the core of the LDL particle are exchanged for triglycerides by the cholesteryl ester transfer protein (CETP). Triglycerides entering the LDL particle are hydrolyzed by hepatic lipase and the core volume of the particle is reduced. The formation of small, dense LDL is limited by the availability of triglyceride-rich lipoproteins, as evidenced by the close positive correlation between plasma triglycerides and small, dense LDL. It is assumed that these processes take quite some time and the end product is therefore an aged particle that has lost its defense against free radical attack. The retention in plasma of the particle is partly due to the fact that small, dense LDL has a lower affinity for the LDL receptor than normal buoyant LDL (Nigon *et al.*, 1991). It is thought that a consequence of the altered chemical composition of the small, dense LDL particle is that it more avidly binds to the subendothelial matrix and upon challenge more easily undergoes oxidative modification thereby triggering foam cell formation (Tribble *et al.*, 1992; Chait *et al.*, 1993; Dejager *et al.*, 1993;).

The presence of triglyceride-rich lipoproteins is a principal modulator of small, dense LDL; the plasma concentration of the latter is strongly and positively related to the concentration of plasma triglycerides. In fact, all examples in which the triglyceride concentration has been altered to observe a change in the LDL profile are consistent: elevation of triglycerides leads to higher abundance of small, dense LDL; the opposite is observed when triglycerides are lowered, treated by diet or pharmacological agents. Low fat diets may lead to increased plasma triglyceride concentration; consequently a reduction in LDL size was observed in a study of 105 men switching from a high fat (46%) to a low fat (24%) diet (Dreon *et al.*, 1994). The total LDL cholesterol concentration was, however, reduced simultaneously, so the net effect on cardiovascular risk is not entirely clear.

In the Quebec Cardiovascular Study the cholesterol concentration in small dense LDL particle may give even more precise information. Again, in the Quebec heart study, the cholesterol concentration in small dense LDL particles showed the strongest association with the risk of CHD. These data suggest that the cholesterol within small dense LDL is particularly harmful. Therefore measurement of LDL particle size and possibly cholesterol content within these particles may enhance our capability to predict cardiovasular events (Lamarche *et al.*, 2001).

5.1.1.3 High-Density Lipoprotein (HDL)

HDL is another lipid profile fraction which is associated to the risk of CVD. Decreased levels of HDL-c correlated to increased risk of CVD. The atheroprotective role for HDL is mainly due to the pathway named *reverse cholesterol transport* (RCT). RCT is defined as the uptake of cholesterol from peripheral tissues back to the liver by HDL. Apo A1 is an apolipoprotein of the HDL that activates the enzyme lecithin-cholesteryl ester acyl-transferase (LCAT). The main function of LCAT is transferring cholesterol from cell to HDL. Both apo C and apo E on HDL are transferred to chylomicrons.

Apo E helps receptors metabolize chylomicron remnants and also inhibits appetite (Gotoh et al., 2006). Therefore high HDL levels are associated with low levels of chylomicrons; *very low density lipoprotein* (VLDL) remnants; and small dense LDLs and subsequently lower atherosclerotic risk. HDL has other potentially atheroprotective properties. The anti-oxidative activity of HDL is typically characterized by its ability to inhibit LDL oxidation. It has also been shown to inhibit the formation of reactive oxygen species. HDL can help to protect endothelial cells from apoptosis induced by mildly oxidized LDL. It can affect platelet function through the promotion of nitric oxide production (Chen et al, 1994; Suc et al 1997) and coagulation by the inhibition of several coagulation factors. There is considerable evidence for a direct protective role of HDL in inflammatory, oxidative, apoptotic, and thrombotic processes.

Major factors that increase HDL cholesterol level are exogenous estrogen, intensive exercise, loss of excess body fat, moderate consumption of alcohol and triglyceride lowering drugs such as fibrates and niacin. Treatment of low serum levels of HDL-C in at risk patients is an important therapeutic intervention and impacts rates of disease progression as well as cardiovascular events (Scanu and Edelstein , 2008).

5.1.2 Inflammation-related factors

Inflammation is a part of atherosclerosis process, beginning with the formation of fatty streak underlying the endothelium of large arteries. The infiltration of monocytes and lymphocytes occurs as a result of the expression of adhesion molecules by endothelial cells lining the artery wall. Several stimuli for the inflammatory response in atherosclerosis have been proposed in which oxidised low-density lipoprotein (LDL), is of most importance. Monocytes that have infiltrated the arterial intima and differentiated into macrophages take up oxidized LDL through scavenger receptors in an unregulated manner, accumulating large amounts of cholesterol and becoming foam cells. Macrophages eventually die, through necrosis and apoptosis, the lipid is deposited within the core of the developing plaque (Figure 3). Cytokines secreted by both lymphocytes and macrophages within the plaque exert pro- and anti-atherogenic effects on components of the vessel wall. Smooth muscle cells migrate from the medial portion of the arterial wall towards the intima and secrete extracellular matrix proteins that form a fibrous cap. The cap separates the highly thrombogenic contents of the plaque lipid core from the potent coagulation system contained within the circulating blood.

This chronic, low-grade inflammation is likely to be the result of cytokines secreted by monocytes and soluble adhesion molecules from the vessel wall into the circulation, where they subsequently act on the liver to induce the secretion of acute phase proteins, including C-Reactive Protein(CRP), fibrinogen and serum amyloid A (Frayn, 2005).

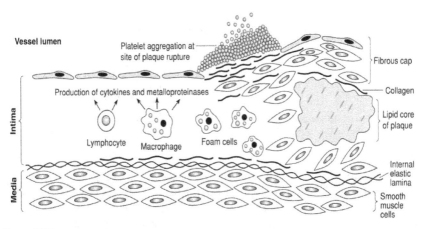

From Frayn 2005

Fig. 3. Schematic representation of the development of an atherosclerotic lesion, showing plaque rupture and platelet aggregation .

5.1.2.1 C-Reactive protein

Multiple studies have demonstrated that elevated levels of high-sensitivity C-reactive protein (hs-CRP) are associated with increased CVD risk (Buckley et al.,2009; Musunuru et al., 2008). hs-CRP, previously considered to be an indicator of systemic inflammation, has recently received much attention in the scientific literature, not only as a potential marker of increased atherosclerotic risk, but also as a potential target of therapy for the prevention of atherosclerotic CVD. Evidence derived mainly from statin trials, supports the potential value of CRP as a therapeutic target for both primary and secondary prevention of CVD and CHD. The largest study to suggest an integral role for CRP as a target for therapy in primary prevention of CVD is the recent Justification for the Use of Statins in Prevention: An Intervention Trial Evaluating Rosuvastatin (JUPITER) trial. The investigators randomized 17,802 men ≥50 years of age and women ≥60 years of age with low LDL cholesterol levels < 130 mg/dL and hs-CRP ≥ 2 mg/L and no history of CVD or diabetes to 20 mg rosuvastatin daily or placebo. The primary end point was the first occurrence of MI, stroke, hospitalization for unstable angina, arterial revascularization, or CV death (Ridker et al; 2008). During the 1.9-year median follow-up duration (maximum follow-up period 5 years), rosuvastatin reduced LDL cholesterol by 50% and hs-CRP by 37%. Thus, JUPITER demonstrated a magnitude of effect larger than that of almost all prior statin trials   (Ridker et al; 2009). Based on the results of the JUPITER study, the U.S. Food and Drug Administration (FDA) in February 2010 agreed to broader labeling for rosuvastatin. Rosuvastatin is currently approved for the reduction of risk for stroke, MI, and revascularization procedures in individuals who have normal LDL cholesterol levels and no clinically evident CHD but who do have an increased risk based on age, CRP levels, and the presence of at least one additional CVD risk factor. Accordingly, JUPITER not only demonstrated that hs-CRP successfully identified a population with "hidden risk" for CVD but also provided additional evidence for the potential utility of hs-CRP as a target for therapy in primary prevention of CVD disease.

Other inflammatory states such as obesity produce elevations in CRP even in young obese children (Blum et al., 2005). Body mass index (BMI) is moderately correlated (r = 0.5) to CRP levels (Rawson et al., 2003). Recently it was demonstrated that weight loss lowers CRP (Tchernof et al., 2002), which provides another physiologic benefit for weight management as a preventive strategy for CHD reduction. Currently it is known that elevated insulin levels in overweight children affect CRP. Physical activity did not appear to be related (Rawson et al., 2003). To date few studies have investigated the effects of dietary variables on CRP. In a cross-sectional study, higher intakes of fruits and vegetables were associated with lower CRP levels (Gao et al., 2004).

5.1.2.2 Fibrinogen

Fibrinogen is the precursor of fibrin. As the major clotting factor in the blood and a pro-inflammatory molecule, fibrinogen plays role in atherosclerosis. It is synthesized in the liver and, like CRP, is an acute phase protein, whose circulating levels can change during acute responses to tissue damage or infection. Thus Fibrinogen (Fg) is a biomarker of inflammation (Ross 1999), which, when elevated, indicates the presence of inflammation and identifies individuals with a high risk for cardiovascular disorders. Increased plasma Fg concentration typically accompanies hypertension development (Lominadze *et al.* 1998) and stroke (D'Erasmo *et al.* 1993). Factors associated with an elevated fibrinogen are smoking, diabetes, hypertension, obesity, sedentary lifestyle, elevated triglycerides, and genetic factors. Recent studies indicate that increased Fg content affects microcirculation by increasing plasma viscosity, RBC aggregation and platelet thrombogenesis (Lominadze et al; 2010). These changes lead to vascular dysfunction and exacerbate microcirculatory complications during cardiovascular diseases (figure 4).

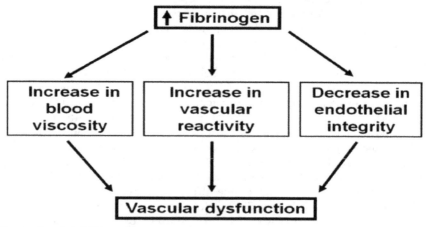

From Lominadze et al. 2010

Fig. 4. Schematic representation of fibrinogen-induced vascular dysfunction.

5.1.2.3 Serum amyloid A

Serum amyloid A (SAA) is a precursor of amyloid A protein and comprises both constitutive (apoSAA1, apoSAA2) and acute phase (apoSAA4) isoforms. The serum amyloid A proteins are a family of inflammatory apolipoproteins with a high affinity for HDL, and their production by the liver and other tissues is thought to be induced by IL-1 and IL 6. Their role in lipid metabolism is unclear, although they may be involved in HDL trafficking. A small number of studies have investigated the association between SAA and the incidence of CHD (Ridker *et al.*, 1998, 2000; Danesh *et al.*, 2000b). Taken together, these studies show that a comparison of individuals with values in the top third with those in the bottom third gives a combined risk ratio of 1.6 for CHD. However, further studies are required to determine whether the association is independent of possible confounders.

5.1.3 Behavioral and lifestyle risk factors

5.1.3.1 Tobacco

There are currently more than 1 billion smokers worldwide. Although use of tobacco products is decreasing in high income countries, it is increasing globally, with more than 80 percent of the world's smokers now living in low and middle income countries (Jha and Chaloupka, 1999).

In the Global Burden of Disease study, Lopez et al. (2006) estimated that in 2000, 880,000 deaths from CHD and 412,000 deaths from stroke were attributable to tobacco. Smoking cessation has been shown to have significant impacts on reducing CHD. In a major review of the evidence, Critchley and Capewell (2003) determined that successful smoking cessation reduced CHD mortality risk by up to 36 percent. Smoking cessation leads to significantly lower rates of reinfarction within 1 year among patients who have had a heart attack and reduces the risk of sudden cardiac death among patients with CHD (Gritz et al., 2007).

Two major trends are of real concern with respect to the future of tobacco-related CVD. First, in most parts of the world, the smoking rates are higher among the poorest populations (WHO, 2008b). The second worrisome trend is in smoking among girls (IOM, 2010).

In addition to active smoking, it has become increasingly apparent that exposure to secondhand smoke significantly increases cardiovascular risk. A recent IOM review of the effects of secondhand smoke exposure concluded that exposure to secondhand smoke significantly increases cardiovascular risk and that public smoking bans can significantly reduce the rate of heart attacks. The report concluded that secondhand smoke exposure increases cardiovascular risk by 25 to 30 percent and that there is sufficient evidence to support a causal relationship between secondhand smoke exposure and acute myocardial infarction (AMIs). This causality was reinforced by the report's conclusion that smoking bans significantly reduce the rate of AMIs, with declines ranging from 6 to 47 percent (IOM, 2009).

5.1.3.2 Dietary factors

The relationship between CVD and diet is one of the most studied relationships in epidemiology. Although nutritional research has traditionally focused on the effect of individual food groups or nutrients on CVD, there has been a shift in recent years toward comparing how different types of dietary patterns in their entirety affect CVD risk (IOM, 2010). The following sections reflect this shift by discussing research on dietary factors that have clear impacts on CVD risk.

5.1.3.2.1 Dietary fat

Healthy oils are those that contain no commercially introduced trans fatty acids, are low in saturated fatty acids, and are high in mono- and polyunsaturated fatty acids.

There is accumulating evidence that it is fat quality (the type of dietary fat), rather than the total amount of fat, that is particularly important for cardiovascular disease (Astrup, 2002).

5.1.3.2.1.1 Saturated Fatty Acids (SFA)

The predominant sources of SFAs are animal foods (meat and dairy). SFAs have the most potent effect on LDL cholesterol, which rises in a dose response fashion when increasing levels of SFAs are consumed. In our study, consumption of habitual hydrogenated fats and full-fat yoghurts (fat content more than 2.5%) increased the risk of CVD (OR = 2.12(1.23-3.64) and 2.35(1.32-4.18), respectively) (Amani et al, 2010). These foods are the major sources of SFAs. SFAs intake is the principal determinant of total cholesterol(TC) and CVD and substitution of 1% carbohydrate calories by SFAs increases TC by 1.5 mg/dL (Joseph et al, 2000). Of all the added fats in the diet, the most hypercholesterolemic promoting are palm kernel, coconut, and palm oils; lard; and butter. SFAs raise serum LDL cholesterol by decreasing LDL receptor synthesis and activity. Regardless of form, all fatty acids lower fasting triglycerides if they replace carbohydrate in the diet. In secondary prevention trials replacement of SFAs with MUFA, α-linolenic acid, and increased fruits and vegetables prevented fatal and nonfatal CVD events in persons with established disease (de Lorgeril, 1999). Thus fatty acids affect disease progression through lipids and other mechanisms and possibly through inflammation and thrombosis (Krummel, 2008).

5.1.3.2.1.2 Monounsaturated Fatty Acids (MUFA)

The American Heart Association (AHA) does not have any recommendation for the *cis* form of MUFAs (Lichtenstein et al., 2006). Oleic acid (C18:1) is the most prevalent MUFA in the American diet. Substituting oleic acid for carbohydrate has almost no appreciable effect on blood lipids; however, replacing SFAs with MUFA lowers serum cholesterol levels, LDL cholesterol levels, and triglyceride levels to about the same extent as polyunsaturated fatty acids (PUFAs) . The effects of MUFAs on HDL cholesterol depend on the total fat content of the diet. When intakes of both MUFA (>15% of total kilocalories) and total fat (>35% of kilocalories) are high, HDL cholesterol does not change or increases slightly compared with levels with a lower-fat diet (Krummel , 2008). Oleic acid as a part of the Mediterranean diet has been shown to have antiinflammatory effects. In epidemiologic studies high-fat diets of people in Mediterranean countries have been associated with low blood cholesterol levels and CHD incidence (Trichopoulou et al., 2003). Among other factors, the main fat source is olive oil, which is high in MUFA. Although higher-fat diets (low in SFA with MUFAs as the predominant fat) can lower blood cholesterol, they should be used with caution because of the caloric density of high-fat diets and the results of clinical trials, which have shown new atherosclerotic lesions in men who consume higher-fat diets. The negative association between the Mediterranean diet and CHD could be the result of factors other than MUFA intake. For example, these populations consume more fruits and vegetables, bread, cereals, fish, and nuts, and less red meat than many populations. Olive oil is the primary source of fat, and eggs are consumed from zero to four times per week (krummel, 2008).

5.1.3.2.1.3 Polyunsaturated Fatty Acids (PUFA)

The essential fatty acid linoleic acid (LA) is the predominant PUFA consumed in the American diet (Krummel, 2008). Population studies have demonstrated a negative correlation between LA intake and CHD rates (Wijendran and Hayes, 2004). Similarly, a meta analysis of 60 controlled human trials found that replacing PUFA for carbohydrate in the diet resulted in a decline in serum LDL cholesterol (Mensink et al., 2003). When SFAs are replaced with PUFAs in a low-fat diet, LDL and HDL cholesterol levels will be lowered. The lipid lowering effects of LA depend on the total fatty acid profile of the diet (Wijendran and Hayes, 2004). When added to study diets, large amounts of LA diminished levels of HDL cholesterol serum levels (Karmally, 2005). Studies suggest that high intakes of n-6 PUFAs may exert adverse effects on the function of vascular endothelium or stimulate production of proinflammatory cytokines. A low ratio of omega-6:omega-3 PUFA is recommended (Basu et al., 2006; Gibauer eial., 2006).

5.1.3.2.1.4 Omega-3 fatty acids

Fish oils, fish oil capsules, and ocean fish are rich source of the two main omega-3 fatty acids (i.e., eicosapentaenoic acid (EPA) and docosahexaenoic acid [DHA]). Many studies have shown that eating fish is associated with a decreased CVD risk. The recommendation for the general population for fish consumption is to eat fish high in omega-3 fatty acids (salmon, tuna, mackerel, sardines) at least twice a week (Psota et al., 2006). For patients who have CVD, 1 g of EPA and DHA combined is recommended from fish if possible but, if not, then from supplements (Lichtenstein et al., 2006). Patients who have hypertriglyceridemia need 2 to 4 g of EPA and DHA per day for effective lowering (Lichtenstein et al.,2006). Omega-3 fatty acids lower triglyceride levels by inhibiting VLDL and apo B-100 synthesis and by decreasing postprandial lipemia.

α-Linolenic acid (ALA), an omega-3 fatty acid from vegetables, has anti-inflammatory effects. CRP levels were reduced when male patients consumed 8 g of ALA daily; similar results have not been observed for fish oil supplementation (Basu et al.,2006). Omega-3 fatty acids also interfere with blood clotting by altering prostaglandin synthesis (Krummel, 2008).

5.1.3.2.1.5 Trans fatty acids

Trans-fatty acids are produced in the hydrogenation process used in the food industry to increase shelf life of foods and to make margarines, firmer (Krummel ,2008). The AHA (Lichtenstein et al., 2006) recommends no more than 1% of calories (about 1-3 g/day) from trans-fatty acids. These fatty acids raise LDL cholesterol; however, effects on inflammation have been conflicting (Basu et al.,2006). Most trans-fatty acids intake comes from partially hydrogenated vegetable oils (krummel, 2008).

Mozaffarian et al (2007) showed that partially hydrogenated oils are extensively being used for cooking in Iranian homes with average per-person intake of 14 g/1000 kcal. Trans fatty acids (TFAs) accounted for 33% of fatty acids in these products, or 4.2% of all calories consumed (12.3 g/day). Consumption of hydrogenated fats was associated with higher

CAD risk (OR = 2.12(1.23-3.64)) in a study performed by Amani et al (2010). On the basis of TC:HDL-cholesterol effects alone, 9% of CHD events would be prevented by replacement of TFA in homes with *cis*-unsaturated fats (8% by replacement with saturated fats). On the basis of relationships of TFA intake with CHD incidence in prospective studies, 39% of CHD events would be prevented by replacement of TFA with *cis*-unsaturated fats (31% by replacement with saturated fats).

5.1.3.2.1.6 Dietary cholesterol

Dietary cholesterol raises total cholesterol and LDL cholesterol but to a lesser extent than SFAs. The AHA dietary patterns contain no more than 200 mg of cholesterol each day (Krummel; 2008). There is a threshold beyond which addition of cholesterol to the diet has minimal effects. When cholesterol intakes reach 500 mg/day, only small increments in blood cholesterol occur. Cholesterol responsiveness also varies widely among individuals. Some people are hyporesponders (i.e., their plasma cholesterol level does not increase after dietary cholesterol challenge), whereas others are hyperresponders (i.e., their plasma cholesterol level responds more strongly than expected to a cholesterol challenge). It has been suggested that hyperresponders may have the apo E-4 allele and poor rates of conversion of cholesterol to bile acids, which causes elevated LDL cholesterol. Feedings cholesterol to animals enriches lipoproteins, which are atherogenic beyond just the rise in serum cholesterol (Krummel, 2008).

SFAs and cholesterol synergistically affect LDL cholesterol level, decrease LDL receptor synthesis and activity, increase VLDLs enriched with apo E, increase all lipoproteins, and decrease chylomicron size (which is associated with CHD risk). The effect of dietary cholesterol on inflammatory factors has been inconsistent (Basu et a1.,2006).

5.1.3.2.2 Dietary sodium

There is evident that excessive sodium intake significantly increases CVD risk and that reduction in sodium intake at the population level decreases CVD burden (He and MacGregor, 2009, IOM, 2010). The most well-established mechanism by which sodium intake increases CVD risk is increasing blood pressure (BP). Numerous studies have found that there is a continuous and graded relationship between salt intake and blood pressure. In their recent major review of sodium trends and impact, He and MacGregor concluded that a reduction in salt from the current global intake of 9 to 12 g/day to the recommended levels of 5-6 g/day would have a major impact on BP and CVD (He and MacGregor, 2009; IOM, 2010). Salt's impact on CVD, however, extends beyond blood pressure. Animal and epidemiological studies have found that a diet high in sodium may directly increase the risk of stroke, which is independent and additive to salt's effect on BP (He and MacGregor, 2009 ; IOM, 2010).

5.1.3.2.3 Soy protein

In recent years, a great deal of interest has emerged in the role of soy-bean isoflavones in reducing heart diseases, and isoflavones might be responsible, in part, for the ability of soybean to lower the risk of CVD and atherosclerosis (Anderson et al, 1995) . Anderson suggested that about 60-70% of the cholesterol lowering effect of soy protein may be due to its isoflavone content (Anderson et al, 1995). Isoflavones are a group of phytoestrogens which occur mainly in soy and it is consumed for the purpose of both promoting health and preventing several chronic diseases, including coronary heart disease, cancers of reproductive organs and osteoporosis (Lichtenstein, 1998 ; Anerson et al, 1999). Aglycone forms of soy isoflavones especially genistein and daidzein have greatly been studied because of their greater estrogenic and antioxidant activities (Arora et al, 1998). Soy isoflavones have been shown to decrease total, VLDL and LDL cholesterol levels while increasing HDL cholesterol levels in peripubertal rhesus monkeys fed soy protein-based diets (Antony et al, 1996). It is claimed that purified isoflavones have no effect on plasma lipid and lipoprotein concentrations in normolipidemic subjects (Nestel et al, 1997; Hodgson et al, 1998). At present, there is no general agreement about the effect of soy protein isoflavones (SPI) on lipid profiles and moreover, it is not clear that which part of the soy protein has lipid-lowering effects. In a study, we designed animal model to assess the effect of SPI on serum lipid, lipoprotein profile, and blood sugar of experimentally- induced hypercholesterolemic rabbits,and to detect any dose-response effect of SPI on the above mentioned variables. In this research, the effect of soy protein containing 200 mg, 100 mg and a trace amount of both glycoside and aglycone forms of soy isoflavones were assessed in hypercholesterolemic male rabbits. Although the rabbits had a cholesterol-rich diet, the serum total and LDL-cholesterol remained unchanged in the SPI+ group (i.e. intact soy protein diet). The results have indicated that soy protein isoflavones maintained the serum lipid and lipoprotein levels in hypercholesterolemic rabbits kept on a high cholesterol diet, but alcohol-extracted (even half-dose isoflavones) soy protein diets do not have positive effect. Moreover, the hypocholesterolemic effect of isoflavones is not in a dose-response manner and it is suggested that isoflavones activity is closely related to soy protein (Amani et al, 2005).

5.1.3.2.4 Fiber

One of the potential ways by which soy protein might exert its effect on blood cholesterol is via its fiber content (about 6 g as non-starch polysaccharide per 100 g boiled beans), which is primarily soluble fiber. Soluble fiber (*e.g.* from oats) has been shown to lower plasma total and LDL-cholesterol, although the effect is small for those consuming moderate amounts (Truswell, 2002). In the meta-analysis by Brown *et al.* (1999) 2–10 g/day of soluble fiber was associated with a small but significant fall in total cholesterol (0.045 mmol/1 per g fiber) and LDL-cholesterol (0.057 mmol/1 per g fiber). Three apples or three (28 g) servings of oatmeal, providing 3 g soluble fiber, decreased total and LDL-cholesterol by about 0.13 mmol/1. The mechanism of this effect remains undefined. Suggestions include bile acid binding, resulting in an up-regulation of LDL receptors and thus increased clearance of LDL-cholesterol; inhibition of hepatic fatty acid synthesis byproducts of fermentation in the large bowel (*e.g.* propionate, acetate, butyrate); changes in motility or satiety; or slowed absorption of macronutrients resulting in improved insulin sensitivity (Brown *et al.*, 1999).

Consumption of diets rich in whole-grain cereals (*e.g.* whole-wheat cereals, whole meal bread and brown rice) has been associated with a lower risk of cardiovascular disease (Pietinen *et al.*, 1996; Jacobs *et al.*, 1999; Liu *et al.*, 1999; Truswell, 2002). Vitamin E, dietary fibre (Richardson, 2000), resistant starch and oligosaccharides (Cummings *et al.*, 1992), as well as plant sterols (Jones *et al.*, 1997) are some of the components of whole-grain cereals that may contribute to a reduced risk of heart disease (Mc Kevith (2004) .

5.1.3.2.5 Antioxidant

Vitamins C, E, and B-carotene have antioxidant roles in the body. Vitamin E is the most concentrated antioxidant carried on LDLs and its major function is to prevent oxidation of

PUFA in the cell membrane (Krummel, 2008). Epidemiologic studies suggest that vitamin E and carotenoids are inversely related to CVD, but randomized trials have not supported these observations (Lee et al., 2005; Lichtenstein et al., 2006). Because data have not shown vitamin E to be protective, the AHA does not recommend vitamin E supplementation for CVD prevention (Lichtenstein et al., 2006). However, RRR-a-tocopherol, the natural form of vitamin E, shows promise as an antiinflammatory agent (Gasu et al., 2006). Foods with concentrated amounts of the phytonutrients catechins, have been found to improve vascular reactivity. These foods are red grapes, red wine, tea (especially green tea), chocolate, and olive oil, and should be worked into any CVD preventive eating plan (Kay et al., 2006). In our case – control study, drinking tea was significantly associated with lower risk of coronary events (Amani et al, 2010).

5.1.3.2.6 Stanols and sterols

Since the early 1950s plant stanols and sterols isolated from soybean oils or pine tree oil have been known to lower blood cholesterol (Lichtensteine et al., 2001). Recently they have been esterified and made into margarines. Consuming between 2 to 3 g/day lowers cholesterol by 9% to 20% (Lichtenstein et al., 2001). The mechanism for cholesterol lowering is by inhibiting absorption of dietary cholesterol. Adult Treatment Panel III (ATP-III) includes stanols as part of dietary recommendations for lowering LDL cholesterol in adults. Because these esters can also affect the absorption of and cause lower β-caroten , a-tocopherol, and lycopene levels, further safety studies are needed for use in normocholesterolemic individuals, children, and pregnant women (Krummel, 2008).

5.1.3.2.7 Dietary patterns

The effect on CVD risk of diets rich in whole grains and low in processed foods that are high in fat, sodium, and sugars has increasingly been investigated in both developed and developing countries. In parallel with economic development, radical dietary shifts toward Westernized diets that are high in animal products and refined carbohydrates and low in whole grains and other plant-based foods have occurred in many developing countries. For example in Iran, the results of Amani et al (2010) study showed that daily consumption of vegetable oils, tea and fish is significantly associated with lower risk of coronary events (odds ratio = 0.55(0.31-0.91), 0.3(0.15-0.65), 0.23(0.13-0.42), respectively). On the other hand, it was indicated that consumption of hydrogenated fats and full-fat yoghurt is associated with higher risk of coronary artery disease (OR = 2.12(1.23-3.64) and 2.35(1.32-4.18), respectively).

Substantial evidence has accumulated to support the notion that the traditional Mediterranean dietary pattern is protective against CVD . This pattern is characterized by an abundance of fruits, vegetables, whole grain cereals, nuts, and legumes; olive oil as the principal source of fat; moderate consumption of fish and lower consumption of red meat. It is important to note, however, that the dominance in research on the Mediterranean diet has come at the cost of research on other diets commonly consumed around the world that may also have heart health benefits (IOM , 2010).

5.1.3.2.8 Therapeutic life style change dietary pattern (TLC)

The ATP-III recommends the TLC dietary pattern for primary and secondary prevention of CHD. AHA recommends diet and lifestyle changes to reduce CVD risk in all people over the age of 2 years (Table 1) (Lichtenstein et al., 2006). SFA recommendations are less than 7% of calories; total fat content has a range of 25% to 35% of calories.

Consuming 30% to 35% of calories from fat while maintaining a low SFA and trans-fatty acid intake is the dietary pattern recommended for individuals with insulin resistance or metabolic syndrome. This higher fat intake, emphasizing PUFAs and monounsaturated fatty acids (MUFA), can be beneficial in lowering triglycerides and raising HDL cholesterol. Also, with a more liberal fat intake, LDL cholesterol can be lowered without exacerbating blood glucose levels. Increasing physical activity and decreasing energy intake to facilitate weight loss are critical to normalize multiple risk factors. Behavioral strategies for weight management to reduce cardiovascular risk have been provided by the AHA (Klein et al., 2004). Learning outcomes include planning meals that fit the TLC plan, reading food labels, modifying recipes, preparing or purchasing appropriate foods, and choosing healthier choices when dining out. Along with the TLC dietary pattern, the Dietary Approaches to Stop Hypertension (DASH) pattern is also appropriate for CVD prevention and treatment . Both of these dietary patterns emphasize grains, cereals, legumes, vegetables, fruits, lean meats, poultry fish, and nonfat dairy products.

Because animal fats provide about two thirds of the SFAs in diet, these foods are limited. High-fat choices are omitted, but low-fat choices can be included. Meat is limited to 5 oz/day, and eggs to four or fewer per week. Lean meats are high in protein, zinc, and iron; thus, patients who wish to consume meat, a 5-oz portion or less can be fit into the dietary plan if other low SFA choices are made. Neither food group has to be omitted; it is a matter of choice. Most people need to add the recommended two servings of fatty fish per week. Meeting sodium guidelines (1500 to 2300 mg daily) can be a challenge because lower-fat processed foods often contain salt to increase palatability. Patients may need to limit processed foods (Krummel 2008).

5.1.3.3 Alcohol

The global burden of diseases attributable to alcohol has recently been summarized; leading to the conclusion that alcohol is one of the largest avoidable risk factors in low and middle income countries (Rehm et al., 2009). Indeed, WHO estimates that the harmful use of alcohol was responsible for 3.8 percent of deaths and 4.5 percent of the global burden of disease in 2004 (WHO, 2009b). Excessive alcohol intake is associated with increased risk for hypertension, stroke, coronary artery disease, and other forms of CVD; however, there is also a robust body of evidence in a range of populations suggesting light to moderate intake of alcohol may reduce the risk of CHD. Indeed, research suggests that the relationship between alcohol intake and CVD outcomes follows a "J" curve, with the lowest rates being associated with low to moderate intakes of alcohol (Beilin and Puddey, 2006; Lucas et al., 2005). It is important to recognize that, as with any discussion of alcohol and health, the key issues are the quantity of alcohol consumed and the risk or benefit conferred by consumption. Although evidence indicates that low to moderate alcohol use can reduce the risk of CHD, excessive and harmful use clearly increases CVD risk (Beilin and Puddey, 2006; Lucas et al., 2005). It is important that approaches to reduce the burden of CVD not neglect the importance of reducing excessive alcohol consumption.

5.1.3.4 Physical activity

WHO and FAO have highlighted the importance of physical activity as a key determinant of obesity, CVD, and diabetes (Joint WHO/FAO Expert Consultation, 2003). For decades, evidences of the relationship between physical activity and CVD, independent of effects on weight and obesity, have been strengthened. Increasing physical activity—including brisk walking—has been shown to decrease the risk of chronic diseases such as CHD, stroke, some cancers (e.g., colorectal and breast cancer), type 2 diabetes, osteoporosis, high blood pressure, and high cholesterol (Physical Activity Guidelines Advisory Committee, 2008)

American Heart Association 2006 Diet Recommendations for Cardiovascular Disease Risk Reduction

- Balance calorie intake and physical activity to achieve or maintain a healthy body weight.
- Consume a diet rich in vegetables and fruits.
- Choose whole grain, high-fiber foods.
- Consume fish, especially oily fish, at least twice a week.
- Limit intake of saturated fat to <7% of energy, *trans*-fat to <1% of energy, and cholesterol to <300 mg/day by:
  - Choosing lean meats and vegetable alternatives.
  - Selecting fat-free (skim), 1%-fat, and low-fat dairy products.
  - Minimizing intake of partially hydrogenated fats.
- Minimize your intake of beverages and foods with added sugars.
- Choose and prepare foods with little or no salt.
- When consuming alcohol, do so in moderation.
- When eating food that is prepared outside of the home, follow the American Heart Association Diet and Lifestyle Recommendations.

Modified from Lichtenstein AH et al: Diet and lifestyle recommendations revision 2006: a scientific statement from the American Heart Association Committee, *Circulation* 114:83, 2006.

Table 1.

Regular physical activity and higher cardiorespiratory fitness are associated with lower overall mortality from CVD. Men and women who are physically active experience a lower risk of cardiovascular disease in general and CHD in particular (US Department of Health and Human Services, 1996; Wannamethee & Shaper, 2002). Furthermore, in the Nurses' Health Study, a large prospective study in the USA, both brisk walking and regular vigorous exercise were associated with a reduction in risk of coronary events by 30–40% (Manson *et al.*, 1999), and sedentary women who became active in middle age or later had a lower risk than their counterparts who remained sedentary . In one study performed among 145 women with central obesity, serum concentration of HDL-c was significantly higher in women who do more physical activity (Sharifi et al,2008). With overall mortality, the epidemiological literature for CHD indicates an inverse association and a dose response gradient between physical activity level or cardiorespiratory fitness and incidence of CHD. It helps to improve several risk factors for cardiovascular disease, including raised blood pressure, adverse blood lipid profile and insulin resistance.

5.1.4 Related diseases/syndrome

5.1.4.1 Overweight and obesity

Traditionally, obesity is defined as a BioPsychoSocial problem but in this chapter we rather intend to present it as an EcoBioPsychoSocioCutural issue.

Overweight and obesity have reached epidemic proportions, not only in developed but also in developing countries (Sassi et al., 2009). Even in low and middle income countries where undernutrition is still highly prevalent, overweight and obesity—especially among women—is a public health problem (Caballero, 2005; Hosseinpanah et al 2009). WHO and FAO reviewed the evidence on the relationship between obesity and the risk of CVD and concluded that overweight and obesity confer a significantly elevated risk of CHD (Joint WHO/FAO Expert Consultation, 2003). Increased body mass index (BMI) is also associated with greater risk of stroke in both Asian and Western populations (WHO/FAO, 2003). The association between obesity and CVD is partly mediated through hypertension, high cholesterol, and diabetes. Abdominal or central obesity measured by waist-to-hip ratio or waist circumference is associated with both CHD and stroke independent of BMI and other cardiovascular risk factors. Even in university educated women, obesity and central fat are also prevalent which increase the risk of heart disease. We studied 101female staff of the university, aged 20-45 years. Based on the bioelectrical impedance analysis (BIA) method, overweight and obesity rates were determined in 34.6 and 40.6 percent of women, respectively, and central obesity was prevalent in 27% of them (Amani, 2007a). It is worthy to note that to prevent erroneous classification, localization of cut-off points can be a more practical way to detect individuals at greater risk of chronic disease. In a sample of 637 married females, it was indicated that subjects in low BMI range tend to have higher fat percentages and they might represent a different category as overfat thin other than normal weight obese in Iranian women. (Amani, 2007b).

Obesity is also an independent risk factor for other cardiovascular outcomes, such as congestive heart failure and sudden cardiac death. Excess energy intake is one of the key contributors to obesity. The lack of data limits policy makers' abilities to focus attention on which dietary components lend to effective interventions that would reduce total calorie intake. One category that has been well studied in developed countries relates to sugar consumption, primarily in the form of sugar-sweetened beverages (including soft drinks, juice drinks, and energy and vitamin drinks). Recent NHANES data shows that up to 5.5 percent of dietary calories come from sugar-sweetened beverages in the United States (Bosire et al., 2009), which has led the American Heart Association to recommend an upper limit of 100 calories per day for women and 150 calories per day for men from added sugars, including soft drinks (Johnson et al., 2009). In some developing countries, consumption of sugar-sweetened beverages has increased dramatically in recent decades. Because of its excess caloric and sugar content, increasing consumption of sugar sweetened beverages may have important implications for obesity and cardiometabolic risk.

5.1.4.2 Hypertension

Hypertension is a risk factor for CHD, stroke, and heart failure. A recent review of the global burden of high blood pressure found that approximately 54 percent of stroke, 47 percent of IHD and 25 percent of other CVDs were attributable to hypertension. Among the major underlying risks for hypertension are sodium, body weight, and access to treatment. Primary prevention focused on sodium reduction, fruit and vegetable intake, weight control, and avoidance of excessive alcohol intake has been shown to make a difference (Krummel, 2008).

5.1.4.3 Diabetes

Around the world, diabetes is increasingly growing and is a significant contributor to CVD risk. People with diabetes have more than two-fold greater risk of CVD compared to non-diabetics (Asia Pacific Cohort Studies Collaboration, 2003). In fact, CVD is the leading cause of morbidity and mortality in people with diabetes (Booth et al., 2006; Kengne et al., 2007, 2009). Individuals without established clinical diabetes, but who are at increased risk of developing diabetes in the future, also have a higher risk of CVD (Asia Pacific Cohort Studies Collaboration, 2007). Women and younger individuals with diabetes have greater risk of CVD. Obesity is the single most important risk factor for type 2 diabetes, but unhealthy diet and physical inactivity also independently raise the population risk for diabetes (Schulze and Hu, 2005). According to the International Diabetes Federation's Diabetes Atlas 2010, the global estimated prevalence of diabetes for 2010 among people aged 20 to 79 years will be approximately 285 million people (6.4 percent of the global population), of which some 70 percent will be living in developing countries (International Diabetes Federation, 2010).

Diabetes is emerging as a particular concern in Asia, where more than 110 million individuals were living with diabetes in 2007, a large proportion of whom were young and middle aged. Asians tend to develop diabetes at a relatively young age and low BMI, and by 2025 the number of individuals with diabetes in the region is expected to rise to almost 180 million (Chan et al., 2009). Intensive glucose control reduces the risk of major cardiovascular events by approximately 10 percent, compared with standard treatment in people with diabetes. Interestingly, this benefit appeared to be independent of other cardiovascular risk factors (Kelly et al., 2009; Turnbull et al., 2009).

To sum up, as with the raising obesity epidemic, the prevalence of diabetes has increased dramatically worldwide. It is associated with serious health consequences and is a major risk factor for CHD and stroke. Therefore, prevention and management of diabetes are critical in reducing the global burden of CVD.

5.1.4.4 Psychosocial risk and mental health

Of all the psychosocial stressors associated with CVD, the link between depression and CVD is probably the best documented. There have been many published reviews and numerous meta-analyses have consistently found that depression and depressive symptoms are associated with an increased likelihood of developing CVD, a higher incidence of CVD events, poorer outcomes after CVD treatment and prevention efforts, and increased mortality from CVD. These associations remain consistent even after controlling for other CVD risk factors (Everson-Rose and Lewis, 2005; Frasure-Smith and Lesperance, 2006; Lesperance and Frasure-Smith, 2007; Lichtman et al., 2008).

Behaviors that increase CVD risks are more common in depressed patients. They are more likely to smoke, have poor diets, and be physically inactive. Furthermore, depression has been found to associate with the risk of non adherence to medical treatment regimens and lifestyle changes, making depressed patients with CVD or high CVD risk less likely to adhere to prevention efforts (Lichtman et al., 2008; Ziegelstein et al., 2000).

Chronic stress, most often studied by examining work-related stress, has been associated with negative behaviors such as low physical activity and poor diet, increased likelihood of recurrent CVD, as well as physiological consequences such as decreased heart rate variability. For instance, we found that the prevalence of overweight and obesity was higher in a sample of firefighters who may have chronic stress. Moreover they had high TC, TG and lipoprotein (a) and low HDL-C concentrations (Azabdaftari et al, 2009).

Acute stress from traumatic life events such as the death of a relative, earthquakes, or terrorist attacks have all been associated with significant temporal increases in the incidence of MI (Everson-Rose and Lewis, 2005; Figueredo, 2009).

It is clear that psychosocial factors play an important role in increasing CVD risk through both direct and indirect pathways. Continued research is needed to further explain the mechanisms by which psychosocial stressors and mental illness affect CVD risk. It is also important that clinicians are made aware of the effect of psychosocial factors on CVD risk, prognosis, and adherence to prevention efforts through improved training and knowledge expanding.

5.2 Nonmodifiable factors

5.2.1 Menopausal status

Loss of estrogen following natural or surgical menopause is associated with increased CVD risk. Endogenous estrogen has a protective role against CVD in premenopausal women, probably by preventing vascular injury. Rates of CHD in premenopausal women are low except in women with multiple risk factors. During the menopausal period total cholesterol, LDL cholesterol, and triglyceride levels increase; and HDL cholesterol level decreases, especially in women who are overweight or obese (Regitz-Zagrosek, 2006).

5.2.2 Age and gender

Age is a nonmodifiable risk factor for CHD. The increased risk for CHD parallels increase in age. Higher mortality rates from CHD are seen in both genders with increasing age.

Being older than 45 years of age is considered a risk factor for men (NCEP, 2002). For women the increased risk comes after the age of 55 years, which is after menopause for most women.

CVD prevalence, incidence, and mortality rates tend to be higher for men than for women. This finding has remained consistent historically (Lawlor et al., 2001) and across countries and regions (Allen and Szanton, 2005; Pilote et al., 2007; WHO, 2009).

Estrogen has a protective effect on the development of CVD risk factors and consequently is the reason most often cited for these gender differences (Regitz-Zagrosek, 2006). Estrogen is thought to contribute to premenopausal women's tendency to have lower systolic blood pressure, higher levels of HDL cholesterol, and lower triglyceride levels than men (Pilote et al., 2007).

The lower prevalence of smoking among women is another factor that could contribute to their decreased CVD incidence and mortality rates. Around the world, the prevalence of female smoking is lower than that of men (Pilote et al., 2007). Although rates of smoking, dyslipidemia, and hypertension are generally lower among women than men, women tend to have less favorable profiles for other key CVD risk factors. Worldwide, women are more likely to be sedentary than men (Guthold et al., 2008). Some researchers have suggested that women's social status in many cultures and their lack of leisure time due to childcare and other familial responsibilities likely contribute to their lower levels of physical activity (Brands and Yach, 2002; Pilote et al., 2007).

Another troubling gender difference is the increased prevalence of obesity among women. WHO data indicate that although overweight (BMI ≥ 25 kg/m2) is more common among men globally; obesity (BMI ≥30 kg/m2) is more common among women.

A number of different reasons have proposed by CVD researchers that why women might delay seeking medical attention, receive delayed treatment, and experience poorer outcomes during and after an MI or stroke. One often-cited reason that women tend to wait longer to seek treatment is that many do not perceive themselves as being at risk (Jensen and Moser, 2008).

Because of the robust evidence indicating gender differences in CVD incidence, morbidity, and outcomes, these differences, as well as the unique needs of women, should be considered when developing CVD research priorities, policies, and health service interventions.

6. Association between early life factors and subsequent risk for CVD

6.1 Low birth weight and adult cardiovascular disease

Ther is growing evidence in developing and developed countries ,based on cohort studies, that fetal and early childhood periods is important in the onset of CVD later in life (Victora et al., 2008; Walker and George, 2007; WHO, 2009c). The influences during this period include maternal factors during pregnancy, such as smoking, obesity, and malnutrition, and factors in infancy and early childhood, such as breastfeeding, low birth weight, and undernutrition.

Maternal smoking during pregnancy has been linked to CVD-related risk factors. It has been consistently associated with increased childhood obesity independent of other risk factors (Oken et al., 2008). A number of studies have examined the effects of maternal obesity on the body weight of their children; however, the evidence is inconsistent. Two cohort studies in the United States found that excessive weight gain or maternal obesity during pregnancy was associated with overweight and obesity in the children at ages 3 and 4 years (Gillman et al., 2008; Whitaker,2004). Similarly, a cohort study in Finland found that mothers' body mass index (BMI) was positively associated with their sons' BMI in childhood (Eriksson et al., 1999).

Another factor that appears to influence risk for long-term cardiovascular health is breastfeeding. Breastfeeding has been found to not only reduce childhood morbidity and mortality but also to be weakly protective against obesity later in life (Bhutta et al., 2008; Gluckman et al., 2008).

Undernutrition in infancy, especially when followed by rapid weight gain, is associated with increased risk of CVD and diabetes in adulthood (Barker and Bagby, 2005; Caballero, 2005; Gluckman et al., 2008). This phenomenon is known as the developmental origins theory of CVD. It means that if disruptions to the nutritional, metabolic, and hormonal environment at critical stages of development are happened, it may lead to permanent "programming" of the body's structure, physiology, and metabolism that translate into pathology and disease, including CVD, later in life (Barker, 1997, 1998, 2007). The exact physiological mechanisms through which this programming occurs are not yet fully elucidated; however, there is evidence that fetal and early postnatal undernutrition can cause metabolic, anatomic, and endocrine adaptations that affect the hypothalamic-pituitary-adrenal axis, lipoprotein profiles, and end organ glucose uptake, among other processes (Prentice and Moore, 2005). Support for the developmental origins theory of CVD comes from a number of retrospective, and more recently prospective, cohort studies in various populations. Studies in the United Kingdom, the United States, Finland, and India found that fetal undernutrition followed by a rapid catch-up growth from childhood to early adolescence was significantly associated with the later development of CVD in both men and women (Barker et al., 2005; Eriksson et al., 1999; Osmond and Barker, 2000). Early undernutrition followed by catch-up growth during childhood has also been associated with subsequent hypertension and type 2 diabetes (Barker, 1998; Osmond and Barker, 2000) This emerging data on the effects of rapid weight gain after early undernutrition have prompted some researchers to suggest a shift from the original "fetal origins" hypothesis to an "accelerated postnatal growth hypothesis" of CVD (Singhal et al., 2003, 2004).

The emerging evidence on the association between low birth weight followed by rapid growth in childhood and subsequent risk for CVD raises important considerations for addressing global CVD because low birth weight and exposure to undernutrition in utero and in infancy are common in many developing countries (Caballero, 2009; Kelishadi, 2007).

The acquisition and accumulation of risk for CVD continues in childhood and adolescence (Celermajer and Ayer, 2006). Unhealthful lifestyle practices such as consumption of high calorie and high fat foods, tobacco use, and physical inactivity begin in childhood, introducing major behavioral risks for CVD. Childhood adversity also influences adult cardiovascular health. In addition, there is also an emerging body of evidence on the presence of biological risk factors in children and youth, including pathophysiological processes associated with heart disease that can be seen as early as childhood.

6.2 Childhood obesity and CVD risk

Childhood obesity is associated with multiple risk factors for CVD, which are amplified in the presence of overweight and persist from childhood into adulthood. These risk factors include hyperlipidemia, high blood pressure, impaired glucose tolerance and high insulin levels, as well as metabolic syndrome. It has been estimated that 60 percent of overweight children possess at least one of these risk factors that can lead to CVD in adulthood (Freedman et al., 1999). This is especially important in terms of implications for global CVD because the prevalence of childhood obesity is increasing in developing countries (WHO, 2008a).

7. Public health approach to cardiovascular disease risk reduction

7.1 Cardiovascular disease as a public health problem

The prevention of cardiovascular disease is a major public health challenge for a number of years around the world. Although death rates have been falling in many westernized countries (*e.g.* USA, Australia, UK), rates are rising rapidly elsewhere.

7.2 Current dietary recommendations for primary prevention

Dietary recommendations tend to be country specific and are based on the available evidence.

The ATP-III recommends the TLC dietary pattern for primary and secondary prevention of CHD. In agreement, the AHA recommends diet and lifestyle changes to reduce CVD risk in all people over the age of 2 years (Lichtenstein et al., 2006).

As is evident, knowledge about the role of diet in risk factor reduction and reducing the risk of cardiovascular events themselves continues to expand. It is now recognized that CVD risk can be mediated through multiple biological pathways other than only serum total and LDL cholesterol or dietary factors. With this in mind, it is necessary to modify the dietary advice offered to those with an increased risk of CVD.

7.3 Health promotion in children and other subgroups of the population

Health aspects present in childhood, such as blood lipids, body weight and blood pressure may track into adulthood. Therefore, a useful health strategy is the adoption of sensible eating habits and an active lifestyle early in childhood. It is important to promote cardiovascular health in childhood by increasing physical activity and preventing or treating obesity, raised blood pressure, insulin resistance and type 2 diabetes (Williams *et al.*, 2002). Current nutritional recommendations for the general population are applicable for most children over 5 years and can be gradually applied from the age of 2 years. It is also recommended that all children and adolescents participate in physical activity for 1 hour daily which should be of at least moderate intensity (Fox & Riddoch, 2000). The implementation of guidelines and success of health strategies require input from the governments, health professionals, the food industry and teachers, as well as the children themselves and their parents. Moreover, social and cultural influences must be recognized when designing and implementing strategies.

8. Summary

- Cardiovascular disease is the leading cause of death worldwide, accounting for around 18 million deaths each year.
- Modifiable risk factors for cardiovascular disease include atherogenic lipoproteins, inflammatory related factors behaviors, lifestyle and chronic diseases such as obesity, diabetes and hypertension.
- Non modifiable risk factors include menopause, age and gender.
- There is evidence that a chronic, low-grade inflammation underlies atherosclerosis, although it is not clear whether this is a cause or effect phenomenon.
- The acute phase proteins, C-reactive protein (CRP), fibrinogen and serum amyloid A, appear to be associated with risk for cardiovascular disease.
- The advantages of a dietary pattern approach rather than individual dietary components can influence plasma cholesterol levels and may also affect other emerging risk factors.
- Physical activity has great impact on CVD risk reduction when it is accompanied by dietary pattern changes.
- Low birth weight and low weight gain during infancy are associated with an increased risk of adult cardiovascular disease, hypertension, type 2 diabetes and the insulin resistance syndrome.

9. Future research

Future research is required to establish the strength of the associations between the emerging risk factors described in this chapter and cardiovascular disease, in order to compare their predictive value with the established risk factors. For example, further work is required to evaluate the independence of many of the novel risk factors for cardiovascular disease and whether these associations are causal. In addition, more information is needed about how these novel risk factors might be modified by different aspects of the diet. As indicated in ancient Traditional Persian Medicine (TPM), understanding the effect of individual foods on the trend of heart disease and hyperlipidemias can be leading fields of study in the near future.

Moreover, local modified risk factors should be defined and addressed to track the patients at greater risks in more applicable ways.

10. References

Allen, J., & S. Szanton. 2005. Gender, ethnicity, and cardiovascular disease. *Journal of Cardiovascular Nursing* 20(1):1-6; quiz 7-8.

Amani R, Baghdadchi J & Zand-Moghaddam A, 2005. Effects of Soy Protein Isoflavones on Serum Lipids, Lipoprotein Profile and Serum Glucose of Hypercholesterolemic Rabbits. *Int J Endocrinol Metab* ; 2:87-92.

Amani R, noorizadeh M, Rahmanian S, Afzali N & Haghighizadeh M, 2010. Nutritional related cardiovascular risk factors in patients with coronary artery disease in IRAN:A case-control study. *Nutrition Journal*, 9:70.

Reza Amani, Fereshteh Boustani. 2007 a. Prevalence of obesity and dietary practices in Jondi-Shapour University female personnel, Ahvaz, Iran Pak J Med Sci;24(4):748-52.

Amani R, 2007 **b**. Comparison between bioelectrical impedance analysis and body mass index methods in determination of obesity prevalence in Ahvazi women. Eur J Clin Nutr ;61(4): 478-82.

Anber V, Millar JS, McConnell M, Shepherd J, Packard CJ& 1997. *Interaction of very-low-density, intermediatedensity, and low-density lipoproteins with human arterial wall proteoglycans. Arteriosclerosis, Thrombosis and Vascular Biology, 17, 2507–14.*

Anderson JW, Johnstone BM and Cook-Newell ME & 1995. Meta-analysis of the effects of soy protein intake on serum lipids. N Engl J Med. 3;333(5):276-82.

Anerson JJB, Anthony M, Messina M & Garner SC, 1999. Effects of phyto-oestrogens on tissues. *Nutr Res Rev.* 12: 75-116.

Anthony MS, Clarkson TB, Hughes CL Jr, Morgan TM & Burke GL, 1996. Soybean isoflavones improve cardiovascular risk factors without affecting the reproductive system of peripubertal rhesus monkeys. J Nutr. 126(1):43-50.

Arora A, Nair MG & Strasburg GM, 1998. Antioxidant activities of isoflavones and their biological metabolites in a liposomal system. *Arch Biochem Biophys.* 356(2):133-41.

Asia Pacific Cohort Studies Collaboration. 2003. The effects of diabetes on the risks of major cardiovascular diseases and death in the Asia Pacific region. *Diabetes Care* 26(2): 360-366.

Asia Pacific Cohort Studies Collaboration. 2007. Cholesterol, diabetes and major cardiovascular diseases in the Asia-Pacific region. *Diabetologia* 50(11):2289-2297.

Astrup A ,2002. *Dietary fat is a major player in obesity – but not the only one. Obesity Reviews, 3, 57– 8.*

Aygun A D et al,2005. Proinflammatoy cytokines and leptin are increased in serum of prepubertal obese children, *Mediators Inflamm* 3 :180.

Azabdaftari N, Amani R, Taha Jalali M, 2009. Biochemical and nutritional indices as cardiovascular risk factors among Iranian firefighters. *Ann Clin Biochem.* Sep;46(Pt 5):385-9

Barker, D. J. 1997. The fetal origins of coronary heart disease. *Acta Paediatrica Supplement* 422:78-82.

Barker, D. J. P. 1998. In utero programming of chronic disease. *Clinical Science* 95(2): 115-128.

Barker, D. J. P., & S. P. Bagby. 2005. Developmental antecedents of cardiovascular disease: A historical perspective. *Journal of the American Society of Nephrology* 16(9): 2537-2544.

Barker, D. J. P. 2007. The origins of the developmental origins theory. *Journal of Internal Medicine* 261(5):412-417.

Basu A et al,2006: Dietary factors that promote or retard inflammation, Arterioscler Thromb Vasc Biol, 26:995.

Beilin, L. J., & I. B. Puddey. 2006. Alcohol and hypertension: An update. *Hypertension* 47(6):1035-1038.

Bhutta, Z. A., T. Ahmed, R. E. Black, S. Cousens, K. Dewey, E. Giugliani, B. A. Haider, B.Kirkwood, S. S. Morris, H. P. S. Sachdev, & M. Shekar. 2008. What works? Interventions for maternal and child undernutrition and survival. *Lancet* 371(9610):417-440.

Blum CA et al,2005. Low-grade inflammation and estimates of insulin resistance during the menstrual cycle in lean and overweight women. *J Clin Endocrinol Metab* 90:3230.

Booth, G. L., M. K. Kapral, K. Fung, & J. V. Tu. 2006. Recent trends in cardiovascular complications among men and women with and without diabetes. *Diabetes Care* 29(1):32-37.

Bosire, C., J. Reedy, & S. M. Krebs-Smith. 2009. *Sources of energy and selected nutrient intakes among the US population, 2005 -06 : A report prepared for the 2010 dietary guidelines advisory committee.* Bethesda, MD: National Cancer Institute.

Brands, A., & D. Yach. 2002. Women and the rapid rise of noncommunicable diseases.*World Health Organization NMH Reader* (1):1-22.

Brown L, Rosner B, Willett WW& Sacks FM ,1999.) *Cholesterol lowering effects of dietary fibre: a meta-analysis.*

Buckley DI, Fu R, Freeman M, Rogers K & Helfand M. (2009). C-reactive protein as a risk factor for coronary heart disease: a systematic U.S. Preventive Services Task Force. *Ann Intern Med , 151,* 483-495.

Caballero, B. 2005. A nutrition paradox – underweight and obesity in developing countries. *New England Journal of Medicine* 352(15):1514-1516.

Caballero, B. 2009. Early undernutrition and risk of CVD in the adult. Presentation at Public Information Gathering Session for the Institute of Medicine Committee on Preventing the Global Epidemic of Cardiovascular Disease, Washington, DC.

Celermajer, D. S., & J. G. Ayer. 2006. Childhood risk factors for adult cardiovascular disease and primary prevention in childhood. *Heart* 92(11):1701-1706.

Chait A, Brazg RL, Tribble DL & Krauss RM ,1993. *Susceptibility of small, dense, low-density lipoproteins to oxidative modification in subjects with the atherogenic lipoprotein phenotype, pattern B. American Journal of Medicine, 94, 350–6.*

Chan, J. C., V. Malik, W. Jia, T. Kadowaki, C. S. Yajnik, K. H. Yoon, F. B. & Hu. 2009. Diabetes in Asia: Epidemiology, risk factors, and pathophysiology. *Journal of the American Medical Association* 301(20):2129-2140.

Chen , L. Y. , & J. L. Mehta . 1994 . Inhibitory effect of high-density lipoprotein on platelet function is mediated by increase in nitric oxide synthase activity in platelets. *Life Sci.* 55 : 1815 – 1821 .

Critchley, J., J. Liu, D. Zhao, W. Wei, and S. Capewell. 2004. Explaining the increase in coronary heart disease mortality in Beijing between 1984 and 1999. *Circulation* 110(10):1236-1244.

Cummings J, Bingham S, Heaton K, Eastwood M ,1992. *Fecal weight, colon cancer risk and dietary intake of non-starch polysaccharide (dietary fibre). Gastroenterology, 103, 1783–7.*

Danesh J, Whincup P, Walker M et al. ,2000. *Low grade inflammation and coronary heart disease: prospective study and update meta-analyses. British Medical Journal, 321, 199–203.*

Davies, A. R., L. Smeeth, and E. M. Grundy. 2007. Contribution of changes in incidence and mortality to trends in the prevalence of coronary heart disease in the UK: 1996-2005. *European Heart Journal* 28(17):2142-2147.

Davignon J, Ganz P, 2004. Role of endothelial dysfunction in atherosclerosis. *Circulation* ,109(23 suppl │):III27.

Dejager S, Bruckert E, Chapman MJ ,1993. *Dense low density lipoprotein subspecies with diminished oxidative resistance predominate in combined hyperlipidaemia. Journal of Lipid Research, 34, 295–308.*

de Lorgeril M et al,1999: Mediterranean diet, traditional risk factors, and the rate of cardiovascular complications after myocardial infarction, *Circulation*, 99 :779.

D'Erasmo E, Acca M, Celi F, Medici F, Palmerini T and Pisani D,1993. Plasma fibrinogen and platelet count in stroke. J Med;24:185-191.

Dreon DM, Fernstrom HA, Miller B, Krauss RM ,1994. Low-density lipoprotein subclass patterns and lipoprotein response to a reduced-fat diet in men. FASEB Journal, 8, 121–6.

Eriksson, J. G., T. Forsen, J. Tuomilehto, P. D. Winter, C. Osmond, and D. J. P. Barker. 1999. Catch-up growth in childhood and death from coronary heart disease: Longitudinal study. *British Medical Journal* 318:7181.

Everson-Rose, S. A., and T. T. Lewis. 2005. Psychosocial factors and cardiovascular diseases. In *Annual Review of Public Health* 26(1):469-500.

Figueredo, V. M. 2009. The time has come for physicians to take notice: The impact of psychosocial stressors on the heart. *American Journal of Medicine* 122(8):704-712.

Foster, R. K., and H. E. Marriott. 2006. Alcohol consumption in the new millennium — weighing up the risks and benefits for our health. *Nutrition Bulletin* 31(4):286-331.

Fox KR, Riddoch CJ (2000) *Charting the physical activity patterns of contempory children and adolescents. Proceedings of the Nutrition Society, 59, 497–504.*

Frasure-Smith, N., and F. Lesperance. 2006. Recent evidence linking coronary heart disease and depression. *Canadian Journal of Psychiatry – Revue Canadienne de Psychiatrie* 51(12):730-737.

Frayn K ,2005. *Cardiovascular disease diet, nutrition and emerging risk factors. Blackwell Publishing.* Oxford,UK.

Gao X et al,2004. Plasma C-reactive protein and homosysteine concentrations are related to frequent fruit and vegetable intake in Hispanic and non-Hispanic white elders . *J Nutr* ,134:913.

Gebauer SK et al, 2006. n-3 fatty acid dietary recommendations and food sources to achieve essentiality and cardiovascular benefits. Am J Clin Nutr 83(6 suppl):15262s.

Gillman, M. W., S. L. Rifas-Shiman, K. Kleinman, E. Oken, J. W. Rich-Edwards, and E. M. Taveras. 2008. Developmental origins of childhood overweight: Potential public health impact. *Obesity* 16(7):1651-1656.

Gluckman, P. D., M. A. Hanson, A. S. Beedle, and D. Raubenheimer. 2008. Fetal and neonatal pathways to obesity. In *Frontiers of hormone research*. Vol. 36. Edited by M. Korbonits. Basel: Karger. Pp. 61-72.

Gotoh K et al, 2006. Apolipoprotein A -IV interacts synergistically with melanocoftins to reduce food intake, *Am J Physiol Regul Integr Comp Physiol* 290 :R202.

Gritz, E. R., D. J. Vidrine, and M. Cororve Fingeret. 2007. Smoking cessation. A critical component of medical management in chronic disease populations. *American Journal of Preventive Medicine* 33(6 Suppl):S414-S422.

Guthold, R., T. Ono, K. L. Strong, S. Chatterji, and A. Morabia. 2008. Worldwide variability in physical inactivity – a 51-country survey. *American Journal of Preventive Medicine* 34(6):486-494.

Hadaegh F, Harati H, Ghanbarian A, Azizi F 2009. Prevalence of coronary heart disease among Tehran adults: Tehran Lipid and Glucose Study. *East Mediterr Health J.*;15(1):157-66.

He, F. J., and G. A. MacGregor. 2009. A comprehensive review on salt and health and current experience of worldwide salt reduction programmes. *Journal of Human Hypertension* 23(6):363-384.

Hodgson JM, Puddey IB, Beilin LJ, Mori TA and Croft KD,1998. Supplementation with isoflavonoid phytoestrogens does not alter serum lipid concentrations: a randomized controlled trial in humans. J Nutr.;128(4):728-32.

Hosseinpanah F, Barzin M, Eskandary PS, Mirmiran P, Azizi F, 2009. Trends of obesity and abdominal obesity in Tehranian adults: a cohort study.*BMC Public Health.* 23;9:426.

Hu, F. B. 2008. Globalization of food patterns and cardiovascular disease risk. *Circulation* 118(19):1913-1914.

IDF (International Diabetes Federation). 2006. The diabetes atlas. Brussels: IDF.

IDF. 2010. *The diabetes atlas.* Brussels: IDF.

IOM (Institute of Medicine). 2009. *Secondhand smoke exposure and cardiovascular effects: Making sense of the evidence.* Washington, DC: The National Academies Press.

IOM. 2010. *Promoting Cardiovascular Health in the Developing World: A Critical Challenge to Achieve Global Health.* Washington, DC: The National Academies Press.

Jacobs DR, Meyer KA, Kushi LH, Folsom AR ,1999. *Is whole grain intake associated with reduced total and cause-specific death rates in older women? The Iowa Women's Health Study. American Journal of Public Health, 89, 322–9.*

Jensen, L. A., and D. K. Moser. 2008. Gender differences in knowledge, attitudes, and beliefs about heart disease. *Nursing Clinics of North America* 43(1):77-104; vi-vii.

Jequier, E. 1999. Alcohol intake and body weight: A paradox. *American Journal of Clinical Nutrition* 69(2):173-174.

Jha, P., and F. J. Chaloupka. 1999. Curbing the epidemic: Governments and the economics of tobacco control. Washington, DC: World Bank.

Johnson, R. K., L. J. Appel, M. Brands, B. V. Howard, M. Lefevre, R. H. Lustig, F. Sacks, L. M. Steffen, J. Wylie-Rosett, P. A. American Heart Association Nutrition Committee of the Council on Nutrition, Physical Activity, and Metabolism, and the the Council on Epidemiology and Prevention. 2009. Dietary sugars intake and cardiovascular health: A scientific statement from the American Heart Association. *Circulation* 120(11):1011-1020.

Joint WHO/FAO Expert Consultation on Diet Nutrition and the Prevention of Chronic Diseases and World Health Organization Department of Nutrition for Health and Development.2003. *Diet, nutrition and the prevention of chronic diseases: Report of a joint WHO/FAO expert consultation, Geneva, January- February 2002, WHO technical report series.* Geneva: World Health Organization.

Jones PJ, MacDougall DE, Ntanios F, Vanstone CA ,1997. *Dietary phytosterols as cholesterol-lowering agents in humans. Canadian Journal of Physiology and Pharmacology, 75, 217–27.*

Joseph A, Kutty VR and Soman CR ,2000. High risk for coronary heart disease in Thiruvananthapuram City: A study of serum lipids and other risk factors. Indian Heart J 2000, 52:29-35.

Karmally W, 2005. Balancing unsaturated fatty acids: what is the evidence for cholesterol lowering ?*J Am Diet assoc* 105:1068.

Kay CD et al, 2006. Effects of antioxidant rich foods on vascular reactivity review of the clinical evidence Curr Atheroscer Rep 8:510.

Kelishadi, R. 2007. Childhood overweight, obesity, and the metabolic syndrome in developing countries. *Epidemiologic Reviews* 29:62-76.

Kelly, T. N., L. A. Bazzano, V. A. Fonseca, T. K. Thethi, K. Reynolds, and J. He. 2009. Glucose control and cardiovascular disease in type 2 diabetes. *Annals of Internal Medicine* 151(6):1-10.

Kengne, A. P., A. Patel, F. Barzi, K. Jamrozik, T. H. Lam, H. Ueshima, D. F. Gu, I. Suh, and M. Woodward. 2007. Systolic blood pressure, diabetes and the risk of cardiovascular diseases in the Asia-Pacific region. *Journal of Hypertension* 25(6):1205-1213.

Kengne, A. P., K. Nakamura, F. Barzi, T. H. Lam, R. Huxley, D. Gu, A. Patel, H. C. Kim, and M. Woodward. 2009. Smoking, diabetes and cardiovascular diseases in men in the Asia Pacific region. *Journal of Diabetes* 1(3):173-181.

Klein S et al, 2004. Clinical implications of obesity with specific focus on cardiovascular disease :a statement for professionals from the American Heart association Council on Nutrition, Physical Activity, and Metabolism: endorsed by the American College of Cardiology Foundation, *Circulation* 110; 2952.

Krummel DA 2008. Medical nutrition therapy for cardiovascular disease, In: *Krauses food & nutrition therapy* (2008). Mahan K & Scott-Stump S,pp(833-864) 12th ed. Philadelphia: Saunders; ISBN: 978-1-4160-3401-8

Lamarche B, St-Pierre AC, Ruel IL, Cantin B, Dagenais GR, Despres JP, 2001. A prospective, population based study of low density lipoprotein particle size as a risk factor for ischemic heart disease in men. Can J Cardiol; 17:859–65.

Lawlor, D. A., S. Ebrahim, and G. Davey Smith. 2001. Sex matters: Secular and geographical trends in sex differences in coronary heart disease mortality. *British Medical Journal* 323(7312):541-545: Erratum 325(7364):580.

Lesperance, F., and N. Frasure-Smith. 2007. Depression and heart disease. *Cleveland Clinic Journal of Medicine* 74(Suppl 1):S63-S66.

Lichtenstein AH,1998. Soy protein, isoflavones and cardiovascular disease risk. J Nutr. Oct;128(10):1589-92.

Lichtenstein AH et al,2001. Stanol/steroel ester-containing foods and blood cholesterol levels, *Circulation* 103:1177.

Lichtenstein AH et al, 2006. Diet and lifestyle recommendations revision 2006: a scientific statement from the American Heart Association Nutrition Committee, *Circulation* 114:82.

Lichtman, J. H., J. T. Bigger Jr., J. A. Blumenthal, N. Frasure-Smith, P. G. Kaufmann, F. Lesperance, D. B. Mark, D. S. Sheps, C. B. Taylor, and E. S. Froelicher. 2008. Depression and coronary heart disease: Recommendations for screening, referral, and treatment—a science advisory from the American Heart Association Prevention Committee of the Council on Cardiovascular Nursing, Council on Clinical Cardiology, Council on Epidemiology and Prevention, and Interdisciplinary Council on Quality of Care and Outcomes Research. *Circulation* 118(17):1768-1775.

Liu S, Stampfer MJ, Hu FB et al. ,1999. *Whole-grain consumption and risk of coronary heart disease: results from the Nurses' Health Study. American Journal of Clinical Nutrition, 70, 412–9.*

Lominadze D, Joshua I and Schuschke D, 1998. Increased erythrocyte aggregation in spontaneously hypertensive rats. Am J Hypertens;11:784–789.

Lominadze D, Dean WL, Tyagi SC and Roberts AM, 2010. Mechanisms of fibrinogen-induced microvascular dysfunction during cardiovascular disease. *Acta Physiol* ;198(1): 1–13.

Lopez, A. D., C. D. Mathers, M. Eszati, D. T. Jamison, and C. J. L. Murray. 2006. *Global burden of disease and risk factors.* Washington, DC: World Bank.

Lucas, D. L., R. A. Brown, M. Wassef, and T. D. Giles. 2005. Alcohol and the cardiovascular system research challenges and opportunities. *Journal of the American College Cardiology* 45(12):1916-1924.

Manson JE, Hu FB, Rich-Edwards JW et al. ,1999. *A prospective study of walking as compared with vigorous exercise in the prevention of CHD in women. New England Journal of Medicine, 341(9), 650–8.*

McKevith B ,2004. *Nutritional aspects of cereals. Nutrition Bulletin, 29, 111–42.*

Mensink RP et al, 2003. Effects of dietary fatty acids and carbohydrates on the ratio of serum total to HDL cholesterol and on serum lipids and apolipoproteins a: meta-analysis of 60 controlled trials, *Am J Clin Nutr* 77 :1146.

Mozaffarian D, Abdollahi M, Campos H, Houshiarrad A, Willett WC, 2007. Consumption of trans fats and estimated effects on coronary heart disease in Iran. *Eur J Clin Nutr*, 61(8):1004-10.

Mukamal, K. J., S. E. Chiuve, E. B. Rimm, K. J. Mukamal, S. E. Chiuve, and E. B. Rimm. 2006. Alcohol consumption and risk for coronary heart disease in men with healthy lifestyles. *Archives of Internal Medicine* 166(19):2145-2150.

Musunuru K, Kral BG, Blumenthal RS, et al. (2008). The use of high-sensitivity assays for C-reactive protein in clinical practice. *Nat Clin Pract Cardiovasc Med* , 5, 621-625.

National Cholesterol Education Program (NCEP): Expert Panel on Detection, Evaluation, and Treatment of High Blood Cholesterol in Adults (Adult Treatment Panel III final report, 2002. *Circulation* 106:3143.

Nestel PJ, Yamashita T, Sasahara T, Pomeroy S, Dart A, Komesaroff P, et al, 1997. Soy isoflavones improve systemic arterial compliance but not plasma lipids in menopausal and perimenopausal women. *Arterioscler Thromb Vasc Biol*; 17 (12):3392-8.

Oken, E., E. B. Levitan, and M. W. Gillman. 2008. Maternal smoking during pregnancy and child overweight: Systematic review and meta-analysis. *International Journal of Obesity* 32(2):201-210.

Osmond, C., and D. J. P. Barker. 2000. Fetal, infant, and childhood growth are predictors of coronary heart disease, diabetes, and hypertension in adult men and women. *Environmental Health Perspectives* 108(Suppl 3):545-553.

Pietinen P, Rimm EB, Korhonen P et al. ,1996. *Intake of dietary fibre and risk of coronary heart disease in a cohort of Finnish men. The Alpha-Tocopherol, Beta carotene Cancer Prevention Study. Circulation, 94, 2720–7.*

Pilote, L., K. Dasgupta, V. Guru, K. H. Humphries, J. McGrath, C. Norris, D. Rabi, J. Tremblay, A. Alamian, T. Barnett, J. Cox, W. A. Ghali, S. Grace, P. Hamet, T. Ho, S. Kirkland, M. Lambert, D. Libersan, J. O'Loughlin, G. Paradis, M. Petrovich, and V. Tagalakis. 2007. A comprehensive view of sex-specific issues related to cardiovascular disease. *Canadian Medical Association Journal* 176(6):S1-S44: Erratum 176(9):1310.

Rawson ES et al, 2001. Body mass index, but not physical activity, is associated with C-reactive protein, *Med Sci Sports Exerc* 35 :1160.=

Regitz-Zagrosek, V. 2006. Therapeutic implications of the gender-specific aspects of cardiovascular disease. *Nature Reviews Drug Discovery* 5(5):425-438.

Rehm, J., C. Mathers, S. Popova, M. Thavorncharoensap, Y. Teerawattananon, and J. Patra.2009. Global burden of disease and injury and economic cost attributable to alcohol use and alcohol-use disorders. *Lancet* 373(9682):2223-2233.

Richardson DP , 2000. *The grain, the wholegrain and nothing but the grain: the science behind the wholegrain and the reduced risk of heart disease and cancer. Nutrition Bulletin, 25, 353–60.*

Ridker PM, Buring JE, Shih J ,1998. *Prospective study of C-reactive protein and the risk of future cardiovascular events among apparently healthy women. Circulation, 97, 425–8*

Ridker PM, Hennekens CH, Buring JE, Rifai N ,2000. *Creactive protein and other markers of inflammation in the prediction of cardiovascular disease in women. N Engl J Med, 342, 836–43.*

Ridker PM, Danielson E, Fonseca FA, et al ,2008. Rosuvastatin to prevent vascular events in men and women with elevated C-reactive protein. *N Engl J Med;359:2195–2207.*

Ridker PM, Danielson E, Fonseca FA, et al ,2009.. Reduction in C-reactive protein and LDL cholesterol and cardiovascular event rates after initiation of rosuvastatin: a prospective study of the JUPITER trial. *Lancet ;373:1175–1182.*

Ross R ,1999. *Mechanisms of disease – atherosclerosis – an inflammatory disease. New England Journal of Medicine, 340, 115–26.*

Rudd JHF et al: Imaging of atherosclerosis-can we predict Plaque rupture?*Trends Cardiovasc Med* 15:17,2005.

Sassi, F., M. Cecchini, J. Lauer, and D. Chisholm. 2009. *Improving lifestyles, tackling obesity: The health and economic impact of prevention strategies.* Paris: OECD.

Scanu AM and Edelstein C, 2008. HDL: bridging past and present with a look at the future. *The FASEB Journal* 22, 4044-54.

Schulze, M. B., F. B. Hu. 2005. Primary prevention of diabetes: What can be done and how much can be prevented? *Annual Review of Public Health* 26:445-467.

Shafey, O., M. Eriksen, H. Ross, and J. Mackay. 2009. *The tobacco atlas.* 3rd ed. Atlanta: American Cancer Society.

Sharifi N, Mahdavi R, Ebrahimi-Mameghani M. Association between physical activity and lipid profile in a sample of women with central obesity. First National Congress of Metabolic Syndrome, Tabriz, Iran. 13-14 June, 2008.

Singhal, A., M. Fewtrell, T. J. Cole, and A. Lucas. 2003. Low nutrient intake and early growth for later insulin resistance in adolescents born preterm. *Lancet* 361(9363):1089-1097.

Singhal, A., T. J. Cole, M. Fewtrell, J. Deanfield, A. Lucas, A. Singhal, T. J. Cole, M. Fewtrell, J. Deanfield, and A. Lucas. 2004. Is slower early growth beneficial for long-term cardiovascularhealth? *Circulation* 109(9):1108-1113.

Skalen K, Gustafsson M, Knutsen Rydberg E et al , 2002. *Subendothelial retention of atherogenic lipoproteins in early atherosclerosis. Nature, 417, 750–4. susceptibility among six low density lipoprotein subfractions of differing density and particle size. Atherosclerosis, 93, 189–99.*

Trichopoulou et al, 2003. Adherence to a Mediterranean diet and survival in a Greek population, *N Engl J Med* 348:2599.

Truswell AS ,2002. *Cereal grains and coronary heart disease. European Journal of Clinical Nutrition, 56, 1–14.*

Turnbull, F. M., C. Abraira, R. J. Anderson, R. P. Byington, J. P. Chalmers, W. C. Duckworth, G. W. Evans, H. C. Gerstein, R. R. Holman, T. E. Moritz, B. C. Neal, T. Ninomiya, A. A. Patel, S. K. Paul, F. Travert, and M. Woodward. 2009. Intensive glucose control and macrovascular outcomes in type 2 diabetes. *Diabetologia.* DOI 10.1007/s00125-00009-01470-00120.

US Department of Health and Human Services ,1996. Physical Activity and Health: A Report of the Surgeon General. US Department of Health and Human Services, Centers for Disease Control and Prevention, Atlanta.

Victora, C. G., L. Adair, C. Fall, P. C. Hallal, R. Martorell, L. Richter, and H. S. Sachdev. 2008. Maternal and child undernutrition: Consequences for adult health and human capital. *Lancet* 371(9609):340-357.

Walker, S., and S. George. 2007. Young@heart. USA: Fox Searchlight Pictures.

Wannamethee SG, Shaper AG , 2002. Physical activity and cardiovascular disease. Seminars in Vascular Medicine, 2, 257–65.

Whitaker, R. C. 2004. Predicting preschooler obesity at birth: The role of maternal obesity in early pregnancy. *Pediatrics* 114(1):e29-e36.

WHO.2003. *The world health report: 2003: Shaping the future.* Geneva: World Health Organization.

WHO.2005.*Preventing chronic diseases: A vital investment.* http://www.who.int/chp/chronic_disease_report/full_report.pdf (accessed April 23, 2009).

WHO. 2008a. *The global burden of disease: 2004 update.* Geneva: World Health Organization.

WHO. 2008b. *WHO report on the global tobacco epidemic, 2008 : The MPOWER package.* Geneva: World Health Organization.

WHO. 2009a. *World health statistics 09 .* Geneva: World Health Organization.

WHO. 2009b. *Global health risks: Mortality and burden of disease attributable to selected major risks.* Geneva: World Health Organization.

WHO. 2009 c. *Aging and life course.* Geneva: World Health Oranization.

WHOSIS (World Health Organization Statistical Information System). 2009. World Health Organization.

Wijendran V and Hayes KC, 2004: Dietary n-6 and n-3 fatty acid balance and cardiovascular health. *Annu Rev Nutr* 24:597.

Willett WC, 1998. *Is dietary fat a major determinant of body fat? American Journal of Clinical Nutrition, 67, 556S–62S.*

Williams CL, Hayman LL, Daniels SR et al., 2002. *Cardiovascular health in childhood: a statement for health professionals from the Committee on Atherosclerosis, Hypertension, and Obesity in the Young (AHOY) of the Council on Cardiovascular Disease in the Young, American Heart Association. Circulation, 106, 143–60.*

Ziegelstein, R. C., J. A. Fauerbach, S. S. Stevens, J. Romanelli, D. P. Richter, and D. E. Bush. 2000. Patients with depression are less likely to follow recommendations to reduce cardiac risk during recovery from a myocardial infarction. *Archives of Internal Medicine* 160(12):1818-1823.

4

French Paradox, Polyphenols and Cardiovascular Protection: The Oestrogenic Receptor-α Implication

Tassadit Benaissa[1], Thierry Ragot[2] and Angela Tesse[1]
*[1]INSERM, UMR 915, Institut de recherche thérapeutique (IRT), Nantes,
[2]CNRS, UMR 8203, Institut de Cancérologie Gustave Roussy, Villejuif,
France*

1. Introduction

Several epidemiological and clinical studies confirm an inverse correlation between a diet rich in vegetables, fruits, and red wine, in cancer development and chronic diseases such as cardiovascular diseases. This is linked to the presence in these aliments of high levels of nutrients of vegetal origin called phytonutrients. They are natural phytochemical compounds contained in plant food; they are not vitamins or minerals but they have beneficial effects on the health, sometimes acting in association with other essential nutrients. Phytonutrients are divided in three families: the terpenes, the sulfuric compounds, and the polyphenols which are the subject of this chapter.

Polyphenols are the most important group of phytonutrients. They are not only present in fruits and vegetables but also in seeds, spices, herbs and teas, at different concentrations and molecular structures in correlation with the aliment involved. The most studied polyphenolic compounds for their vascular action are resveratrol, delphinidin, quercetin and tannins contained in red wine. Indeed, the red wine is the beverage the most correlated to cardiac and vascular protection. It could reduce of 40% the risk of myocardial infarction, and of 25% the risk of vascular thrombotic events in brain.

Elevated content in polyphenols of red wine seems to play a benefic role in the mechanism of vascular and cardiac protection, not only by its anti-oxidant but also by its anti-thrombotic properties. Thus, more recently, research works were focused to study the vascular and cardiac effects of non-alcoholic fractions of red wine and have identified the oestrogenic receptor-α (ERα), as the preferential endothelial target of these molecules.

First, this chapter is focused on the "French Paradox" history. Then, we have described successively the composition and content of these compounds in food and beverages, and the epidemiological and fundamental studies showing how red wine polyphenolic compounds (RWPC) are able to improve endothelial function and cardiovascular protection. Finally, we explain the effects of oestrogens on the cardiovascular system and the implication of ERα in the beneficial cardiovascular effects of these natural molecules that could be used to prevent or treat cardiovascular diseases.

2. French paradox history

For a long time, it was suggested that a high fat intake is associated with an elevated risk of mortality for cardiovascular diseases in Anglo-Saxon populations. In contrast, several epidemiological studies have revealed a relatively low incidence of coronary heart diseases (CHD) in the French population, despite a high dietary intake of saturated fats. This was potentially attributable to the consumption of red wine (Renaud et al., 1999).

One of the first epidemiological studies conducted on 100,000 subjects in 1970 by Doctor Arthur Klatsky, a cardiologist of the Oakland Hospital in California, clearly evidenced that people following a diet with moderated consumption of red wine (1-3 glasses per day), showed a very little risk of death by CHD (Renaud et al., 1999). This was confirmed in 1979 by Doctor Saint-Léger which evidenced a negative correlation between wine consumption and mortality for CHD in men and women (from 55 to 64 years old), in more than 18 developed countries. Furthermore, Italy and France showed a lower level of mortality by myocardial infarction (about 3 or 5 folds less) compared to Anglo-Saxon populations such as Irish, North-American, and Scottish (Renaud et al., 1999). On the other hand, it has been demonstrated that to drink one glass of wine per day reduced death risk by CHD, but to drink more than three glasses of wine per day was associated with an increased death rate (Thun et al., 1997). In wine drinkers, the lower all-cause mortality was associated with a significant reduction in mortality from CHD, for about 45-48%, and other cardiovascular diseases (CVD), for about 39-40% (Renaud et al., 1999). Other studies have also suggested that both non-drinkers and heavy-drinkers have a higher risk of cardiovascular mortality than those who drink wine moderately (Providencia, 2006).

Then, numerous correlation studies concerning the strict relation between consumption of fat and CHD mortality have been conducted in various countries. In one of the most interesting ones, Artaud-Wild and colleagues examined the relation between CHD mortality and the intake of foodstuffs and nutrients in 40 different countries. After they have defined a cholesterol–saturated fat index (CSI), they studied this correlation in 100,000 men (aged 55 to 64 years) in all the countries studied. The findings of this epidemiological study evidenced that France had a CSI of 24 per 1000 kcal and a CHD mortality rate of 198; whereas Finland had a CSI of 26 per 1000 kcal and a CHD mortality rate of 1031 (Ferrières, 2004). The high consumption of saturated fatty acids suggests that French subjects could be exposed to a high risk of CHD (Renaud 1992), but it is in fact not the case considering the low rate of CHD mortality observed. Then, much attention has been focused on the possible superior protective effect of red wine consumption relative to those of other alcoholic beverages. So, the differential effects of wine, beer, and spirits have been examined. European research carried out in France and Denmark has shown that wine consumption was associated with a decrease of 24 up to 31% of all cause mortality; little to moderate wine drinking leads to a lower mortality rate from CVD than having an equivalent consumption of beer or spirits (Ferrières, 2004).

Nevertheless, alcohol consumption, from whatever sources, appears to have a J-shaped curve, whereby a modest intake is beneficial and either no intake or excess is harmful. This is confirmed by several studies: the Framingham study (Fuchs et al., 1995), the British Doctors study (Doll et al., 1994), the Cancer Prevention study of Thun and coworkers, conducted on about 490,000 persons (Thun et al., 1997), the Nurse Health study (Emberson et al., 2005), and other epidemiological investigations (Gaziano et al., 2000; Suh et al., 1992). It would take too long to report on all the studies dealing with the relations between alcohol and CHD.

The mechanisms involved in the protective role of red wine include anti-platelet, anti-coagulatory, improved glucose control, and anti-inflammatory effects as shown in MONICA (multinational MONItoring of trends and determinants in CArdiovascular disease) study (Imhof et al., 2004). The World Health Organization had collected all the results of these data, evidencing the protective role of moderated red wine consumption in cardiovascular disease development. Despite the high consumption of saturated fatty acids, why the French people do not develop a high CHD risk? This is the central question behind the "French Paradox" concept. The French epidemiologist Serge Renaud evidenced for the first time this "Paradox", which is defined as the light level of incidence of CVD in people following a diet containing a high quantity of saturated fatty acids, but also having a moderated red wine consumption (Pechanova et al., 2006, Renaud et al., 1999).

The results of Criqui and colleagues (Criqui & Ringel, 1994) were found in agreement with the French Paradox. In 21 developed countries, subjects in an age range of 35 to 74, without differences linked to gender, were studied and assessed at four time periods: 1965, 1970, 1980, and 1988, respectively. The independent variables chosen were: consumption of wine, beer, spirits, animal fats, vegetables, and fruits. Ischemic heart disease and all-cause mortality were finally assessed. Wine was the beverage most strongly negatively correlated with coronary diseases. Animal fat had a tendency to positive correlation, while fruits were negatively correlated. On the light of the numerous epidemiological studies, a protective activity of wine against CVD has been widely described, suggesting that moderated consumption of wine could reduce the risk of myocardial infarction and the risk of vascular thrombosis of brain vessels.

So many questions arose next. What were the elements that differentiate the wine (especially red wine) of other spirits? What were the processes responsible for the beneficial effect of wine consumption? What, in wine, promoted this effect?

3. Differences in polyphenolic compositions in food and beverages

Polyphenolic compounds are the biggest group of phytochemicals characterized by one or more phenolic rings associated with one or more hydroxyl groups, free or implicated in an ester, ether or eteroside function (Richter, 1993). This family of substances includes more than 8000 phenolic structures currently known, and among them, over 4000 flavonoids have been yet identified in plants and the list is constantly growing (Bravo, 1998; Cheynier, 2005; Harborne & Williams, 2000). Flavonoids contain a structural backbone C6-C3-C6, characterized by two C6 units of phenolic nature; while the non-flavonoids are phenolic acids divided in two main types, benzoic acid and cinnamic acid derivatives, based on C1-C6 and C3-C6 backbones, respectively (Tsao, 2010). The phenolic acids are usually contained as free molecules in fruits and vegetables. Phenolic acids could be also found in the bound form in grains and seeds (Chandrasekara & Shahidi, 2010).

Polyphenols are enrolled in numerous physiological functions in vegetal organisms: cell development, latent buds, blooming, and tuber formation. These substances are involved in the color of fruits, in particular they play a main role to confer the red color of ripe fruits, and in the savor and properties of food (Bahorun, 1997). Polyphenols include yellow, orange, red and blue pigments and various compounds implicated also in bitterness and astringency of unripe fruits, resulting from interaction of tannins with salivary proteins. Moreover, some volatile polyphenols, in particular vanillin and eugenol, are potent odorants and are responsible of the characteristic odor of cloves (Cheynier, 2005).

The content of polyphenolic compounds is particularly elevated in red wine but also in skin of red grapes, red fruits, cereals, several vegetables such as red onions, chocolate, tea, and coffee with different polyphenolic composition and percentage according to the kind of vegetal food or beverage (see Table 1) (Bravo, 1998; Tsao, 2010). Considering the diversity and wide distribution of polyphenols, they have been classified by their source of origin, biological function, and chemical structure. In plants, the majority of polyphenols exists as glycosides associated to sugar units or acylated sugars linked at different positions of the polyphenolic skeletons (Tsao, 2010).

Food	Total polyphenols (mg/100 g of dry mutter)	Food	Total polyphenols (mg/100 g of fresh mutter)
Cereals:		Vegetables:	
Barley	1200-1500	Onion	100-2025
Millet	590-1060		
Legumes:		Fruits:	
Black gram	540-1200	Apple	27-298
Green gram	440-800	Blackcurrant	140-1200
Pigeon peas	380-1710	Grapes	50-490
		Raspberry	37-429
Beverages	Total polyphenols (mg/L)	Beverages	Total polyphenols (mg/L)
Orange juice	370-7100	Tea	750-1050
Red wine	1000-6500	Coffee	1330-3670
White wine	200-300		

Table 1. Plant food and beverages with high levels of total polyphenolic compounds (from Bravo, 1998).

Some flavonoids such as the isoflavones are mostly found in plants of the leguminous family. Genistein and daidzein are the two main isoflavones found in soybeans and red clovers (Tsao et al., 2006). The flavonoid subgroup of the neoflavonoids is rarely present in food plants, but the open-ring chalcones are still found in fruits, in particular in apples and hops of beers (Tsao et al., 2003; Zhao et al., 2005). In contrast, other flavonoid subgroups such as flavones, flavonols, flavanones and flavanonols are most common and ubiquitous in the plant kingdom and in particular quercetin and kaempferol (Tsao, 2010). Flavanols or flavan-3-ols, also called catechins, are found in many fruits, the skin of grapes, apple and blueberries (Tsao et al., 2003). Catechin, epicatechin (isomer of catechin with *cis* configuration), and their derivatives, gallocatechins, are the major flavonoids contained in tea leaves and cacao beans and thus in chocolate (Si et al., 2006; Prior et al., 2001).

The red, blue and purple pigments of the majority of flower petals, fruits and vegetables and certain varieties of grains, for instance black rice, mainly contain anthocyanidins and in particular cyanidin, delphinidin, pelagonidin, and their methylated derivatives (composed up to 90% of anthocyanins). The color of these kinds of molecules can change with the pH and temperature: they are red in acidic and blue in basic conditions (Tsao, 2010). In grapes and apples, anthocyanins are found only in the red varieties (Cheynier, 2005).

Polyphenols are highly unstable species and, accordingly, their chemical structure can change during food and beverage processing and storage, leading to new compounds with different properties compared to their precursors (Xu et al., 2011). In particular, total catechin contents of fresh fruits can decrease of about 26% up to 58% after home preparation or industrial transformations (Cheynier, 2005).

Wine is a hydro-alcoholic acid solution. Indeed, its major component is water (80-90%) and ethanol (10-14%) implicated in the solubilization of polyphenols. The fraction of polyphenolic compounds contained in wine is high in red wine and its composition depends of the kind of wine. More precisely, generally red wine contains 1.2 gr/L of polyphenolic compounds while white wine contains only 0.2 gr/L of these compounds and, besides, does not contain the molecules involved in the red color such as the anthocyanidins and in particular delphinidin (see Table 2) (Pellegrini et al., 2000; Soleas et al., 1997). Interestingly, the level of these compounds in red wine is modified by the fermentation process used during wine production. Vinification variations and techniques are known to affect the phenolic composition of red wines. The fermentation of grape juice into wine is a

Compounds (mg/L)	White young wine	White aged wine	Red young wine	Red aged wine
Total phenols	215	190-290	1300	955-1215
Non flavonoides	175	160-260	235	240-500
Flavonoides	30	25	1060	705
Catechins	25	15	200	150
Anthocyanins	0	0	200	20
Soluble tannins	5	10	550	450

Table 2. Polyphenolic compound contents in several types of wine (from Soleas et al., 1997).

complex microbial reaction, traditionally due to the sequential development of various species of yeast and lactic acid bacteria. In the past, wine was produced by natural fermentation of grape juice by yeasts originating from grapes and winery equipment (Ribereau-Gayon et al., 2000). Nowadays, another kind of fermentation process, the carbonic maceration, is more and more used to produce wine. With this method, freshly harvested bunches of grapes are allowed to ferment in carbonic anaerobiosis, in an atmosphere saturated with carbon dioxide (Navarro et al., 2000). The absence of oxygen is important to reduce the oxidation of polyphenolic compounds, especially the monomeric anthocyanidins such as malvidin and delphinidin. The preservation of these molecules by this new carbonic process increases their final levels in wine compared to the traditional maceration of grapes (Pellegrini et al., 2000). Furthermore, the wine ageing could modify polyphenol composition and levels in white and red wines with a time-dependent reduction of catechins and anthocyanidins contents (see Table 2) (Pellegrini et al., 2000; Soleas et al., 1997).

It is interesting to note that, after food or beverage intake, the degradation and absorption of polyphenols within the gastrointestinal tract depend on the nature of the polyphenolic compound but also of the intestinal microflora, with subsequent fermentative effect on other dietary components. Thus, these molecules are modified by intestinal bacteria but they can influence in return microflora and its fermentative capacity (Bravo, 1998). Several recent studies are focused in how processing and beverage composition might influence phenolic profiles and bioavailability of an individual polyphenol. Specifically, they showed the impact of beverage formulations and the influence of digestion on stability, bioavailability, and metabolism of bioactive polyphenolic compounds from food and beverages. For example, the co-formulation with ascorbic acid and other phytochemicals may improve absorption of these health-promoting phytochemicals (Ferruzzi, 2010). Thus, it is critical to develop beverage products designed to deliver specific health benefits.

4. Beneficial effects of RWPC in cardiac and vascular functions

Evidences from different experimental studies has suggested the presence of molecules with anti-oxidant properties in red wine, such as tannins and other flavonoids. These molecules could be key factors in the protective effects observed (Vidavalur et al., 2006). Red wine, might provide, through the polyphenols (non-flavonoids and flavonoids), an anti-oxidant role, leading to additional protection mechanisms in coronary arteries (Liu et al., 2007). Thus, RWPC are able to decrease oxidative stress, enhance cholesterol efflux from the vascular wall, and inhibit lipoprotein oxidation. These components may also increase nitric oxide (NO) bioavailability, thereby antagonizing the development of endothelial dysfunction. Thus, RWPC are able to modify several factors involved in the development of CDV by a direct action on vascular cells and in particular in endothelium, thus playing a preventive role in the development of atherosclerosis, hypertension and myocardial infarction. One of the most studied molecules, the resveratrol, found in grapes and wine in significant amounts, is implicated in this beneficial action because of its ability to act as an anti-oxidant and an inhibitor of platelet aggregation (Kopp, 1998; Providencia, 2006).

On the light of several recent major studies, the consumption of RWPC reduces the incidence of CVD probably by their ability to change many factors and intermediate markers implicated in these diseases. A beneficial association between consumption of food rich in polyphenols, especially flavonoids, and other chronic diseases was also investigated. People with very low consumption of flavonoids showed a higher risk to develop chronic and degenerative diseases including cardiovascular disorders, diabetes, obesity and neurodegenerative disorders compared to people with a diet rich in polyphenols (Mojzisova and Kuchta, 2001). Thus, it is important to better identify factors that may affect the bioavailability of specific phenolic components from food and beverages and to better understand how these molecules are able to act positively on organism.

4.1 Role on nitric oxide production

RWPC are able to improve NO production and vascular endothelium-dependent relaxation. This is possible through their action to increase endothelial nitric oxide synthase (eNOS) expression and activation *in vitro* on endothelial cells and *ex vivo* on rodent vessels.

One of the earliest works on this purpose was conducted in 1993 by Fitzpatrick and coworkers. They found that extracts from grapes and wine containing polyphenols were able to induce an endothelial-dependent vasorelaxation, probably by NO production and elevated accumulation of guanosine 3',5'-cyclic monophosphate (cGMP) (Fitzpatrick et al., 1993). The mechanisms and the identification of the molecules involved in these vascular effects were still unknown. These findings were confirmed later by another study, in which it was evidenced an endothelial and NO-dependent relaxation induced by a non-alcoholic red wine extract, RWPC, and leucocyanidol administrated directly at low concentrations (from 10^{-4} to 10^{-2} g/L) *ex vivo* on noradrenaline pre-contracted rat aortic rings (Andiambeleson et al., 1997). This was associated with an enhanced NO generation and a seven-fold increase in cGMP accumulation. A non-relevant relaxant effect was found using the structurally closely related polyphenol, catechin, at the same concentrations on the same vessels. To better determine which group(s) of polyphenols were able to cause endothelial-dependent vasorelaxation, the same team separated RWPC by chromatography in 10 fractions. These fractions were tested separately for their capacity to induce the vascular relaxation on rat aortic rings with and without endothelium. In this study, it was shown that fractions containing high polymeric condensed tannins produced a moderate vasorelaxation, at relatively high concentrations (10^{-2} to 10^{-1} g/L) and flavan-3-ol, (+)-epicathechin, also failed to produce endothelium-dependent vasorelaxation. In contrast, oligomeric condensed tannins and fractions containing anthocyanins, and in particular delphinidin, displayed strong vasorelaxant properties (maximal relaxation in the range of 59–77%) comparable to the original RWPC mixture (Andriambeloson et al., 1998).

The same endothelial-dependent relaxation was also found in small mesenteric arteries, but it was due to both NO and endothelium-derived hyperpolarizing factor (EDHF) and it was absent in vessels without endothelium. The NO component of the relaxation was linked to eNOS activity and absent when the NOS inhibitor, the N^G-nitro-L-arginine methyl ester (L-NAME), was used, while the EDHF component was abolished by partial depolarization with KCl. Thus, NO and EDHF are both required to promote endothelium-dependent relaxation produced by RWPC in mesenteric resistance arteries (Duarte et al. 2004).

Several studies conducted *in vitro* confirmed these results. In bovine aortic endothelial cells (BAECs) treated with RWPC (10^{-2} g/L), it was found an increased Ca^{2+}-dependent eNOS activation and a subsequent increased NO production. These required the presence of extracellular Ca^{2+}, although polyphenolic compounds were able to mobilize Ca^{2+} from intracellular stores and were also able to activate phospholipase C (PLC) and tyrosine kinase (TK) pathways. Provinols™, which contain similar types of polyphenols compared to the RWPC used by Andriambeloson and coworkers, and delphinidin displayed differences in the process leading to this increase in endothelial intracellular Ca^{2+}, thus illustrating multiple cellular targets of natural dietary polyphenolic compounds (Martin et al., 2002). This effect of RWPC in this cell model is associated with an increased superoxide ion (O_2^-) production in order to promote Ca^{2+} signaling (Duarte et al., 2004). Most recently, it was found that resveratrol, a stilbenoid contained in wine, used at nanomolar concentrations, rapidly activated extracellular-signal-regulated kinase (ERK)1/2 in BAECs and, in turn, activated eNOS (Klinge et al., 2005). The same effect of resveratrol was confirmed later in another model of endothelial cells, the human umbilical endothelial cells (HUVECs). The implication of ERα in the eNOS-pathway activation by resveratrol was also evoked (Klinge et al., 2008).

Interestingly, beneficial effects on hemodynamic parameters and on endothelial function were confirmed *in vivo* after a short-term oral administration of RWPC in normotensive rats at the dose of 20 mg/kg for 7 days. Indeed, these rats, after only 4 days of treatment, showed a significant decrease in blood pressure (129 ± 4 mmHg versus 141 ± 2 mmHg for control non-treated rats). This effect was associated, *ex vivo*, with an increased endothelium-dependent relaxation to acetylcholine in aortic rings, that was related to the enhanced endothelial NO activity. Nevertheless, RWPC induced at the same time gene expression of inducible NOS (iNOS) and inducible cyclooxigenase (COX-2), with subsequent endothelial thromboxane A_2 release in the arterial wall, maintaining unchanged agonist-induced contractility (Diebolt et al., 2001). The *in vivo* effects of Provinols™ (40 mg/kg per day) on hemodynamic and functional cardiovascular changes were also investigated during the inhibition of NO synthesis by L-NAME (40 mg/kg per day for 4 weeks) in rats. This model of hypertension evidenced that RWPC partially prevent L-NAME-induced hypertension, cardiovascular remodeling, and vascular dysfunction or accelerate the decrease of systolic blood pressure after L-NAME administration. These beneficial effects were mediated by the increased NO-synthase activity and the oxidative stress prevention (Bernatova et al., 2002; Pechanova et al., 2004). Nevertheless, most recently, the anti-hypertensive effects of RWPC, orally administered for 5 weeks at the dose of 40 mg/kg by gavage, was confirmed in female spontaneously hypertensive rats (SHR). The authors suggested that a chronic treatment with RWPC reduced hypertension and vascular dysfunction in this model of hypertension, rather through reduction in vascular oxidative stress (Lopez-Sepulveda et al., 2008). This findings revealed a major preventive role of these substances in cardiovascular complications linked to hypertension.

Polyphenol vascular activity in human vessels after food or beverage intake was confirmed by several studies that detected these molecules in human plasma at individual levels in the range of 0.5 to 1.6 µmol/L, comparable to the concentration required to induce 50% of the maximal relaxation, comprised between 1 and 10 µmol/L of active fractions (Paganga and Rice-Evans, 1997). Polyphenols detected in human plasma are in the range of 2.5 µg/ml after a 100 ml red wine intake (Duthie et al., 1998). Most interestingly, the vasorelaxant effect of polyphenols from red wine was confirmed also in men in which NO and normalized flow-mediated dilation were measured before and 30, 60, and 120 minutes after red wine consumption (Boban et al., 2006; Papamichael et al., 2004). Moreover, RWPC are not only able to improve NO production, for their anti-oxidant and anti-inflammatory properties but also increase the NO bioavailability in the vascular wall, by decreasing its transformation in peroxynitrite induced by O_2^- during oxidative stress.

Altogether, these findings suggest a possible beneficial effect of a diet rich in these vasoactive polyphenolic compounds to prevent hypertension as the effective concentrations of these molecules can be reached in human plasma and they might act on the endothelium *in vivo*. The RWPC responsible of this effect (resveratrol, delphinidin and tannins) could be used for hypertension treatment.

4.2 Protective role in cardiac function and ischemic diseases

RWPC, administrated in a preventive purpose way, are able to reduce cardiac or cerebral ischemic injuries in rat models of myocardial infarct and stroke, respectively. Left ventricular hypertrophy, myocardial fibrosis and vascular remodeling were investigated in rats during chronic inhibition of NOS activity by L-NAME. The *in vivo* treatment of rats with Provinols™ (40 mg/kg per day) reduced not only the increase in blood pressure caused by L-NAME treatment, but also protein synthesis in the heart and aorta caused by the chronic inhibition of NO synthesis, finally reducing myocardial fibrosis. These effects were associated with an increase of NOS activity, a moderate enhancement of eNOS expression and a reduction of oxidative stress in the left ventricule and aorta (Pechanova et al. 2004).

The protective cardiac effect of polyphenols was confirmed by another study, conducted in rats and observing, *ex vivo*, the effects of short-term oral administration of RWPC (20 mg/kg per day for one week) on cardiac responsiveness and ischaemia-reperfusion injury. The involvement of NO in the cardiac effects of RWPC was evaluated using L-NAME (2 mg/kg per day for one week), a dose which did not affect blood pressure, in a group of rats previously treated with polyphenols. Heart reactivity was studied in perfused isolated hearts by the Langendorff method. The hearts harvested from RWPC-treated rats showed a lower basal pressure, a greater heart rate and decreased inotropic responses to either isoprenaline or carbachol, the agonists of beta-adrenoceptors or muscarinic receptors, respectively. RWPC treatment did not modify cardiac expression of eNOS or Cu/Zn superoxide dismutase, a protein involved in oxidative stress protection. However, it was found increased nitrite levels in the coronary effluent from hearts harvested from RWPC-treated rats, suggesting an increased NO production. Most interestingly, in ischaemia-reperfusion protocols, RWPC treatment reduced infarct size, oxidative stress, and the myocardial content of end products resulting from lipid peroxidation, malondialdehyde and 4-hydroxynonenal, without affecting post-ischaemic contractile dysfunction. All these observed effects were prevented by L-NAME treatment, suggesting the involvement of NO in this protective role of RWPC on heart. In conclusion, these data showed that short-term treatment with RWPC could prevent the heart injury caused by cardiac ischemia through oxidative stress decrease and NO pathway improvement (Ralay-Ranaivo et al., 2004).

The presence of melatonin in red wine was demonstrated in most recent studies. Lamont and co-workers investigated the cardio-protective role of both melatonin and resveratrol. These molecules improve heart protection via the activation of the newly discovered survivor activating factor enhancement (SAFE) pathway. This pro-survival signaling pathway involves the activation of pro-inflammatory molecules such as tumor necrosis factor alpha (TNFα) and interleukin 6 (IL6) and the signal transducer and activator of transcription 3 (STAT3). They realized *ex vivo* studies in isolated perfused hearts from either wild type or total TNFα receptor 2-knockout or cardiomyocyte-specific STAT3-deficient mice. The protocols of heart injury by ischemia-reperfusion showed that both resveratrol and melatonin, at concentrations found in red wine, significantly reduced infarct size in wild-type mice (25% ± 3% versus 69 ± 3% in the control non treated mice) but failed to protect hearts in both knockout mice. Perfusion with either melatonin or resveratrol increased STAT3 phosphorylation prior to ischemia by 79% and 50% versus the control, respectively. These findings suggest that both melatonin and resveratrol contained in red wine, protect heart via the SAFE pathway, in an experimental model of myocardial infarction (Lamont et al., 2011).

Concerning cerebral ischemia, Ritz and co-workers investigated the beneficial effects of chronic or acute treatment of RWPC in rats submitted to an experimental model of stroke. Rats were treated for the chronic treatment with RWPC (30 mg/kg per day) dissolved in drinking water for one week, before being subjected surgically to a transient middle cerebral artery occlusion followed by reperfusion. The volume of the ischemic lesions was assessed 24 h after reperfusion and a proteomic analysis of brain tissues was performed, to study the effects of RWPC on expression of proteins involved in cerebral stroke injury. Treatment with RWPC partially or completely prevented the increased levels of excitatory amino acids (aspartate, glutamate and taurine) that characterized the response to ischemia in control rats, significantly reduced brain infarct volumes, and enhanced residual cerebral blood flow after brain ischemia. This was associated to lower basal concentrations of energy metabolites including glucose, lactate, and free radical scavengers such as ascorbate, in the brain parenchyma, compared with untreated rats. No difference in uric acid levels was found. These effects resulted in arterial vasodilatation, as the internal diameters of several arteries were significantly enlarged after RWPC treatment. Proteomic analysis revealed that RWPC could be able to modulate *in vivo* the expression of proteins involved in maintenance of neuronal caliber and axon formation, in protection against oxidative stress, and in energy metabolism (Ritz et al., 2008a). These data were confirmed in the second work of the same team, about the protective effects of an acute treatment with RWPC (a bolus of 0.1 mg/kg), realized by an intracerebral microdialysis started at the beginning of the stroke. In this study, RWPC induced increased residual blood flow after 10 minutes of the reperfusion following ischemia and reduced size of the cerebral ischemic infarct in both cortex and striatum. The acute treatment of rats with RWPC dramatically decreased the extracellular concentrations of excitatory amino acids and, concomitantly, increased the levels of free radical scavengers such as uric and ascorbic acids (Ritz et al., 2008b). Altogether these findings provide an experimental evidence of the advantage to use RWPC for the prevention, in patients with high risk to developing ischemic events, or in the acute treatment of patients during stroke.

Angiogenesis is a main process involved in the repair of ischemic injury. The role of RWPC in angiogenesis was also investigated and several studies evidenced that these molecules are able to modulate, at the molecular and cellular levels, several actors of the pivotal pathways involved in vascular cell proliferation and migration. Previous studies had demonstrated an anti-angiogenic role of polyphenols both *in vitro* and *in vivo* (Fotsis et al., 1998; Igura et al., 2001). In contrast, most recently, Baron-Menguy and co-workers evidenced a dose-dependent effect on angiogenesis of RWPC, and in particular of delphinidin, in a model of post-ischaemic neovascularization in rats submitted to femoral artery ligature. Indeed, high doses of RWPC (i.e. 7 glasses of red wine) reduced arterial, arteriolar, and capillary densities and blood flow, inhibited the phosphoinositol 3-kinase (PI3-K)/Akt/eNOS pathway, decreased vascular endothelial growth factor (VEGF) expression, and reduced metalloproteinase-2 (MMP-2) activation. In contrast, low doses of RWPC (i.e. 1/10th glass of red wine) increased neovascularisation in ischemic legs compared to control level in association with an increased blood flow. The angiogenic effect was linked to the overexpression of PI3-K/Akt/eNOS pathway and to increased VEGF production, without effect on MMP-2 activation. These anti- or pro-angiogenic effects of RWPC were reproduced when they used delphinidin, administrated alone at low or high doses. This dual dose-dependent effect of polyphenols in angiogenesis is particular interesting because of its potential applications both in the therapy of diseases requiring the block of angiogenesis such as in some cancers, and in the treatment of post-ischemic injuries to improve angiogenesis and ameliorate reperfusion of tissues, at high and low doses, respectively.

4.3 Role in metabolic diseases

It has been extensively evidenced the strict correlation between metabolic dysfunctions and the development of cardiovascular diseases. Endothelial dysfunction, an independent predictor of cardiovascular events, has been consistently associated with obesity and the metabolic syndrome in a complex interplay with insulin resistance. Deficiency of eNOS is considered as the primary defect that links insulin resistance and endothelial dysfunction (Cersosimo and Defronzo, 2006; Defronzo, 2006; Fornoni and Raij, 2005). Furthermore, several epidemiological studies have shown that patients affected by metabolic diseases are often also affected by hypertension and other cardio-vascular complications such as atherosclerotic plaque formation and increased levels of pro-thrombotic factors, associated to an elevated risk of mortality by vascular thrombotic events (Kopelman, 2000).

More recently, we have suggested a protective role of RWPC in metabolic syndrome (Agouni et al., 2009). In our study, Zuker fatty (ZF) rats (Fa/Fa), an experimental model of metabolic syndrome, or their "lean" littermates, received normal diet or a diet supplemented with Provinols™ for 8 weeks in food. This treatment significantly reduced the plasmatic levels of metabolic products such as glucose, fructosamine, total and LDL-cholesterol, and triglycerides, and finally improved cardiac and endothelial vascular functions. Regarding vascular function, Provinols™ corrected endothelial dysfunction in aortas and mesenteric arteries from ZF rats by improving endothelium-dependent relaxation in response to acetylcholine. This beneficial effect in endothelium was associated to an enhanced NO bioavailability due to increased NO production and eNOS activity, and reduced oxidative stress and O_2^- release. The effect on eNOS activity was associated to a decreased expression of caveolin-1, a protein known to inactivate eNOS by cell membrane sequestration, while the reduction of free radical production was linked to a decrease of Nox-1 (NADPH oxidase membrane sub-unit) expression (Agouni et al., 2009). In agreement with our work, this protective effect of RWPC in plasmatic metabolic parameters and oxidative stress linked to metabolic disorders was confirmed recently in hamsters submitted to high-fat diet (Suh et al., 2011).

Because of these interesting results, polyphenols might be good candidates for prevention and treatment of metabolic syndrome and cardiovascular risk reduction. This was previously suggested by another study of Napoli and coworkers who have shown that red wine consumption improved insulin resistance in type 2 diabetic patients (Napoli et al., 2005). Thus, RWPC could represent a new class of medicinal products against obesity-associated diseases.

5. The oestrogenic receptors in cardiovascular protection

Several epidemiological studies suggested a protective effect of oestrogens in premenopausal women in vascular and metabolic diseases development. These numerous studies showed that the incidence of hypertension and other cardiovascular diseases is significantly lower in premenopausal females compared to males and that, after the onset of menopause, the incidence increases dramatically, eventually approaching the level observed in age-matched males (Mendelsohn and Karas, 1999). This effect has been attributed to the fall in circulating oestrogen levels, contributing to a menopause-related increase in blood pressure, and thus to a greater predisposition to cardiovascular disease. Consistent with this, oestrogen replacement therapy has been reported to reduce the risk of cardiovascular disease, and in particular of hypertension and atherosclerosis, in postmenopausal women to that observed in premenopausal women (Barton et al., 2007; Mendelsohn and Karas, 1999). Oestrogens have been shown to have direct vasodilatory and anti-atherosclerotic effects via the oestrogen receptors expressed on human and rat arteries (Haas et al., 2007; Shaw et al., 2001). The mechanisms involved in the protective role played by these hormones is associated to vascular inflammation reduction (Nilsson, 2007), increased endothelial NO production (Chen et al., 1999) and the prevention of smooth muscle vascular cell proliferation (Pareet al., 2002). But the ability of oestrogens to elicit effects on autonomic functions involved in cardiac control appears also to constitute a major part of its beneficial effects (Spary et al., 2009). Despite wealth of evidences for its central autonomic role, the sites and mechanisms of oestrogenic action on the neural pathways of cardiovascular regulation are still poorly understood.

Oestrogens act on specific receptors which are transcription factors, the nuclear oestrogenic receptors (ERs). Two ERs have been described, ERα and ERβ, with several structurally and functionally conserved domains, and involved in genomic signaling mechanism or associated to plasma membrane, influencing cytosolic non-genomic signaling. ERα was first characterized in mid-1980 and the cloning of ERβ following in late 1995 (Kuiper et al., 1996). In addition, as a result of alternative splicing of the eight exons encoding rat ERβ, five different isoforms of this ER exist (β1, β2, β1δ3, β2δ3 and β1δ4) with a not yet completely determined role (Maruyama et al., 1998; Petersen et al., 1998; Price et al., 2000). It has been suggested that ERβ may modulate ERα gene transcription, acting in some conditions by opposite actions to ERα (Lindberg et al., 2003; Maruyama et al., 1998; Zhao et al., 2008).

In the absence of oestrogens, the receptors are conserved in an inactive state in a complex with one of the several chaperone molecules, such as heat shock protein 90 (Beato and Klug, 2000). Following binding to oestrogens, the receptor undergoes a conformational change, activating an intracellular cascade leading to the ER release from the chaperone. ER can forms homo- or hetero-dimers that interact with target gene promoters, inducing the up- or the down-regulation of several genes (Figure 1) (Hall et al, 2001). The ER subtypes have also been shown to interact differently with a range of other transcription factors, including activating protein-1 (Paech et al., 1997; Webb et al., 1999; Zhao et al., 2008). This genomic response usually occurs within hours after oestrogen exposure and is believed to be the result of a direct action, not involving the second messenger signaling pathways. In contrast, the non-genomic oestrogenic signaling is also possible but less well understood. It is associated to the cytosolic pathways with classical second messengers and occurs considerably faster than the genomic signaling (Kang et al., 2010). It is possible that these rapid non-genomic events are mediated by cytoplasmic, rather than nuclear ERα and ERβ, suggesting the involvement of another plasma membrane receptor, a particular G protein-coupled receptor (GPCR) which is not related to ERα or ERβ. To confirm this hypothesis more recently, another membrane-bound ER was emerged. This GPCR, the G protein coupled oestrogen receptor 1 (GPER1), also called GPR30, is able to bind with a high affinity to 17β-estradiol (E2), mediating oestrogenic signals in cardiovascular and metabolic regulations (Nilsson et al., 2011). GPER1 is expressed in different vascular segments and in the heart of several species. In rats, the mRNA of this receptor was found both in endothelial and in smooth muscle cells; but in mice and humans, it seems to be expressed primarily in endothelial cells of small systemic arteries, suggesting a direct role of GPER1 in endothelial function regulation, while the effects of its activation in vascular smooth muscle cells and vascular tone are indirect, via the endothelium (Nilsson et al., 2011). GPER1 is located to the endoplasmic reticulum of vascular cells mediating the rapid oestrogen signaling (Revankar et al., 2005).

The role of GPER1 activation by its specific agonist, G-1, on vascular tone was investigated in rat vessels. Several studies showed the involvement of this receptor in vascular relaxation by reducing angiotensin II (AngII) and/or endothelin-1 (ET-1)-induced vascular contractions. This was not influenced by the endogenous oestrogenic levels and it was gender independent (Haas et al, 2009, Lindsey et al., 2009; Meyer et al., 2010). This effect was not found in serotonin-dependent vascular contraction, suggesting a direct effect of GPER1 activation on the renin-angiotensin system, probably independent of NO production (Nillson et al, 2011). In contrast, another study suggests that GPER1 causes arterial relaxation via an endothelial and a NO-dependent mechanism (Broughton et al., 2010). Thus, the involvement of endothelial NO in this vascular relaxation cannot be excluded. Moreover, an hypotensive effect of GPER1 activation was observed in ovariectomized animals, in agreement with the hypertensive phenotype of GPER1 knock-out mice (Martensson et al., 2009). Furthermore, GPER1 activation could play a protective role in atherosclerosis and/or excessive angiogenesis during cancer, reducing vascular smooth muscle or endothelial cell proliferation, respectively (Haas et al., 2009; Holm et al., 2011).

If the non-genomic effects of E2 are realized through GPER1, ERα is the receptor implicated in the anti-atherogenic effects of oestrogens. Indeed, the ERα, when stimulated by E2, induces endothelial cell proliferation, vascular re-endothelialization, endothelial NO production, vascular inflammation attenuation, and reduction of smooth muscle cell proliferation (Brouchet et al., 2001; Pare et al., 2002; Vegeto et al., 2003). Nevertheless, studies conducted on vessels harvested from ERα or ERβ knockout mice showed that both these ERs are responsible for E2-dependent vascular relaxation (Guo et al., 2005). It was previously evidenced the association of a subpopulation of ERα with the endothelial membrane and the complex structure of caveolae (Chambliss and Shaul, 2002). The binding of E2 with ERα in caveolae leads to the MAPK/Akt pathway activation, resulting in eNOS phosphorylation and activation, and subsequent increased NO production (Figure 1) (Chambliss and Shaul, 2002). This beneficial effect on vascular function played by oestrogens was confirmed by epidemiological studies, in which the presence of endogenous oestrogens and their effect on cardiovascular homeostasis appear to be closely related to the degree of atherosclerosis progression throughout a woman's life (Clarkson 2007). Experimental studies suggest that in the mouse, ERα appears to be largely responsible for the protective effects of oestrogens against atherosclerotic vascular disease (Hodgin et al., 2001). In turn, according to some studies, the abundance of both ER subtypes, ERα and ERβ, in human aorta, decreases with the progression of atherosclerosis, aggravating the endothelial dysfunction of atherosclerotic vessels by the reduction of oestrogenic-dependent eNOS activation and NO release (Losordo et al., 1994; Nakamura et al., 2004).

On the light of the effect of E2 via ERα in eNOS pathway activation and NO production, a vascular role of oestrogens, similar to that evidenced for RWPC on endothelium, was evoked. Some researchers and our studies started to investigate if RWPC or one of the polyphenolic compounds contained in red wine, resveratrol or delphinidin, could play a role of phytoestrogens, interacting at high affinity with ERs and inducing their beneficial vascular effects via these endothelial receptors.

6. Oestrogenic receptor alpha and polyphenols

After the description of these encouraging findings, nobody exactly identified the pivotal compound responsible of RWPC vascular effects and, most important, how this molecule was able to interact with the vascular endothelium, thus improving endothelial function. It was previously described that resveratrol is able to enhance eNOS expression and activity, but the mechanisms by which this polyphenol induced these effects were still not well known (Wallerath et al., 2002). In a study conducted *in vitro* in BAECs, nanomolar concentrations of resveratrol induced ERK1/2 signaling activation, similar to that of E2, since this was dependent of ER activity triggering eNOS activation and NO release (Klinge et al., 2005). The same team, in another study *in vitro* (in HUVECs), better determined the mechanisms by which resveratrol was able to improve eNOS activation pathway. The authors of this work demonstrated for the first time that resveratrol increased interaction between ERα, Caveoline-1 (Cav-1) and proteins involved in eNOS activation such as Src, by a Gα-protein-coupled mechanism. A main role for ERα in the NO production induced by resveratrol in endothelial cells was suggested because they observed attenuated effects of resveratrol in cells in which ERα was depleted using a siRNA. Resveratrol and E2 did not stimulate ERβ/Cav-1 interaction (Klinge et al., 2008). Moreover ERα is 4.5 times more expressed then ERβ in HUVECs and no effect of a siRNA directed versus ERβ was found on resveratrol action in endothelium. This study implies that dietary intake of resveratrol might offer possible vascular protective effects via the activation of ERα *in vivo*.

In contrast, experiments conducted in rats did not evidence a role of oestrogen receptors in aorta endothelium-dependent relaxation to RWPC (Kane et al., 2009). The authors of this work showed that RWPC caused redox-sensitive PI3-K/Akt-dependent eNOS activation and NO-mediated relaxation in rat aortas *ex vivo*. This vascular effect was more pronounced in the aorta of female than male rats, but it was due most likely to increased expression levels of eNOS rather than activation of oestrogen receptors, because the inhibition of ER by the oestrogen antagonist, ICI 182780, did not modify the ability of RWPC to induce their vascular effects (Kane et al., 2009). Interestingly, another study conducted in female SHR rats evidenced that the chronic treatment with RWPC of ovariectomized rats induced reduction of arterial pressure and vascular dysfunction characterizing this hypertensive model in a manner independent of the ovarian function (Lopez-Sepulveda et al., 2008).

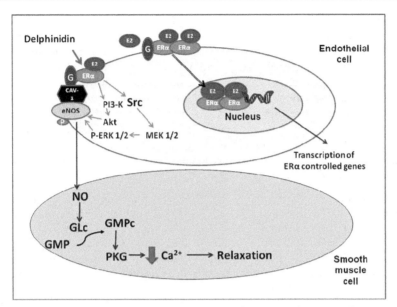

Fig. 1. ERα activation by polyphenols or oestrogens induces eNOS increased activity and NO production. Signaling pathway by which delphinidin or E2 interacting with ERα, activates rapidly eNOS and increases NO production in endothelial cells by PI3-K/Akt or via Src/ERK1/2 pathways. ERα is associated in endothelial cells caveolae with Cav-1 which links to the membrane the inactive form of eNOS. When ERα binds E2 or polyphenols, eNOS is phosphorylated in its active site, thus improving NO release. The same pathways implicated in delphinidin-ERα activation were proposed by Klinge and coworkers for endothelial cell stimulation by resveratrol at nanomolar concentrations (Klinge et al., 2008). NO is able to activate guanilyl-cyclase (GLc) in smooth muscle cells inducing increased levels of cyclic-GMP (GMPc) with subsequent protein-kinase G activation (PKG), reducing intracellular calcium and inducing vascular relaxation. On the right of the figure, is represented the homo-dimer formation and nuclear translocation of E2-activated ERα, inducing the genomic response.

Conversely, we investigated the hypothesis that ERα is one of the key targets involved *in vivo* in the vasculoprotective effects of RWPC (and in particular of delphinidin) interacting with the endothelium. Thus, the ERα implication in the French Paradox was first tested using ERα-deficient mice (Chalopin et al., 2010). We have shown the necessity of this oestrogenic receptor in the Provinols™- or delphinidin-induced endothelial-dependent relaxation, eNOS activation, and NO release. Indeed, no effect of these products on endothelium were observed in vessels harvested from ERα-deficient mice or in wild-type vessels without endothelium. The activation of ERα by RWPC or delphinidin alone induced the activation of the same pathway, evidenced by the previously described *in vitro* work of Klinge and colleagues with resveratrol. Indeed, E2 and the selective agonist of ERα, 1,3,5-tris(4-hydroxyphenyl)-4-propyl-1H-pyrazole (PPT), as well as Provinols™ and delphinidin, are able to activate molecular pathways involving Src, ERK1/2, eNOS and caveolin-1 phosphorylations (see Figure 1). The mechanism involved required ERα activation because of the absence of effect in vessels or cells from ERα-deficient mice, and after silencing, in wild-type endothelial cells, ERα activity or expression either with a pharmacological inhibitor (fulvestran) or with a siRNA, respectively. Moreover, using a binding assay and a docking study, we have shown that delphinidin fits on ERα's activation site, exerting 73% of specific inhibition against E2 on ERα, in the binding assay. Most importantly, ERα is also implicated in the *in vivo* effects observed in mice treated with Provinols™ administrated in the food, with respect to the improvement in endothelial function given by the concomitant increase in NO and decrease in O_2^- release in vessels. Indeed, these vascular and anti-oxidant effects of the *in vivo* treatment with Provinols™ were not found in ERα-deficient mice (Chalopin et al., 2010). Then, we have demonstrated for the first time the physiological relevance of ERα in the *in vivo* vascular effects of RWPC.

It is important to note that ERα, ERβ, and GPER-1 are all expressed in the arterial wall of both women and men (Meyer et al., 2006; Haas et al., 2007), and that E2 has potent dilator effects on vascular tone of human coronary and internal mammary arteries harvested from patients without gender differences (Haas et al., 2007; Mugge et al., 1993). These findings suggest a potential function for oestrogen receptor also in male cardiovascular system. Thus, RWPC could have the same protective vascular properties in both women and men through ERα. In line with the fact that ERα mediates atheroprotective effects, in a man with a disruptive mutation in the ERα gene, it was noted an impaired vascular function and a premature coronary artery disease (Sudhir et al., 1997). Thus, not only the female but also the male cardiovascular system appears to be an important target for oestrogens affecting vascular disease development (Haas et al., 2007; Meyer et al., 2008). Nevertheless, studies in humans comparing oestrogen plasma concentrations and the progression of cardiovascular diseases have revealed conflicting results (Meyer et al., 2008). Actually, there is doubt about the interest to treat male patients with oestrogen receptor agonists to interfere with atherosclerosis progression.

Finally, further works are needed to confirm if ERs are implicated in all the vascular and metabolic effects of RWPC or if ERα activation by RWPC induces only the eNOS pathway improvement. For instance, the role of ERs activation by RWPC in inhibition of endothelial cell proliferation and cell cycle progression or in angiogenesis has not been investigated yet.

7. Conclusion

The first epidemiological studies played a main role in the demonstration of a French Paradox existence, leading to the start of about forty years of scientific findings concerning the protective properties of polyphenols and, more particularly, those contained in red wine. Currently, the numerous data obtained *in vitro*, *ex vivo*, and *in vivo*, on their beneficial effects in heart and vessels, validly suggest a therapeutic potential for RWPC.

The last findings have identified in delphinidin and resveratrol some of the key molecules involved in the vascular effects of RWPC via ERα activation, adding a new piece to the puzzle explaining the French Paradox (Chalopin et al., 2010; Klinge et al., 2008). Indeed, despite a previous study (Kane et al., 2008), which evidenced no implication of ERs in RWPC-dependent vascular relaxation in rats, the last studies clearly showed that the beneficial endothelial effects of RWPC require ERα activation. This is followed by a rapid response to the polyphenolic stimuli in endothelial cells, involving the pathways associated to eNOS activation and subsequent NO release. Furthermore, the phytoestrogenic role of RWPC, and especially of delphinidin, was confirmed by binding experiences which found high affinity of delphinidin against ERα compared to its natural agonist E2 (Chalopin et al., 2010). Similar mechanisms and a phytoestrogenic role on ERα activation were suggested also for resveratrol on endothelial cells by Klinge and coworkers (Klinge et al., 2005, 2008).

In this chapter, we have focalized our attention on the red wine because it contains both, delphinidin and resveratrol, the main vasoactive compounds contained in non-alcoholic red wine extract. In particular, we wanted to explain the main mechanisms by which these compounds are able to induce cardiovascular protection against hypertension, cardiac ischemia, stroke and atherosclerotic plaque formation as one of the complications linked to metabolic syndrome. It is important to note that the effects of these substances could be different according to the concentrations employed as evidenced in experimental models of angiogenesis (Baron-Menguy et al., 2007). It is also relevant to remember of other beneficial properties of RWPC, as anti-oxidant, anti-inflammatory, anti-tumor or antithrombotic agents, that we have not extensively described here. Indeed, RWPC are also able to modulate the apoptotic, proliferative or migration processes in cells (Martin et al., 2003) by acting directly on vascular remodeling and angiogenesis (Brownson et al., 2002; Favot et al., 2003). Here, we have chosen to stress on strong properties of RWPC as vasodilators inducing endothelial NO production, because this effect implicates ERα activation as demonstrated in the last studies.

Furthermore, despite the favorable effect of some molecules contained in red wine in the prevention of several cardiovascular pathologies, alcohol is a serious problem of public health and, actually, it is important to remenber that these beneficial effects are due to the non-alcoholic fractions of red wine. Interestingly, in multinational studies it was shown an increased risk of mortality by myocardial infarction, especially in women who take no alcohol, but compared to moderate drinkers (Yusuf et al., 2004). Moreover, on the light of other epidemiological data, it seems to be developed the view that modest alcohol but neither zero nor more than modest intake reduces total mortality and cardiovascular risk by cardio and neuroprotection (Collins et al., 2009; Opie and Lecour, 2007).

According with the French Paradox, the moderate intake of wine (1 or 2 glasses per day) could be beneficial for health by reducing the risk of CVD mortality. As evidenced in Table 1, the content of these vasoactive substances is more relevant in red wine compared to other food and beverages. Finally on the light of all the epidemiological and fundamental studies analyzed in this chapter, and our works, we can suggest that RWPC, and in particular delphinidin and resveratrol, could be used for their therapeutic potential in the prevention and treatment of cardiovascular pathologies. We think that ERα activation might be the main molecular target triggering the beneficial effects of dietary supplementation of RWPC. Nevertheless, further studies are needed to verify the implication of ERα in other physiological effects of polyphenols and not only in NO release and vascular relaxation.

8. References

Agouni A., Lagrue-Lak-Hal A.H., Mostefai H.A., Tesse, A., Mulder P., Rouet, P., Desmoulin, F., H;eymes, C., Martinez, M.C., & Andriantsitohaina, R. (2009). Red wine polyphenols prevent metabolic and cardiovascular alterations associated with obesity in Zucker fatty rats (Fa/Fa). *PloS one*, Vol.4, No.5, (May 2009), pp. e5557.

Andriambeloson, E., Kleschyov, A.L., Muller, B., Beretz, A., Stoclet, J.C., & Andriantsitohaina, R. (1997). Nitric oxide production and endothelium-dependent vasorelaxation induced by wine polyphenols in rat aorta. *British J. Pharmacol.*, Vol.120, No. 6, (Mars 1997), pp. 1053-1058.

Andriambeloson, E., Magnier, C., Haan-Archipoff, G., Lobstein, A., Anton, R., Beretz, A., Stoclet, J.C., & Andriantsitohaina, R. (1998). Natural dietary polyphenolic compounds cause endothelium-dependent vasorelaxation in rat thoracic aorta. *J. Nutr.*, Vol.128, No.12, (December 1998), pp. 2324-2333.

Bahorun, T. (1997). Substances naturelles actives : La Flore Mauricienne, Une source d'aprovisionnement potentielle. In : *Proceedings of the Second Annual Meeting of Agricultural Scientists (AMAS)*, pp. 83-94, Food and Agricultural Research Council, Réduit, Mauritius, August 1997.

Baron-Menguy, C., Bocquet, A., Guihot, A.L., Chappard, D., Amiot, M.J., Andriantsitohaina, R., Loufrani, L., & Henrion, D. (2007). Effects of red wine polyphenols on postischemic neovascularization model in rats: low doses are proangiogenic, high doses anti-angiogenic. *FASEB J.*, Vol.2, No.13, (November 2007), pp. 3511-3521.

Barton, M., Meyer, M.R., & Haas, E. (2007). Hormone replacement therapy and atherosclerosis in postmenopausal women: does aging limit therapeutic benefits? *Arterioscler. Thromb. Vasc. Biol.*, Vol.27, No.8, (August 2007), pp. 1669-1672.

Beato, M., & Klug, J. (2000). Steroid hormone receptors: an update. *Hum. Reprod. Update*, Vol.6, No.3, (May-June 2000), pp. 225-236.

Bernatova, I., Penchanova, O., Babal, P., Kysela, S., Stvrtina, S., & Andriantstohaina, R. (2002). Wine polyphenols improve cardiovascular remodeling and vascular function in NO-deficient hypertension. *Am. J. Physiol. Heart Circ. Physiol.*, Vol. 282, No.3, (March 2002), pp. 942-948.

Boban, M., Modun, D., Music, I., Vukovic, J., Brizic, I., Salamunic, I., Obad, A., Palada, I., & Dujic, Z. (2006). Red wine induced modulation of vascular function: separating the role of polyphenols, ethanol, and urates. *J. Cardiovasc. Pharmacol.*, Vol.47, No.5, (May 2006), pp. 695-701.

Bravo, L. (1998). Polyphenols: chemistry, dietary sources, metabolism, and nutritional significance. *Nutr. Rev.*, Vol.56, No.11, (November 1998), pp. 317-33.

Brouchet, L., Krust, A., Dupont, S., Chambon, P., Bayard, F., & Arnal, J.F. (2001). Estradiol accelerates reendothelialization in mouse carotid artery through estrogen receptor-alpha but not estrogen receptor-beta. *Circulation*, Vol. 103, No.3, (January 2001), pp. 423-428.

Broughton, B.R., Miller, A.A., & Sobey, C.G. (2010). Endothelium-dependent relaxation by G protein-coupled receptor 30 agonists in rat carotid arteries. *Am. J. Physiol. Heart Circ. Physiol.*, Vol.298, No.3, (March 2010), pp. H1055-H1061.

Brownson, D.M., Azios, N.G., Fuqua, B.K., Dharmawardhane, S.F., & Mabry, TJ. (2002). Flavonoid effects relevant to cancer. *J. Nutr.*, Vol.132, No.11, (November 2002), pp. 3482S-3489S.

Cersosimo, E., & Defronzo, R.A. (2006). Insulin resistance and endothelial dysfunction: the road map to cardiovascular diseases. *Diabetes Metab. Res. Rev.*, Vol.22, No.6, (November-December 2006), pp. 423-436.

Chalopin, M., Tesse, A., Martínez, M.C., Rognan, D., Arnal, J.F., & Andriantsitohaina, R. (2010) Estrogen receptor alpha as a key target of red wine polyphenols action on the endothelium. *PLoS One*, Vol.5, No.1, (January 2010), pp. e8554.

Chambliss, K.L., & Shaul, P.W. (2002). Rapid activation of endothelial NO synthase by estrogen: evidence for a steroid receptor fast-action complex (SRFC) in caveolae. *Steroids*, Vol.67, No.6, (May 2002), pp. 413-419.

Chandrasekara, A., & Shahidi, F. (2010). Content of insoluble bound phenolics in millets and their contribution to antioxidant capacity. *J. Agric. Food Chem.*, Vol.58, No.11, (June 2010), pp. 6706-6714.

Chen, Z., Yuhanna, I.S., Galcheva-Gargova, Z., Karas, R.H., Mendelsohn, M.E., & Shaul, P.W. (1999). Estrogen receptor alpha mediates the nongenomic activation of endothelial nitric oxide synthase by estrogen. *J. Clin. Invest.*, Vol.103, No.3, (May 1999), pp. 401-406.

Cheynier, V. (2005). Polyphenols in foods are more complex than often thought. *Am. J. Clin. Nutr.*, Vol.81, No.1, (January 2005), pp. 223S-229S.

Clarkson, T.B. (2007). Estrogen effects on arteries vary with stage of reproductive life and extent of subclinical atherosclerosis progression. *Menopause*, Vol.14, No.3, (May-June 2007), pp. 373-384.

Collins, M.A., Neafsey, E.J., Mukamal, K.J., Gray, M.O., Parks, D.A., Das, D.K., & Korthuis, R.J. (2009). Alcohol in moderation, cardioprotection, and neuroprotection: epidemiological considerations and mechanistic studies. *Alcohol Clin. Exp. Res.*, Vol.33, No.2, (February 2009), pp. 206-219.

Criqui, M.H., & Ringel, B.L. (1994). Does diet or alcohol explain the French paradox? *Lancet*, Vol.344, No.8939-8940, (December 1994), pp. 1719-1723.

Defronzo, R.A. (2006). Is insulin resistance atherogenic? Possible mechanisms. *Atheroscler. Suppl.*, Vol.7, No.4, (August 2006), pp. 11–15.

Duarte, J., Andriambeloson, E., Diebolt, M., & Andrantsitohaina, R. (2004). Wine polyphenols stimulate superoxide anion production to promote calcium signaling and endothelial-dependent vasodilatation. *Physiol. Res.*, Vol.53, No.6, (2004), pp. 595-602.

Diebolt, M., Bucher, B., & Andriantsitohaina, R. (2001). Wine polyphenols decrease blood pressure, improve NO vasodilatation, and induce gene expression. *Hypertension*, Vol.38, No.2, (August 2001), pp. 159-165.

Doll, R., Peto, R., Hall, E., Wheatley, K., & Gray, R. (1994). Mortality in relation to consumption of alcohol: 13 years' observations on male British doctors. *B.M.J.*, Vol.309, No.6959, (October 1994), pp. 911-918.

Duthie, G.G., Pedersen, M.W., Gardner, P.T., Morrice, P.C., Jenkinson, A.M., McPhail, D.B., & Steele, G.M. (1998). The effect of whisky and wine consumption on total phenol content and antioxidant capacity of plasma from healthy volunteers. *Eur. J. Clin. Nutr.*, Vol.52, No.10, (October 1998), pp. 733-736.

Emberson, J.R., Shaper, A.G., Wannamethee, S.G., Morris, R.W., & Whincup, P.H. (2005). Alcohol intake in middle age and risk of cardiovascular disease and mortality: accounting for intake variation over time. *Am. J. Epidemiol.*, Vol.161, No.9, (May 2005), pp. 856-863.

Favot, L., Martin, S., Keravis, T., Andriantsitohaina, R., & Lugnier, C. (2003). Involvement of cyclin-dependent pathway in the inhibitory effect of delphinidin on angiogenesis. *Cardiovasc. Res.*, Vol.59, No.2, (August 2003), pp. 479-487.

Ferrières, J. (2004). The French paradox: lessons for other countries. *Coronary disease*, Vol.90, No.1, (January 2004), pp. 107-111.

Ferruzzi, M.G. (2010). The influence of beverage composition on delivery of phenolic compounds from coffee and tea. *Physiol. Behav.*, Vol.100, No.1, (April 2010), pp. 33-41.

Fitzpatrick, D.F., Hirschfield, S.L., & Coffey, R.G. (1993). Endothelium-dependent vasorelaxing activity of wine and other grape products. *Am. J. Physiol.*, Vol.265, No.2, (August 1993), pp. H774-H778.

Fornoni, A., & Raij, L. (2005). Metabolic syndrome and endothelial dysfunction. *Curr. Hypertens. Rep.*, Vol.7, No.2, (April 2005), pp. 88–95.

Fotsis, T., Pepper, M.S., Montesano, R., Aktas, E., Breit, S., Schweigerer, L., Rasku, S., Wähälä, K., & Adlercreutz, H.(1998). Phytoestrogens and inhibition of angiogenesis. *Baillieres Clin. Endocrinol. Metab.*, Vol.12, No.4, (December 1998), pp. 649-666.

Fuchs, C.S., Stampfer, M.J., Colditz, G.A., Giovannucci, E.L., Manson, J.E., Kawachi, I., Hunter, D.J., Hankinson, S.E., Hennekens, C.H., & Rosner, B. (1995). Alcohol consumption and mortality among women. *N. Engl. J. Med.*, Vol.332, No.19, (May 1995), pp. 1245-1250.

Gaziano, J.M., Gaziano, T.A., Glynn, R.J., Sesso, H.D., Ajani, U.A., Stampfer, M.J., Manson, J.E., Hennekens, C.H., & Buring, J.E. (2000). Light-to-moderate alcohol consumption and mortality in the Physicians' Health Study enrollment cohort. *J Am Coll. Cardiol.*, Vol.35, No.1, (January 2000), pp. 96-105.

Guo, X., Razandi, M., Pedram, A., Kassab, G., & Levin, E.R. (2005). Estrogen induces vascular wall dilation: mediation through kinase signaling to nitric oxide and estrogen receptors alpha and beta. *J. Biol. Chem.*, Vol.280, No.20, (May 2005), pp. 19704-19710.

Haas, E., Bhattacharya, I., Brailoiu, E., Damjanović, M., Brailoiu, G.C., Gao, X., Mueller-Guerre, L., Marjon, N.A., Gut, A., Minotti, R., Meyer, M.R., Amann, K., Ammann, E., Perez-Dominguez, A., Genoni, M., Clegg, D.J., Dun, N.J., Resta, T.C., Prossnitz, E.R., & Barton, M. (2009). Regulatory role of G protein-coupled estrogen receptor for vascular function and obesity. *Circ. Res.*, Vol.104, No.3, (February 2009), pp. 288-291.

Haas, E., Meyer, M.R., Schurr, U., Bhattacharya, I., Minotti, R., Nguyen, H.H., Heigl, A., Lachat, M., Genoni, M., & Barton, M. (2007). Differential effects of 17beta-estradiol on function and expression of estrogen receptor alpha, estrogen receptor beta, and GPR30 in arteries and veins of patients with atherosclerosis. *Hypertension*, Vol.49, No.6, (June 2007), pp. 1358-1363.

Hall, J.M., Couse, J.F., & Korach, K.S. (2001). The multifaceted mechanisms of estradiol and estrogen receptor signaling. *J. Biol. Chem.*, Vol.276, No.40, (October 2001), pp. 36869-36872.

Harborne, J.B. & Williams, C.A. (2000). Advances in flavonoid research since 1992. *Phytochemistry*, Vol.55, No.6, (November 2000), pp.481-504.

Hodgin, J.B., Krege, J.H., Reddick, R.L., Korach, K.S., Smithies, O., & Maeda, N. (2001). Estrogen receptor alpha is a major mediator of 17beta-estradiol's atheroprotective effects on lesion size in ApoE−/− mice. *J. Clin. Invest.*, Vol.107, No.3, (February 2001), pp. 333-340.

Holm, A., Baldetorp, B., Olde, B., Leeb-Lundberg, L.M., & Nilsson, B.O. (2011). The GPER1 agonist G-1 attenuates endothelial cell proliferation by inhibiting DNA synthesis and accumulating cells in the S and G2 phases of the cell cycle. *J. Vasc. Res.*, Vol.48, No.4, (January 2011), pp. 327-335.

Igura K, Ohta T, Kuroda Y, & Kaji K. (2001). Resveratrol and quercetin inhibit angiogenesis in vitro. *Cancer Lett.*, Vol.171, No.1, (Septembre 2001), pp. 11-16.

Imhof, A., Woodward, M., Doering, A., Helbecque, N., Loewel, H., Amouyel, P., Lowe, G.D., & Koenig, W. (2004). Overall alcohol intake, beer, wine, and systemic markers of inflammation in western Europe: results from three MONICA samples (Augsburg, Glasgow, Lille). *Eur. Heart J.*, Vol.25, No.23, (December 2004), pp. 2092-2100.

Kane, M.O., Anselm, E., Rattmann, Y.D., Auger, C., & Schini-Kerth, V.B. (2009). Role of gender and estrogen receptors in the rat aorta endothelium-dependent relaxation to red wine polyphenols. *Vascul. Pharmacol.*, Vol.51, No.2-3, (August-September 2009), pp. 140-146.

Kang, L., Zang X, Xie, Y., Tu, Y., Wang, D., Liu, Z., & Wang, Z.Y. (2010). Involvement of estrogen receptor variant ER-alpha36, not GPR30, in nongenomic estrogen signaling. *Mol. Endocrinol.*, Vol.24, No.4, (April 2010), pp. 709-721.

Klinge, C.M., Blankenship, K.A., Risinger, K.E., Bhatnagar, S., Noisin, E.L., Sumanasekera, W.K., Zhao, L., Brey, D.M., & Keynton, R.S. (2005). Resveratrol and estradiol rapidly activate MAPK signaling through estrogen receptors alpha and beta in endothelial cells. *J. Biol. Chem.*, Vol.280, No.9, (March 2005), pp. 7460-7468.

Klinge, C.M., Wickramasinghe, N.S., Ivanova, M.M., & Dougherty, S.M. (2008). Resveratrol stimulates nitric oxide production by increasing estrogen receptor α-Src-caveolin-1 interaction and phosphorylation in human umbilical vein endothelial cells. *F.A.S.E.B. J.*, Vol.22, No.7, (July 2008), pp. 2185-2197.

Kopelman, P.G. (2000). Obesity as a medical problem. *Nature*, Vol.404, No.6778, (April 2000), pp. 635–643.

Kopp, P. (1998). Resveratrol, a phytoestrogen found in red wine. A possible explanation for the conundrum of the French paradox? *Eur. J. Endocrinol.*, Vol.138, No.6, (June 1998), pp. 619–620

Kuiper, G.G., Enmark, E., Pelto-Huikko, M., Nilsson, S., & Gustafsson, J.A. (1996). Cloning of a novel receptor expressed in rat prostate and ovary. *Proc. Natl. Acad. Sci. U.S.A.*, Vol.93, No.12, (June 1996), pp. 5925-5930.

Lamont, K.T., Somers, S., Lacerda, L., Opie, L.H., & Lecour S. (2011). Is red wine a SAFE sip away from cardioprotection? Mecanisms involved in resveratrol and melatonin-induced cardioprotection. *J. Pineal Res.*, Vol.50, No.4, (May 2011), pp. 374-380.

Lindberg, M.K., Movérare, S., Skrtic, S., Gao, H., Dahlman-Wright, K., Gustafsson, J.A., & Ohlsson, C. (2003). Estrogen receptor (ER)-beta reduces ERalpha-regulated gene transcription, supporting a "ying yang" relationship between ERalpha and ERbeta in mice. *Mol. Endocrinol.*, Vol.17, No.2, (February 2003), pp. 203-208.

Lindsey, S.H., Cohen, J.A., Brosnihan, K.B., Gallagher, P.E., & Chappell, M.C. (2009). Chronic treatment with the G protein-coupled receptor 30 agonist G-1 decreases blood pressure in ovariectomized mRen2.Lewis rats. *Endocrinology.*, Vol.150, No.8, (August 2009), pp. 3753-3758.

Liu, B.L., Zhang, X ., Zhang, W., & Zhen, H.N. (2007). New enlightenment of French paradox resveratrol's potential for cancer chemoprevention and anti-cancer therapy. *Cancer Biology & Therapy,* Vol.6, No.12, (December 2007), pp. 1833-1836.

López-Sepúlveda, R., Jiménez, R., Romero, M., Zarzuelo, M.J., Sánchez, M., Gómez-Guzmán, M., Vargas, F., O'Valle, F., Zarzuelo, A., Pérez-Vizcaíno, F., & Duarte, J. (2008) Wine polyphenols improve endothelial function in large vessels of female spontaneously hypertensive rats. *Hypertension,* Vol.51, No.4, (April 2008), pp. 1088-1095.

Losordo, D.W., Kearney, M., Kim, E.A., Jekanowski, J., & Isner, J.M. (1994).Variable expression of the estrogen receptor in normal and atherosclerotic coronary arteries of premenopausal women. *Circulation,* Vol.89, No.4, (April 1994), pp. 1501-1510.

Maruyama. K., Endoh, H., Sasaki-Iwaoka, H., Kanou, H., Shimaya, E., Hashimoto, S., Kato, S., & Kawashima, H. (1998). A novel isoform of rat estrogen receptor beta with 18 amino acid insertion in the ligand binding domain as a putative dominant negative regular of estrogen action. *Biochem. Biophys. Res. Commun.,* Vol.246, No.1, (May 1998), pp. 142-147.

Martensson, U.E., Salehi, S.A., Windahl, S., Gomez, M.F., Swärd, K., Daszkiewicz-Nilsson, J., Wendt, A., Andersson, N., Hellstrand, P., Grände, P.O., Owman, C., Rosen, C.J., Adamo, M.L., Lundquist, I., Rorsman, P., Nilsson, B.O., Ohlsson, C., Olde, B., & Leeb-Lundberg, L.M. (2009). Deletion of the G protein-coupled receptor 30 impairs glucose tolerance, reduces bone growth, increases blood pressure, and eliminates estradiol-stimulated insulin release in female mice. *Endocrinology,* Vol.150, No.2, (February 2009), pp. 687-698.

Martin, S., Andriambeloson, E., Takeda, K., & Andriantsitohaina, R. (2002). Red wine polyphenols increase calcium in bovine aortic endothelial cells: a basis to elucidate signalling pathways leading to nitric oxide production. *Br. J. Pharmacol.,* Vol.135, No.6, (March 2002), pp. 1579-1587.

Martin, S., Giannone, G., Andriantsitohaina, R., & Martinez, M.C. (2003). Delphinidin, an active compound of red wine, inhibits endothelial cell apoptosis via nitric oxide pathway and regulation of calcium homeostasis. *Br. J. Pharmacol.,* Vol.139, No.6, (July 2003), pp.1095-1102.

Mendelsohn, M.E., & Karas, R.H. (1999). The protective effects of estrogen on the cardiovascular system. *N. Engl. J. Med.,* Vol.340, No.23, (June 1999), pp. 1801-1811.

Meyer, M.R., Baretella, O., Prossnitz, E.R., & Barton, M. (2010) Dilation of epicardial coronary arteries by the G protein-coupled estrogen receptor agonists G-1 and ICI 182,780. *Pharmacology,* Vol.86, No.1, (July 2010), pp. 58-64.

Meyer, M.R., Haas, E., & Barton, M. (2008). Need for research on estrogen receptor function: importance for postmenopausal hormone therapy and atherosclerosis. *Gend. Med.,* Vol.5, No.Suppl.A, (2008), pp. S19-S33.

Meyer, M.R., Haas, E., & Barton, M. (2006). Gender differences of cardiovascular disease: new perspectives for estrogen receptor signaling. *Hypertension,* Vol.47, No.6, (June 2006), pp. 1019-1026.

Mojzisová, G., & Kuchta, M. (2001). Dietary flavonoids and risk of coronary heart disease. *Physiol. Res.,* Vol.50, No.6, (2001), pp. 529-535.

Mügge, A., Riedel, M., Barton, M., Kuhn, M., & Lichtlen, P.R. (1993). Endothelium independent relaxation of human coronary arteries by 17 beta-oestradiol in vitro. *Cardiovasc. Res.*, Vol.27, No.11, (November 1993), pp. 1939-1942.

Nakamura, Y., Suzuki, T., Miki, Y., Tazawa, C., Senzaki, K., Moriya, T., Saito, H., Ishibashi, T., Takahashi, S., Yamada, S., & Sasano, H. (2004). Estrogen receptors in atherosclerotic human aorta: inhibition of human vascular smooth muscle cell proliferation by estrogens. *Mol. Cell. Endocrinol.*, Vol.219, No.1-2, (April 2004), pp. 17-26.

Napoli, R., Cozzolino, D., Guardasole, V., Angelini, V., Zarra, E., Matarazzo, M., Cittadini, A., Saccà, L., & Torella, R. (2005). Red wine consumption improves insulin resistance but not endothelial function in type 2 diabetic patients. *Metabolism*, Vol.54, No.3, (March 2005), pp. 306-313.

Navarro, S., Oliva, J., Barba, A., Navarro, G., Garcia, M.A., & Zamorano, M. (2000). Evolution of chlorpyrifos, fenarimol, metalaxyl, penconazole, and vinclozolin in red wines elaborated by carbonic maceration of Monastrell grapes. *J. Agric. Food Chem.*, Vol.48, No.8, (August 2000), pp. 3537-3541.

Nilsson, B.O. (2007). Modulation of the inflammatory response by estrogens with focus on the endothelium and its interactions with leukocytes. *Inflamm. Res.*, Vol.56, No.7, (July 2007), pp. 269-273.

Nilsson, B.O., Olde, B., & Leeb-Lundberg, L.M. (2011). G protein-coupled oestrogen receptor 1 (GPER1)/GPR30: a new player in cardiovascular and metabolic oestrogenic signalling. *Br. J. Pharmacol.*, Vol.163, No.6, (July 2011), pp. 1131-1139.

Opie, L.H., & Lecour, S. (2007). The red wine hypothesis: from concepts to protective signaling molecules. *European Heart Journal*, Vol.28, No.14, (July 2007), pp. 1683-1693.

Paech, K., Webb, P., Kuiper, G.G., Nilsson, S., Gustafsson, J., Kushner, P.J., & Scanlan, T.S. (1997). Differential ligand activation of estrogen receptors ERalpha and ERbeta at AP1 sites. *Science*, Vol.277, No.5331, (September 1997), pp. 1508-1510.

Paganga, G., & Rice-Evans, C.A. (1997). The identification of flavonoids as glycosides in human plasma. *F.E.B.S. Lett.*, Vol.401, No.1, (January 1997), pp.78-82.

Papamichael, C., Karatzis, E., Karatzi, K., Aznaouridis, K., Papaioannou, T., Protogerou, A., Stamatelopoulos, K., Zampelas, A., Lekakis, J., & Mavrikakis, M. (2004). Red wine's antioxidants counteract acute endothelial dysfunction caused by cigarette smoking in healthy nonsmokers. *Am. Heart J.*, Vol.147, No.2, (February 2004), pp. E5.

Pare, G., Krust, A., Karas, R.H., Dupont, S., Aronovitz, M., Chambon, P., & Mendelsohn, M.E. (2002). Estrogen receptor-alpha mediates the protective effects of estrogen against vascular injury. *Circ. Res.*, Vol.90, No.10, (May 2002), pp. 1087-1092.

Pechánová, O., Bernátová, I., Babál, P., Martínez, M.C., Kyselá, S., Stvrtina, S., & Andriantsitohaina, R. (2004). Red wine polyphenols prevent cardiovascular alterations in L-NAME-induced hypertension. *J. Hypertens.*, Vol.22, No.8, (August 2004), pp. 1551-1559.

Pechanova. O., Rezzani, R.., Babal, P., Bernatova, I., & Andriantsitohaina R. (2006). Beneficial effects of provinols: cardiovascular system and kidney. *Physiol. Res.*, Vol.55, No.Suppl.1, (2006), pp. 17-30.

Pellegrini, N., Simonetti, P., Gardana, C., Brenna, O., Brighenti, F., & Pietta, P. (2000). polyphenol content and total antioxidant activity of *vini novelli* (young red wines). *J. Agric. Food Chem.*, Vol.48, No.3, (March 2000), pp. 732–735.

Petersen, D.N., Tkalcevic, G.T., Koza-Taylor, P.H., Turi, T.G., & Brown, T.A. (1998). Identification of estrogen receptor beta2, a functional variant of estrogen receptor beta expressed in normal rat tissues. *Endocrinology*, Vol.139, No.3, (March 1998), pp. 1082-1092.

Price, R.H. Jr, Lorenzon, N., & Handa, R.J. (2000). Differential expression of estrogen receptor beta splice variants in rat brain: identification and characterization of a novel variant missing exon 4. *Brain Res. Mol. Brain Res.*, Vol.80, No.2, (September 2000), pp. 260-268.

Prior, R.L., Lazarus, S.A., Cao, G., Muccitelli, H., & Hammerstone, J.F. (2001). Identification of procyanidins and anthocyanins in blueberries and cranberries (Vaccinium spp.) using high-performance liquid chromatography/mass spectrometry. *J. Agric. Food Chem.*, Vol.49, No.3, (March 2001), pp. 1270-1276.

Providencia, R. (2006). Cardiovascular protection by alcoholic beverages: scientific basis of the French paradox. *Rev. Port. Cardiol.*, Vol.25, No.11, (November 2006), pp. 1043-1058.

Ranaivo H.R., Diebolt M., & Andriantsitohaina R. (2004). Wine polyphenols induce hypotension, and decrease cardiac reactivity and infarct size in rats: involvement of nitric oxide. *British J. Pharmacol.*, Vol.142, No.4 (June 2004), pp. 671–678.

Renaud, S.C. (1992). What is the epidemiologic evidence for the thrombogenic potential of dietary long-chain fatty acids? *Am. J. Clin. Nutr.*, Vol.56, No.Suppl.4, (October 1992), pp. 823S-824S.

Renaud, S.C., Guéguen, R., Siest, G., & Salamon, R. (1999). Wine, beer, and mortality in middle-aged men from eastern France. *Arch. Intern. Med.*, Vol.159, No.16, (September 1999), pp. 1865-1870.

Revankar, C.M., Cimino, D.F., Sklar, L.A., Arterburn, J.B., & Prossnitz, E.R. (2005). A transmembrane intracellular estrogen receptor mediates rapid cell signaling. *Science*, Vol.307, No.5715, (March 2005), pp. 1625-1630.

Ribereau-Gayon, P., Dubourdieu, D., Donèche, B., & Lonvaud, A. (2000). Cytology, taxonomy and ecology of grape and wine yeast, In: *Handbook of Enology*, Vol.1, pp. 1–49, John Wiley & Sons.

Richter G. (1993). *Métabolisme des végétaux. Physiologie et biochimie*, Presses Polytechniques et Universitaires Romandes.

Ritz, M.F., Curin, Y., Mendelowitsch, A., & Andriantsitohaina, R. (2008b). Acute treatment with red wine polyphenols protects from ischemia-induced excitotoxicity, energy failure and oxidative stress in rats. *Brain Res.*, Vol.1239, (November 2008), pp. 226-234.

Ritz, M.F., Ratajczak, P., Curin, Y., Cam, E., Mendelowitsch, A., Pinet, F., & Andriantsitohaina, R. (2008a). Chronic treatment with red wine polyphenol compounds mediates neuroprotection in a rat model of ischemic cerebral stroke. *J. Nutr.*, Vol.138, No.3, (March 2008), pp. 519-525.

Shaw, L., Taggart, M., & Austin, C. (2001). Effects of the oestrous cycle and gender on acute vasodilatory responses of isolated pressurized rat mesenteric arteries to 17 beta-oestradiol. *Br. J. Pharmacol.*, Vol.132, No.5, (March 2001), pp. 1055-1062.

Si, W., Gong, J., Tsao, R., Kalab, M., Yang, R., & Yin, Y. (2006). Bioassay-guided purification and identification of antimicrobial components in Chinese green tea extract. *J. Chromatogr. A.,* Vol.1125, No.2, (September 2006), pp. 204-210.

Soleas, G.J., Diamandis, E.P., & Goldberg, D.M. (1997). Wine as a biological fluid: History, production, and role in disease prevention issue. *J. Clinical Laboratory Analysis,* Vol.11, No.5, (December 1998), pp. 287-313.

Spary, E.J., Maqbool, A., & Batten, T.F. (2009). Oestrogen receptors in the central nervous system and evidence for their role in the control of cardiovascular function. *J. Chem. Neuroanat.,* Vol.38, No.3, (November 2009), pp. 185-196.

Sudhir, K., Chou, T.M., Chatterjee, K., Smith, E.P., Williams, T.C., Kane, J.P., Malloy, M.J., Korach, K.S., & Rubanyi, G.M. (1997). Premature coronary artery disease associated with a disruptive mutation in the estrogen receptor gene in a man. *Circulation,* Vol.96, No.10, (November 1997), pp. 3774-3777.

Suh, I., Shaten, B.J., Cutler, J.A., & Kuller, L.H. (1992). Alcohol use and mortality from coronary heart disease: the role of high-density lipoprotein cholesterol. The Multiple Risk Factor Intervention Trial Research Group. *Ann. Intern. Med.,* Vol.116, No.11, (June 1992), pp. 881-887.

Suh, J.H., Virsolvy, A., Goux, A., Cassan, C., Richard, S., Cristol, J.P., Teissèdre, P.L., & Rouanet, J.M. (2011). Polyphenols prevent lipid abnormalities and arterial dysfunction in hamsters on a high-fat diet: a comparative study of red grape and white persimmon wines. *Food Funct.,* Vol.2, No.9, (September 2011), pp. 555-561.

Tsao, R. (2010). Chemistry and biochemistry of dietary polyphenols. *Nutrients,* Vol.2, No.12, (December 2010), pp. 1231-1246.

Tsao, R., Papadopoulos, Y., Yang, R., Young, J.C., & McRae, K. (2006). Isoflavone profiles of red clovers and their distribution in different parts harvested at different growing stages. *J. Agric. Food Chem.,* Vol.54, No.16, (August 2006), pp. 5797-5805.

Tsao, R., Yang, R., Young, J.C., & Zhu, H. (2003). Polyphenolic profiles in eight apple cultivars using high-performance liquid chromatography (HPLC). *J. Agric. Food Chem.,* Vol.51, No.21, (Octobre 2003), pp. 6347-6353.

Thun, M.J., Peto, R., Lopez, A.D., Monaco, J.H., Henley, S.J., Heath, C.W., & Doll, R. (1997). Alcohol consumption and mortality among middle-aged and elderly U.S. adults. *N. Engl. J. Med.,* Vol.337, No.24, (December 1997), pp. 1705–1714.

Vegeto, E., Belcredito, S., Etteri, S., Ghisletti, S., Brusadelli, A., Meda, C., Krust, A., Dupont, S., Ciana, P., Chambon, P., & Maggi, A. (2003). Estrogen receptor-alpha mediates the brain antiinflammatory activity of estradiol. *Proc. Natl. Acad. Sci. U.S.A.,* Vol.100, No.16, (August 2003), pp. 9614-9619.

Vidavalur, R., Otani H., Singal, P.K., & Maulik N. (2006). Significance of wine and resveratrol in cardiovascular disease: French paradox revisited. *Exp. Clin. Cardiol.,* Vol.11, No.3, (Fall 2006), pp. 217-225.

Wallerath T., Deckert G., Ternes T., Anderson H., Li H., Witte K., & Förstermann U. (2002). Resveratrol, a polyphenolic phytoalexin present in red wine, enhances expression and activity of endothelial nitric oxide synthase. *Circulation,* Vol.106, No.13, (September 2002), pp. 1652-1658.

Webb, P., Nguyen, P., Valentine, C., Lopez, G.N., Kwok, G.R., McInerney, E., Katzenellenbogen, B.S., Enmark, E., Gustafsson, J.A., Nilsson, S., & Kushner, P.J. (1999). The estrogen receptor enhances AP-1 activity by two distinct mechanisms with different requirements for receptor transactivation functions. *Mol. Endocrinol.*, Vol.13, No.10, (October 1999), pp.1672-1685.

Xu, Y., Simon, J.E., Welch, C., Wightman, J.D., Ferruzzi, M.G., Ho, L., Passinetti, G.M., & Wu, Q. (2011). Survey of polyphenol constituents in grapes and grape-derived products. *J. Agric. Food Chem.*, Vol.59, No.19, (October 2011), pp. 10586-10593.

Yusuf, S., Hawken, S., Ounpuu, S., Dans, T., Avezum, A., Lanas, F., MacQueen, M., Budaj, A., Pais, P., Varigos, J., & Lisheng, L. (2004). Effect of potentially modifiable risk factors associated with myocardial infarction in 52 countries (the INTERHEART study); case-control study. *Lancet*, Vol.364, No.9438, (September 2004), pp. 937-952.

Zhao, C., Dahlman-Wright, K., & Gustafsson, J.A. (2008). Estrogen receptor beta: an overview and update. *Nucl. Recept. Signal.*, Vol. 6, (February 2008), pp. e003.

Zhao, F., Watanabe, Y., Nozawa, H., Daikonnya, A., Kondo, K., & Kitanaka, S. (2005). Prenylflavonoids and phloroglucinol derivatives from hops (Humulus lupulus). *J. Nat. Prod.*, Vol.68, No.1, (January 2005), pp. 43-49.

5

Importance of Dermatology in Infective Endocarditis

Servy Amandine, Jones Meriem
and Valeyrie-Allanore Laurence*
*Department of Dermatology,
Hôpital Henri Mondor, Créteil,
France*

1. Introduction

Infective endocarditis (IE) is a rare affection with an annual incidence of between 15 to 60 cases per million. If untreated, IE is fatal, and the overall mortality is evaluated above 20%. IE is an endovascular microbial infection of intracardiac structures. The early characteristic lesion corresponds to variable sized vegetation leading to valvular destruction and abscess formation.

Epidemiologic profile evolved progressively with decreasing proportion of IE on abnormal native valve compensated by an increased proportion of prosthetic valve IE and native valve IE with previously unrecognized predisposing conditions. Among causative microorganisms, the responsibility of staphylococci is more frequently observed. Diagnosing IE remains a clinical challenge because evolution is insidious and symptoms are polymorphous. This diagnosis must be systematically considered in the presence of purpura, distal necrosis but also in patients who had have chronic dermatosis which correspond to an underestimated potential source of IE.

2. Pathophysiology

Secondary to damage of endothelium, extracellular matrix proteins are exposed leading to development of non-bacterial thrombotic endocarditis (NBTE) with fibrin and platelets. Endothelial damage can occur after mechanical lesions (devices, repeated intravenous injection of particulate material), turbulent blood flow (congenital heart disease, prosthetic valves...), inflammation (chronic rheumatic fever) or degenerative lesions (European society of cardiology [ESC], 2009). NBTE facilitates micro-organism adherence and infection of endothelium (Figure 1).

International specialists (American Heart Association [AHA], 2007; ESC, 2009) no longer differentiate acute, subacute and chronic IE based on usual progression of untreated disease. Indeed, although clinical manifestations are more insidious in subacute IE, severe

---

*Corresponding Author

complications can occur and it is currently difficult to determine the onset of the disease. Presently, IE are classified depending on the type of valve damage (right/left-sided, native/prosthetic valve).

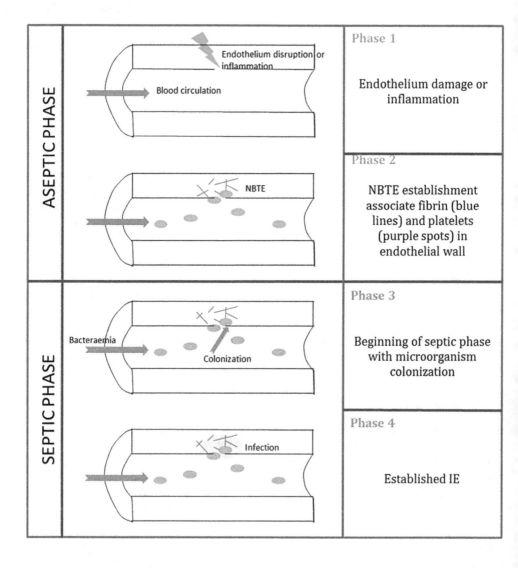

Fig. 1. Pathophysiology of IE with aseptic and septic phases (A. Servy; August 2011). NBTE: non- bacterial thrombotic endocarditis

3. Epidemiology

3.1 Incidence

IE is a rare disease with 2 to 6 per 100 000 persons affected per year (Que, 2011). Classically described in young patients after chronic rheumatic heart disease. Its incidence in industrialized countries is more elevated in at-risk groups, mainly persons older than 65 years old (15 per 100 000 per year). At present, the average is 57 years old (Que, 2011; ESC, 2009).

Native valve IE is the most frequent. Left-sided native valve IE represents 70% of disease incidence and the mortality is evaluated at 15% (25-45% with healthcare-associated). 5-10% of IE affect right-sided native valve, mainly in intravenous-drug users, and patients with congenital heart disease or devices. *Staphylococcus spp* is most frequently involved in right-sided native valve IE and mortality is less than 10% (Que, 2011).

Prosthetic valve IE is also increasing (10-30% of IE), mechanical and bioprosthetic equally. The prevalence of valve prostheses IE is above 6% (0.3-1.2% per year). Left-sided prosthetic valve endocarditis (20% of IE) is the most severe with 20 to 40% mortality. The main germs involved in early prosthetic valve IE (less than one year after cardiac surgery) include staphylococci, fungi and Gram-negative bacilli, whereas late IE is associated with staphylococci, oral streptococci, *S. bovis* and enteroccoci (ESC, 2009).

3.2 Risk factors

3.2.1 Characteristics of patient

The main risk factor is age (median age above 60) (Murdoch, 2009) due to degenerative valve, immunosuppressive conditions and multiple comorbidities. However, edentate people have a lower risk of IE. Digestive portal of entry is frequent in this population, mainly in *S. bovis* and enterococcus IE and should be researched.

Many comorbidities increase the risk of IE, leading to heart diseases. At present, in industrialized countries, chronic rheumatic heart disease has become exceptional and the proportion of degenerative valve lesion and congenital heart disease is more important as well as their responsibility for IE (Moreillon, 2004). Chronic immunosuppressive therapy (chemotherapy, topical corticosteroid…) or affections are predisposing conditions, mainly diabetes mellitus (16% of IE), hemodialysis (8%), cancer (8%) and HIV infection (2%) (Murdoch, 2009). Physicians should be aware of the risk of EI in cases of acute or chronic dermatosis. Chronic bacteria carriers, wounds, and percutaneous invasive procedure increase significantly the risk of bacteremia.

3.2.2 Situations at risk

All iatrogenic invasive procedures are at risk of bacteremia such as catheter, urinary surgery, and endoscopy (Table 1). Nevertheless, intravenous drug users are more at risk (10% of IE) due to poor hygiene. Indeed 55% of active heroin, cocaine and methamphetamine injection drug users report a lifetime history of skin infection mainly in cases of intramuscular injection or frequent heroin or speedball injection (Phillips, 2010). In these cases, *S. aureus* and fungi must be suspected and treated. Dental treatments are too easily suspected (AHA, 2007; Strom, 1998) whereas most of the time, no procedure or situation at risk are identified and daily bacteremia is often involved (AHA, 2007). In a recent French study (Association pour l'Etude et la Prévention de l'Endocardite Infectieuse [AEPEI], 2002), 63% of IE cases had no situation at risk identified.

Risk factors of IE		
Patient characteristics		Situations at risk
Age		Invasive procedures:
Comorbidities	Heart disease and prosthetic valve Diabetes mellitus Chronic renal failure Immunosuppressive affection	- percutaneous (drug, catheter...) or - dental Daily bacteremia - Brushing teeth - Chewing ...
Treatment	Immunosuppressive therapy	

Table 1. Procedures and situations at risk of bacteremia.

3.3 Causal microorganisms

Distribution of causative microorganisms of IE is different, depending on the patient's characteristics (Table 2) and portal of entry. Gram-positive bacteria are the most frequent microorganisms. They are responsible for more than 80% of IE because they have greatest ability to adhere and colonize damaged valves (Que, 2011).

Microorganisms (%)	Valve affected			
	Native valve IE		Intracardiac device IE	
	Drug abusers	Others patients	Prosthetic valve	Others
Staphylococcus aureus	68	28	23	35
Coagulase-negative staphylococcus	3	9	17	26
Viridans group streptococci	10	21	12	8
Streptococcus bovis	1	7	5	3
Enterococcus ssp	5	11	12	6
HACEK	0	2	2	1
Fungi	1	1	4	1
Polymicromial	3	1	0.8	0
Negative culture findings	5	9	12	11

Table 2. Microbiologic etiology of IE depend on patient's characteristics (Murdoch, 2009). HACEK: Haemophilus (parainfluenzae, aphrophilus, paraphrophilus and influenza), Actinobacillus actinomycetemcomitans, Cardiobacterium hominis, Eikenella corrodens, Kingella (kingae and dentrificans).

Although increasing involvement of oral streptococci, streptococcaceae remain the main pathogen (nearly 60% of IE). In streptococci group, group D (*S. bovis*...) are found in 25%, oral streptococci in 17% and pyogenic streptococci (*S. agalactiae, S. pyogenes*) in 6% of IE.

Enterococci (mainly *E. faecalis*) are also frequent (8%), mainly in elderly people and prosthetic valve carriers (AEPEI, 2002). Urinary and digestive portal of entry (including colon cancer, and diverticulitis) must be researched with colonoscopy and imaging. Presence of *S. bovis* equally implies digestive portal of entry.

The role of Staphylococcaceae is increasing (20-34% of IE) with 23% of IE due to *S. aureus* and 6% to coagulase-negative staphylococci (AEPEI, 2002; Miro, 2005). Staphylococcus IE is more frequent in intravenous drug users, HIV patients, right-sided IE and iatrogenic infection. The prevalence of IE in patients with *Staphylococcus aureus* bacteremia is elevated (22%) and some authors recommend a systematic echocardiography in this situation (Rasmussen, 2011).

The responsibility of others germs is lesser and unusually several microorganisms are associated in rare instances (less than 5%). No germ is identified in 5% of cases (AEPEI, 2002).

3.4 Portals of entry

Any site of infection can be responsible of IE. However, some portals of entry are more frequent and must be investigated. Cutaneous portal of entry is frequent (20%) and often misdiagnosed by physicians. In these cases, IE mainly developed on traumatic or chronic wounds, infected or inflammatory dermatosis, intravenous drug use, percutaneous iatrogenic procedures... Dental portal of entry is observed in 9% of cases (poor dental condition, dental procedure). Genitourinary and digestive portal of entry are observed respectively in above 2-11% and 5-9% (AEPEI, 2002; Tornos, 2005).

4. Diagnosis

4.1 Clinical manifestations

Clinical diagnosis of IE is often difficult because of various clinical manifestations and insidious evolution. Moreover, atypical presentation is usual in elderly, immunocompromised patients (lack of fever) and carriers of prosthetic valve, mainly in earlier phase (less than one 1 year after surgery). In fact, in this last group, blood cultures are frequently negative, echocardiography is difficult (ESC, 2009) and inflammatory syndrome and fever is classical even in absence of IE. So, clinical suspicion of IE should be systematically discussed in these cases, and complementary investigations performed.

4.1.1 General signs

Fever is the most frequent sign (approximately 90%) and usually temperature normalizes within 1 week (5-10 days) under adaptive antibiotherapy. An impaired general health condition can be observed with weight loss, fatigue and anorexia.

4.1.2 Cardiological signs

Cardiological manifestations are nearly constant. Heart murmurs are found in up 85% of IE (ESC, 2009) but occurrence of new ones (48%) or increasing of an older murmur (20%) are more evocative (Murdoch, 2009). Clinical manifestations of heart complications can be added (mainly heart failure).

4.1.3 Extracardiac manifestations

Extracardiac manifestations are also frequent, particularly in right-sided IE (78% versus 52% in left-sided IE) with 68% of pulmonary embolism (AEPEI, 2002).

If IE is suspected, dermatological manifestations should be systematically searched and discussed despite rarity (5 to 25% of IE present skin manifestations) not only for diagnosis but also for prognostic (Table 5). They can easily lead to suspicion of IE. In our recent study (unpublished data), we demonstrated a link between the presence of cutaneous signs and embolic events (18.4% of embolic events in lack of cutaneous sign versus 33%) without higher mortality. Dermatological manifestations (Figures 2 and 3) seem to be also less frequently observed with enteroccoci infection (14.5% versus 27.1%) (Martínez-Marcos, 2009).

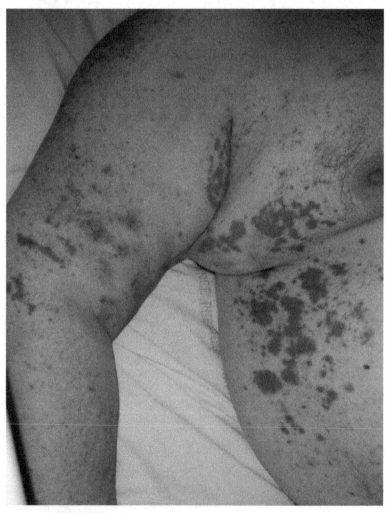

Fig. 2. Vascular purpura on trunk and arms during IE.

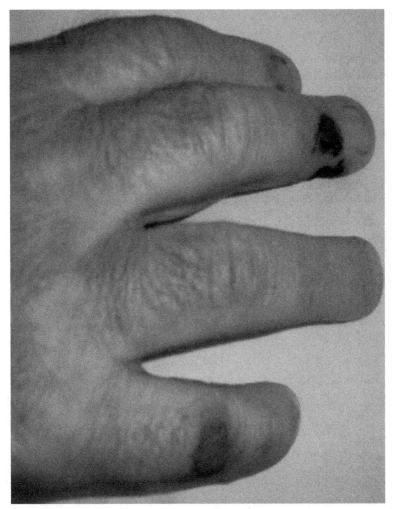

Fig. 3. Necrotic lesions of fingers (same patient): old Janeway lesion or purpura lesion.

-   **Osler's lesions** are specific and described as purple painful nodes on palms, soles, fingertips, pulp of the toes or sometimes on ears (Farrior, 1976). Unfortunately, prevalence is low (3-3.6%) (AEPEI, 2002; Murdoch, 2009) and lesions disappear in a few days without sequelae. In a study including 43 intravenous-drug users IE, Osler's nodes were observed in 50% of left-sided IE whereas none were noticed in right-sided IE (33 right-sided). Moreover, bacteriological study of nodes revealed the same microorganisms as in blood (*S. aureus*).
-   **Janeway lesions** are small non tender erythematous and painless macular (sometimes nodular!) localized on palms or soles (2-5% of IE) (AEPEI, 2002; Murdoch, 2009). These lesions are equally specific and their differenciation difference with Osler nodes is often as difficult, clinically as histologically.

- **Purpura** is more frequent (7.3%) (AEPEI, 2002) but not specific. Its pathophysiology is still unclear including often septic embolism and/or leucocytoclastic cutaneous vasculitis by complex immune depositions (Lévesque 1999). Vascular purpura is characterized by red lesions that don't blanch on applying pressure, caused by erythrocyte extravasation. Lesions are localized on lower parts of the body (legs, back). In IE, lesions are also described on the neck and near the clavicles. IE mucosal purpura is often observed on conjunctivae and mouth (Heffner, 1979).
- **Splinter haemorrhages** are common in many diseases and found in 8 to 14% of IE (Konstantinou, 2009; Murdoch, 2009).

30% of IE (ESC, 2009) has at least one vascular or immunological phenomenon. Vascular phenomenon includes systemic arterial embolism (17-33%) (AEPEI, 2002; Murdoch, 2009), infectious embolism (septic pulmonary infarct, infectious aneurysm) and classically Janeway lesions. Immunological manifestations are mainly represented by Osler's nodes and Roth spots (2%) (Murdoch, 2009).

Musculoskeletal symptoms are common with mainly arthralgia (14%) (Murdoch, 2009), myalgia and back pain. In the presence of, spondylodiscitis (3-15%) (ESC, 2009) mainly observed in streptococci IE must be systemically discussed. Splenomegaly is less frequently noticed (11%) (Murdoch, 2009).

4.2 Laboratory studies

4.2.1 Biology findings

- Inflammatory syndrome

In most cases, unspecific inflammatory syndrome is observed, including neutrophils hyperleucocytosis, elevated erythrocyte sedimentation rate (ESR) and C-reactive protein.

- Microbiological diagnosis

Three sets of blood cultures, including at least one aerobic and one anaerobic samples and spaced of at least 30 minutes, should be obtained from a peripheral vein before beginning any antimicrobial therapy. The blood cultures are positive in 85% of cases (ESC, 2009). However, blood culture can be negative in cases of prior antibiotherapy or specific microorganisms (Table 3). In this last case, other bacteriological investigations are performed, such as serologies, specific PCR and culture on surgical material, catheter and device (pacemaker, defibrillator…) or embolus samples.

Negative blood culture	
Frequently	Constantly: bacteria intracellular
Fastidious Gram-negative bacilli of HACEK group Nutritionally variant streptococci Brucella Fungi	Coxiella burnetii Bartonella Chlamydia Trophynema whipplei

Table 3. Microorganisms and negative blood culture. HACEK group: Haemophilus (parainfluenzae, aphrophilus, paraphrophilus and influenza), Actinobacillus actinomycetemcomitans, Cardiobacterium hominis, Eikenella corrodens, Kingella (kingae and dentrificans).

- Rheumatoid factor is an immunological phenomenon, not specific but found in 5% of IE (Murdoch, 2009).

4.2.2 Histologic findings

Valvular histology after cardiac surgery is the gold standard for diagnosis of IE and observed vegetations, microorganisms and/or valvular inflammation (Greub, 2005).

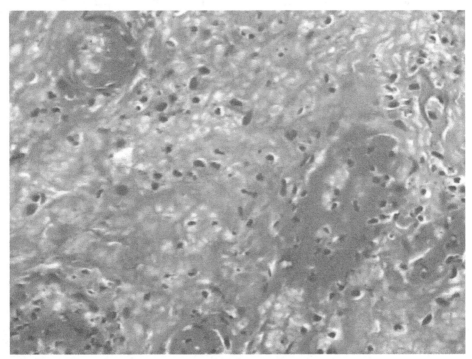

Fig. 4. Cutaneous leucocytoclastic vasculitis (H&E stain; x200).

Kidney fragments can reveal different unspecific lesions including glomerulonephritis or interstitial lesions.

Skin biopsies for histological study are often performed. Osler's nodes are classically explained by immune complex deposition, mainly responsible of leucocytoclastic vasculitis. Janeway lesions are associated with septic emboli; however, all histological findings can be observed in both lesions (Cardullo, 1990; Kerr, 1979; Loewe, 2009; Espinosa Parra, 2002).

4.3 Imaging studies

4.3.1 Echocardiography

Echocardiography is the second fundamental examination for IE diagnosis and its heart complications. In first-line, transthoracic echocardiography (TTE) must be systematically performed in case of suspicion. Its sensibility only ranges from 40 to 63%. So, in cases with negative examination, poor quality of the exam, prosthetic valve... transoesophageal echocardiography (TEE) is recommended if there is high clinical suspicion. In the other cases, a second echocardiography must be performed 7-10 days later if suspicion remains (ESC, 2009). Evocative signs of IE are vegetations (mobile echogenic masses implanted in the endothelium in the trajectory of valvular regurgitation or implanted in prosthetic material), abscess and new dehiscence of a valvular prosthesis (Evangelista, 2004). However, echocardiography does not permit differentiation between septic and aseptic vegetations; so lesions persisting after effective treatment must not be interpreted as a clinical recurrence of the disease unless supported by clinical features and bacteriological evidence.

Echocardiography is repeated as soon as new complications are suspected or at completion of antibiotic therapy for evaluation of cardiac and valve function.

4.3.2 Other imaging

Computed tomography can be used in second intention to diagnose (good evaluation of valvular abnormalities) IE (Feuchtner, 2009) and its systemic complications.

Magnetic resonance imaging is also useful for detection of complications such as cerebral emboli.

4.4 Duke criteria

Various manifestations of IE exist and diagnosis is often difficult. Therefore, the Duke criteria combining clinical and biological criteria have been proposed (Table 4) (Li, 1999).

5. Differential diagnoses

IE is an insidious disease associated with a clinical polymorphism. Differential diagnoses are multiple and it is impossible to give an exhaustive list. Suspicion of IE must be systematically discussed in cases of unexplained fever until proof of contrary. Note echocardiographic differential diagnoses: aseptic vegetations in Libman-Sacks endocarditis (in systemic lupus erythematosus and antiphospholipid syndrome) and marantic endocarditis associated with gastric and pulmonary adenocarcinoma.

6. Severe complications

6.1 Morbidity

6.1.1 Heart complications

Heart failure is the most frequent complication (50 to 60% of IE) mainly on aortic native valve IE (29%). It can be explained by valve insufficiency after native valve destruction causing acute regurgitation (chordal rupture, leaflet rupture or perforation) or prosthesis dehiscence. Other causes of heart failure include intracardiac fistulae, myocarditis, pericarditis (in *S. aureus* infection mainly) or valve obstruction by big vegetations. Surgery is often indicated (Table 5) in emergency because this complication is the worst predictive factor of in-hospital and 6-month mortality.

Definition of term used			
Pathologic criteria	**Microorganisms** demonstrated by culture or histologic examination of a vegetation, a vegetation that has embolized, or an intracardiac abscess specimen		
	Pathologic lesions showing active IE: vegetation or intracardiac abscess confirmed by histologic examination		
Clinical criteria	Major criteria	Blood culture positive for IE	Typical microorganisms consistent with IE from 2 separate blood culture	• Viridans streptocci • *Streptococcus bovis* • HACEK group • *Staphylococcus aureus* • Community-acquired enteroccoci in the absence of a primary focus
			Microorganisms consistent with IE from persistently positive blood culture	At least 2 positive cultures of blood samples drawn > 12h apart
				All of 3 or a majority of ≥ 4 separate cultures of blood (with first and last sample drawn at least 1h apart)
			Single positive blood culture for *Coxiella burnettii* or antiphase I IgG antibody titer >1:800	
		Evidence of endobacterial involvment	Echocardiogram positive for IE TEE recommended in patients with prosthetic valves rated at least "possible IE" by clinical criteria or complicated IE (paravalvular abscess) TTE as first test in others patients	Oscillating intracardiac mass on valve or supporting structures in the path of regurgitant jets or on implanted material in the absence of an alternative anatomic explanation
				Abscess
				New partial dehiscence of prosthetic valve
			New valvular regurgitation (worsening or changing of pre-existing murmur not sufficient)	
	Minor criteria	Predisposition, predisposing heart condition or injection drug use		
		Fever, temperature >38°C		
		Vascular phenomena, major arterial emboli, septic pulmonary infarcts, mycotic aneurysm, intracranial hemorrhages, Janeway's lesion		
		Immunologic phenomena: glomerulonephritis, Osler's nodes, Roth's spots, rheumatic factor		
		Microbiological evidence: positive blood culture but does not meet a major criterion, serological evidence of active infection with organism consistent with IE		
Definition of IE			
Definite IE	Pathologic criteria	≥1	
	Clinical criteria	2 major criteria	
		1 major + 3 minor criteria	
		5 minor criteria	
Possible IE	1 major + 1 minor criteria		
	3 minor criteria		
Rejected	Firm alternative diagnosis explaining evidence of IE		
	Resolution of IE syndrome with antibiotic therapy for ≤ 4 days		
	No pathologic evidence of IE at surgery or autopsy, with antibiotic therapy for ≤ 4 days		
	Does not meet criteria for possible IE as above		

Table 4. Modified Duke criteria (Li, 1999) (TEE: transesophageal echocardiography; TTE: transthoracic echocardiography)

Perivalvular complications should be suspected in case of persistent fever, unexplained or occurrence of atrioventricular block. They included abscess (most common in aortic and prosthesis IE), pseudoaneurysms, fistulae and signed uncontrolled infection. *Staphylococcus aureus* is most often implicated. Despite surgical treatment, 41% of patients die during hospitalization (ESC, 2009).

6.1.2 Uncontrolled infection

Resistant microorganisms, persisting systemic infection, other sites of infection, septic shock etc … can explain locally uncontrolled infection leading to acute coronary syndrome and third degree atrioventricular block. Indication of surgery should be discussed in these cases. Persisting fever, after 7-10 days of antibiotherapy, may discuss uncontrolled infection, adverse reaction to antibiotic, perivalvular complication, thrombosis, emboli… A complete infectious investigation with blood sample examination and intravenous line replacement and cultures, should be performed as well as echocardiography.

6.1.3 Systemic embolism

Migration of cardiac vegetations is responsible for systemic embolism (20-50% of IE) mainly in brain and spleen in left-sided IE and lung in native right-sided and pacemaker lead IE (ESC, 2009). However, all organs can be affected in case of patent foramen ovale. Embolisms are not uncommonly silent (20%) and often life-threatening. The incidence of embolic events increases during the first 2 weeks after the onset of antibiotherapy. Risk factors of embolism are individualized (Table 5) and prompt antibiotherapy can limit its occurrence (Thuny, 2005). Addition of antithrombotic therapy (thrombolytic drugs, anticoagulant or antiplatelet therapy) doesn't appear helpful in preventing whereas cardiac surgery during the first week of antibiotherapy (embolic risk peak) seems beneficial.

Risk factors of embolism		
Vegetation characteristics	Location	Mitral valve
		Multivalvular IE
	Size	>10mm
	Mobility	Increasing or decreasing under antibiotherapy
Microorganisms	Bacteria	Staphylococci
		Streptococcus bovis
	Fungi	*Candida spp*
Past history	Previous embolism	
Biology	Elevated C-reactive protein	

Table 5. Risk factors of embolism in IE (Durante Mangoni, 2003; ESC, 2009)

6.1.4 Neurological complications

Neurological damages after vegetation embolism are observed in 20 to 40 % of IE, mainly due to *Staphylococcus aureus* infection. These complications include stroke, infectious aneurysm (or mycotic aneurysm), brain abscess, meningitis, toxic encephalopathy and seizure and are associated with poor prognosis (mainly ischaemic or haemorragic strokes) (ESC, 2009; Thuny, 2007). Cerebral imaging (computed tomography or better magnetic resonance imaging) should be performed in the presence of neurological signs or headaches (infectious aneurysm).

Only poor neurological prognostic factors (coma, severe comorbidities and severe brain damage) can prohibit cardiac surgery (Table 5). In case of haemorragic stroke, cardiac surgery must be postponed for at least 1 month. In emergency cardiac situation, cooperation with neurosurgeon is mandatory. The best way to prevent these complications is to quickly start antibiotherapy (ESC, 2009).

For patients with previous antithrombotic treatment and in the absence of stroke, oral anticoagulant therapy should be replaced by unfractionned heparin for a period of 2 weeks, mainly in case of *S. aureus* IE (higher risk of bleeding). In case of an ischaemic stroke, the same schema of replacement is proposed. Anticoagulation has to be stopped in case of a haemorragic stroke and a mechanical valve; unfractionned heparin should be reinitiated as soon as possible. Previous antiplatelet therapy must be stopped only in the occurrence of major bleeding (ESC, 2009).

6.1.5 Metastatic infection

Infectious aneurysms (3% of IE) (AEPEI, 2002) are secondary to arterial septic embolism, mainly in the brain. Most of them are silent but rupture is associated with poor prognosis. No predicting factor has been individualized, however treatment (neurosurgery or endovascular surgery) is proposed in case of large, enlarging or already ruptured aneurysms. After specific antibiotherapy, most of unruptured infectious aneurysms resolve.

Systemic abscesses (other than cerebral) are rare and should be suspected in case of persistent fever and bacteremia. Clinical criteria and imaging investigation help to find the site of the infection s (tomography, ultrasound etc). Treatment can be completed by surgery or percutaneous drainage in case of partial response to antibiotics. All organs can be affected: spleen, bone (spondylodiscitis 3-15%) etc (ESC, 2009).

6.1.6 Renal complications

Acute renal failure is frequent (30%) but often reversible. Causes are multiple: glomerulonephritis by immune complex deposition, renal infarction, haemodynamic impairment and antibiotic or contrast agent toxicity (ESC, 2009).

6.1.7 Recurrences: Relapses and re-infections

Relapse is mainly observed after inadequate antibiotic treatment (insufficient duration, resistant microorganisms, empirical antibiotherapy in IE with negative blood culture) or persistent focus of infection. Conversely, re-infection is a new IE with different microorganism(s) and mainly includes patients with previous IE, intravenous drug abusers, prosthetic valve carriers and chronic dialysis patients. Re-infection increases risk of death and of valve surgery (ESC, 2009).

6.2 Mortality

In-hospital mortality varies from 9.6 to 26%. Prognosis is influenced by many factors (Table 6) but the mortality is higher (79%) in presence of heart failure associated with periannular complications and Staphylococcus infection (Chu, 2004; ESC, 2009). Operative mortality is also significant (16%) mainly in patients with prosthetic valves (Fayad, 2011).

Predictors of a poor prognostic			
Patient characteristics	Presence of complications	Microorganisms	Echocardiographic findings
- Older age - Prosthetic valve IE - Previous IE (= reinfection) - Insulin-dependent diabetes mellitus - Comorbidities	- Heart failure - Renal failure - Stroke - Septic chock - Periannular complications	- *S. aureus* - Fungi - Gram-negative bacilli	- Periannular complications - Severe left-side valve regurgitation - Low left-ventricular ejection fraction - Large vegetation - Severe prosthetic dysfunction - Premature mitral valve closure and other signs of elevated diastolic pressure

Table 6. Predictors factor of a poor prognosis in IE (ESC, 2009)

7. Treatment: Prolonged antimicrobial therapy and infectious source eradication

7.1 Medical treatment

Medical treatment should be started quickly after carrying out of bacteriological samples, in particular blood cultures (3 independent sets at 30 minutes intervals). Antimicrobial therapy is first empirical (Table 7) and as soon as possible, it is adapted to micro-organism sensitivity (ESC, 2009). In all the cases, this treatment should be prolongated for several weeks and toxicity should be followed-up. As soon as possible, portal of entry and complications should be found and treated. Symptomatic care is usual and classical.

7.2 Surgical treatment

Cardiac surgery is often necessary to treat or prevent complications or eradicate infectious sites (Table 8). Surgery is more frequently necessary in some types of IE such as native valve IE (87% of IE operated with 57% in aortic IE and 50% for mitral IE), Staphylococci and Streptococci IE (respectively 35 and 33% of IE operated) (Fayad, 2011).

With the exception of an emergency, extracardiac infections must be eradicated before surgery. Coronary angiography is also recommended in patients at risk (men older than 40, post-menopausal women, patients with at least one cardiovascular risk factor or a history of coronary disease) excluding emergency or cases with large aortic vegetation (risk of dislodgment during examination). Repair and replacement of the valve are possible but the last technique is preferred in complex cases. Intra operative transoesophageal echocardiography is precious to guide surgeons. The operative mortality is moderate (16%) and is more frequent with prosthetic valve carriers (ESC, 2009).

Characteristics of patient		Antibiotherapy suggested for adults patients		
		Association of antibiotics	Dosage	Duration (weeks)
• Native valve or • Prosthetic valve since more than 12 months		Ampicillin-sulbactam IV	12g/day (in 4 doses)	4-6
		Gentamicin IV or IM	3mg/kg/day (in 2 or 3 doses)	4-6
	Allergy to β-lactams	Vancomycin IV	30mg/kg/day (in 2 doses)	4-6
		Gentamicin IV or IM	3mg/kg/day (in 2 or 3 doses)	4-6
		Ciprofloxacin	1000 mg/day (in 2 doses) po or 800mg/day (in 2 doses) IV	4-6
Prosthetic valve since less than 12 months		Vancomycin IV	30mg/kg/day (in 2 doses)	6
		Gentamicin IV or IM	3mg/kg/day (in 2 or 3 doses)	2
		Rifampicin po	1200mg/day (in 2 doses)	2

Table 7. Proposed antibiotic regimens for initial empirical treatment (po: *per os*/ IM: intramuscular/ IV intravenous). Be careful with chronic use of gentamicin and vancomycin. Serum levels of these antibiotics should be measured once a week for both and additional renal function testing should be performed for gentamicin.

7.3 Follow-up

Complications are usual and should be searched for regularly. This requires a daily clinical examination during the first weeks. Electrocardiogram should be performed frequently (mainly in aortic or prosthesis IE) looking for new atrioventricular block or ischemia signs. Bacteriological samples should be analyzed until their negativity. Heart failure and death can occur after several months, so echocardiography is recommended in case of cardiological signs but also after antibiotic treatment and should be repeated regularly during the first year (at 1, 3, 6 and 12 months) (ESC, 2009).

Recurrence is frequent. Consequently, patients should be informed about this risk and prevention rules should be applied closely.

8. Prevention

8.1 Antibiotic prophylaxis

In recent years, antibiotic prophylaxis has become more and more limited. In fact, no antibiotic permit disappearance of bacteremia after at-risk at-risk procedures. Until now, no study has proven the benefit of prophylactic treatment in the prevention of IE. At present, only antibiotic prophylaxis is recommended by ESC (ESC, 2009) for highest risk dental procedures in patients with highest risk cardiac conditions (Table 9). AHA (AHA, 2007) also recommends antibiotic prophylaxis for procedures on the respiratory tract or on infected skin in patients with highest risk of IE. Prophylaxis is associated with a small risk of death by anaphylaxis but no case has been reported to date and the main risk is microbial resistance development.

Indications	Location of IE		
	Left-sided native valve IE	Prosthetic valve IE (PVE)	Right-sided IE
Heart complications — Heart failure — **+**	Severe acute regurgitation or valve obstruction causing refractory oedema pulmonary or cardiogenic shock	Severe prosthetic dysfunction (dehiscence or obstruction)	Right heart failure secondary to severe tricuspid regurgitation with poor response to diuretic therapy
	Emergency	*Emergency*	
	Fistula into a cardiac chamber or pericardium causing refractory pulmonary oedema or shock		
	Emergency		
	Severe acute regurgitation or valve obstruction and persisting heart failure or echocardiographic signs of poor haemodynamic tolerance (early mitral closure or pulmonary hypertension)	Severe prosthetic dysfunction and persisting heart failure	
	Urgent	*Urgent*	
−	Severe regurgitation and no heart failure	Severe prosthetic dehiscence without heart cardiac	
	Elective	*Elective*	
Uncontrolled infection	Locally uncontrolled infection (abscess, false aneurysm, fistula, enlarging vegetation)		Microorganisms difficult to eradicate (persistent fungi…) or bacteremia for > 7 days (*S. aureus, P. aeruginosa…*)
	Urgent		
	Persisting fever and positive blood cultures > 7-10 days		
	Urgent		
	Fungi or multiresistant organisms		
	Urgent / Elective		
		Staphylococci or Gram negative bacteria (most of cases of early PVE)	
		Urgent/Elective	
Prevention of embolism	Large vegetation (>10mm) following one or more embolic episodes despite appropriate antibiotic therapy	Recurrent emboli despite appropriate antibiotic treatment	Persistent tricuspid valve vegetation > 20mm after recurrent pulmonary emboli with or without concomitant heart failure
	Urgent	*Urgent*	
	Large vegetation (>10mm) and other predictors of complicated course (heart failure, persistent infection, abscess)		
	Urgent		
	Isolated very large vegetation (>15mm)		
	Urgent		

Table 8. Indications and timing of surgery (ESC, 2009). Emergency: within 24 hours. Urgent: within a few days. Elective: after 1-2 weeks of antibiotic treatment.

Cardiac conditions at highest risk of IE	Dental procedures at high risk	

• Prosthetic cardiac valve or material used for cardiac valve repair
• Previous IE
• Some congenital heart disease (CHD)
  • Cyanotic CHD
- without surgical repair or
- with residual defects, palliative shunts or conduits
  • CHD with complete repair with prosthetic material whether placed by surgery or by cutaneous technique, up to 6 months after the procedure
  • CHD when a residual defect persists at the site of implantation of a prosthetic material or device by cardiac surgery or percutaneous technique
	• Manipulation of gingival region
	• Manipulation of periapical region of the teeth
	• Perforation of oral mucosa	

	Antibiotic prophylaxis	
	Single dose 30-60 minutes before procedure	

	• Adults
	  • Amoxicill in 2g po or IV
	  • If allergy: Clindamy cin 600mg po or IV
		• Children
		  • Amoxicilli n 50mg/kg po or IV
		  • If allergy: Clindamy cin 20mg/kg po or IV

Table 9. Recommendations for antibiotic prophylaxis of IE for patients undergoing dental procedures (ESC, 2009) (po: *per os*/ IV: intravenous)

8.2 Hygienic rules

Most IE occurs without history of procedure more at-risk situation of bacteremia (Strom, 1998).

Daily activities like chewing or tooth brushing carry transient but significant bacteremia and can cause IE (AHA, 2007). Consequently, it is recommended to maintain a good oral hygiene for all population.

For patients and drug users, disposable intravenous material is mandatory.

8.3 Others rules

In medical practice, percutaneous iatrogenic procedures should be avoided especially on skin injuries and topical corticosteroid should be used with caution. Regular bacteriological skin analysis is recommended during the follow-up of erosive dermatosis because it allows quick adapted antibiotherapy in the case of secondarily advent IE. Of course, all prospective portals of entry and all comorbidities have to be searched and supported.

9. Conclusion

Infective endocarditis (IE) is a severe disease the diagnosis of which remains difficult due to clinical polymorphism and frequent insidious evolution over several days or months. Skin manifestations are very useful for diagnosis but should alert practitioners for presence of embolic complications. Epidemiologic profile of IE has changed in recent years and so has prophylactic and therapeutic recommendations. IE concerns all practitioners and we have to keep it in mind with any patient.

10. Acknowledgment

Thank you to Pr Olivier Chosidow (Department of dermatology, Hôpital Henri Mondor, Créteil; France) and Dr Nicolas Ortonne (Department of pathology, Hôpital Henri Mondor, Créteil; France) for histological pictures.

11. References

Cardullo, AC.; Silvers, DN. & Grossman, ME. (1990). Janeway lesions and Osler's nodes: a review of histopathologic findings. *J Am Acad Dermatol,* Vol.22, No.6, (June 1990), pp. 1088-90, ISSN 2370335

Chu, VH. et al (2004). Early predictors of in-hospital death in infective endocarditis. *Circulation,* Vol.109, No.14, (March 2004), pp. 1745-9, ISSN 1503 7538

Durante Mangoni, E. et al (2003). Risk factors for "major" embolic events in hospitalized patients with infective endocarditis. *Am Heart J,* Vol.146, No.2, (August 2003), pp. 311-6, ISSN 1289 1201

Espinosa Parra, FJ. et al (2002). Diagnostic utility of Osler's nodules in infectious endocarditis among parenteral drug users. *An Med Interna,* Vol. 19, No.6, (June 2002), pp. 299-301, ISSN 1215 2389

Evangelista, A. & Gonzalez-Alujas, MT. (2004). Echocardiography in infective endocarditis. *Heart,* Vol.90, No.6, (June 2004), pp. 614-7, ISSN 1514 5856

Farrior, JB. & Silverman, ME. (1976). A consideration of the differences between a Janeway's lesion and an Osler's node in infectious endocarditis. *Chest,* Vol.70, No.2, (August 1976), pp. 239-43, ISSN 947688

Fayad, G. et al (2011). Characteristics and prognosis of patients requiring valve surgery during active infective endocarditis. *J Heart Valve Dis,* Vol.20, No.2 (March 2011), pp. 223-8, ISSN 2156 0826

Feuchtner, GM. et al (2009). Multislice computed tomography in infective endocarditis: comparison with transesophageal echocardiography and intraoperative findings. *J Am Coll Cardiol,* Vol.53, No.5, (February 2009), pp. 436-44, ISSN 1917 9202

García-Porrúa, C. & González-Gay, MA. (1999). Bacterial infection presenting as cutaneous vasculitis in adults. *Clin Exp Rheumatol,* Vol.17, No.4, (July 1999), pp. 471-3, ISSN 1046 4561

Greub, G. et al (2005). Diagnosis of infectious endocarditis in patients undergoing valve surgery. *Am J Med,* Vol.118,No.3, (March 2005), pp. 230-8, ISSN 1574 5720

Habib, G. et al; ESC Committee for Practice Guidelines (2009). Guidelines on the prevention, diagnosis, and treatment of infective endocarditis (new version 2009): the Task Force on the Prevention, Diagnosis, and Treatment of Infective Endocarditis of the European Society of Cardiology (ESC). Endorsed by the European Society of Clinical Microbiology and Infectious Diseases (ESCMID) and the International Society of Chemotherapy (ISC) for Infection and Cancer. *Eur Heart J ,* Vol.30, No.19, (October 2009), pp. 2369-413, ISSN 1971 3420

Heffner, JE. (1979). Extracardiac manifestations of bacterial endocarditis. *West J Med*, Vol.131, No.2, (August 1979), pp. 85-91, ISSN 516715

Hoen, B. et al; Association pour l'Etude et la Prévention de l'Endocardite Infectieuse (AEPEI) Study Group (2002).Changing profile of infective endocarditis: results of a 1-year survey in France. *JAMA*, Vol.288, No.1, (July 2002), pp. 75-81, ISSN 1209 0865

Kerr, A Jr. & Tan, JS. (1979). Biopsies of the Janeway lesion of infective endocarditis. J Cutan Pathol, Vol.6, No.2, (April 1979), pp. 124-9, ISSN 479431

Konstantinou, MP. et al (2009). Infective endocarditis in dermatological unit. Ann Dermatol Venereol, Vol.136, No.12, (December 2009), pp. 869-75, ISSN 2000 4311

Lévesque, H. & Marie, I. (1999). Infection and vascular purpura. *J Mal Vasc*, Vol.24, No.3, (June 1999), pp. 177-82, ISSN 1046 7526

Li, JS. et al (2000). Proposed modifications to the Duke criteria for the diagnosis of infective endocarditis. *Clin Infect Dis*, Vol.30, No.4, (April 2000), pp. 633-8, ISSN 1077 0721

Loewe, R.; Gattringer, KB. & Petzelbauer, P. (2009). Janeway lesions with inconspicuous histological features. *J Cutan Pathol*, Vol.36, No.10, (October 2009), pp. 1095-8, ISSN 1918 7106

Martínez-Marcos, FJ. et al; Grupo para el Estudio de las Infecciones Cardiovasculares de la Sociedad Andaluza de Enfermedades Infecciosas (2009). Enterococcal endocarditis: a multicenter study of 76 cases. *Enferm Infecc Microbiol Clin*, Vol.27, No.10, (December 2009), pp. 571-9, ISSN 1947 7041

Miro, JM. et al; International Collaboration on Endocarditis Merged Database Study Group (2005). Staphylococcus aureus native valve infective endocarditis: report of 566 episodes from the International Collaboration on Endocarditis Merged Database. *Clin Infect Dis*, Vol.41, No.4, (August 2005), pp. 507-14, ISSN 1602 8160

Moreillon, P. & Que, YA. (2004) Infective endocarditis. *Lancet*, Vol.363, No.9403, (January 2004), pp. 139-49, ISSN 1472 6169

Murdoch, DR. et al; International Collaboration on Endocarditis-Prospective Cohort Study (ICE-PCS) Investigators(2009). Clinical presentation, etiology, and outcome of infective endocarditis in the 21st century: the International Collaboration on Endocarditis-Prospective Cohort Study. *Arch Intern Med, Vol. 169, No.5, (March 2009)*, pp. 463-73, ISSN 1927 3776

Phillips, KT. & Stein, MD. (2010). Risk practices associated with bacterial infections among injection drug users in Denver, Colorado. *Am J Drug Alcohol Abuse*, Vol.36, No.2, (March 2010), pp. 92-7, ISSN2033 7504

Que, YA. & Moreillon, P. (2011). *Infective endocarditis. Nat Rev Cardiol*, Vol.8, No.6, (June 2011), pp. 322-36, ISSN 2148 7430

Rasmussen, RV. et al (2011). Prevalence of infective endocarditis in patients with Staphylococcus aureus bacteraemia: the value of screening with echocardiography. *Eur J Echocardiogr*, Vol.12, No.6, (June 2011), pp. 414-20, ISSN 2168 5200

Strom, BL. et al (1998). Dental and cardiac risk factors for infective endocarditis. A population-based, case-control study. *Ann Intern Med*, Vol.129, No.10, (November 1998),pp. 761-9, ISSN9841581

Strom, BL. et al (2000). Risk factors for infective endocarditis: oral hygiene and nondental exposures. *Circulation*, Vol.102, No.23, (December 2000), pp. 2842-8, ISSN 1110 4742

Thuny, F.et al. (2005). Risk of embolism and death in infective endocarditis: prognostic value of echocardiography: a prospective multicenter study. *Circulation*, Vol.112, No.1, (July 2005), pp. 69-75, ISSN .1598 3252

Thuny, F.et al. (2007). Impact of cerebrovascular complications on mortality and neurologic outcome during infective endocarditis: a prospective multicentre study. *Eur Heart J*, Vol.28, No.9, (May 2007), pp. 1155-61. ISSN 1736 3448

Tornos, P. et al (2005). Infective endocarditis in Europe: lessons from the Euro heart survey. *Heart*, Vol.91, No.5, (May 2005), pp. 571-5, ISSN 1583 1635

Wilson, W. et al; American Heart Association Rheumatic Fever, Endocarditis and Kawasaki Disease Committee, Council on Cardiovascular Disease in the Young; Council on Clinical Cardiology; Council on Cardiovascular Surgery and Anesthesia; Quality of Care and Outcomes Research Interdisciplinary Working Group; American Dental Association (2007). Prevention of infective endocarditis: guidelines from the American Heart Association: a guideline from the American Heart Association Rheumatic Fever, Endocarditis and Kawasaki Disease Committee, Council on Cardiovascular Disease in the Young, and the Council on Clinical Cardiology, Council on Cardiovascular Surgery and Anesthesia, and the Quality of Care and Outcomes Research Interdisciplinary Working Group. *J Am Dent Assoc*, Vol.138, No.6, (June 2007), pp. 739-45 and 747-60, ISSN 1754 5263

6

Cardiovascular Risk Factors: Implications in Diabetes, Other Disease States and Herbal Drugs

Steve Ogbonnia
Department of Pharmacognosy,
University of Lagos, Lagos,
Nigeria

1. Introduction

The danger and the increasing prevalence of heart diseases world wide are now of a great concern and are attributed to the cardiovascular risk factors. Cardiovascular risk factors have been identified to be the underlying latent or potent causes of death in all heart diseases and also in many other disease states such as diabetes. Reduction in the risk factors with synthetic drugs or drugs of natural products origin in the course of treatment of some disease states where implicated has been found to improve tremendously the health of the patient.

Cardiovascular risk factors include triacylglycerols (triglycerides), cholesterol, cholesteryl esters, very low density lipoprotein–cholesterol (VLDL-c), low density lipoprotein-cholesterol (LDL-c), and anti-athrogenic high density lipoprotein–cholesterol (HDL-c) and are collectively referred to as plasma lipids. An increase in plasma lipids concentrations beyond certain level give rise to physiological condition known as "Hyperlipidemia". Hyperlipidemia is, therefore, characterized by abnormal elevation in plasma triglyceride, cholesterol and low density lipoprotein-cholesterol (LDL-c) and very low lipoprotein - cholesterol (VLDL-c) and has also been reported to be the most prevalent indicator for susceptibility to atherosclerotic heart disease (Maruthapan and Shree, 2010). Managing cardiovascular disease states, therefore, requires drugs that would be capable of lowering blood plasma lipids in order to reduce mortality and morbidity associated with the cardiovascular complications (Hasimun et al., 2011). It has been reported in epidemiological studies that a strong positive correlation exists between increase in the blood cholesterol level and incidence of cardiovascular heart disease (CHD) (Hamed et al., 2010; Imafidon 2010; Maruthapana and Shree 2010), and also increase in the incidence of atherosclerosis(Hasimun et al., 2011). A strong relationship between increase in C-reactive protein (CRP) and cardiovascular risk factors has also been reported as well as increase in myocardial infection and coronary artery disease among individuals with angina pectoris (Ghayour –Mobarhan et al. 2007).

Atherosclerosis arises from the deposition of fatty substances, cellular waste products, calcium and fibrin in the arteries, resulting in clotting (Lewis et al., 2002) and is considered one of the major causes of coronary heart disease. It is recognized as a common threat to life, usually seen in individuals consuming high quantities of cholesterol and saturated fats in their diets. It has also been established in animal studies that raising dietary cholesterol alone could increase atherosclerosis susceptibility (Madhumathi et al., 2006). Atherosclerosis is characterized by endothelia dysfunction, muscular inflammation resulting from build up of plasma lipids which tantamount to vascular remodeling, acute and chronic luminal obstruction, abnormalities in the blood flow and diminished oxygen supplies to target organs (Madhumathi et al., 2006). The development of atherosclerosis could also be attributed to other factors such as oxidative stress which is responsible for the oxidation of low-density lipoprotein-cholesterol (LDL-c) and is considered as one of the first steps of atherosclerotic pathogenesis. Local inflammatory processes have also been identified to play a crucial role in the transition from reversible accumulation of cholesterol in the arterial wall to irreversible damage of the arteries (Brunner-La Rocca1, et al., 2005). Many factors contributing to etiology of atherosclerosis in addition to diet include diabetes mellitus, psychological factors and the presence of glucocorticoids.

Diabetes mellitus (DM) is a major degenerative disease in the world today afflicting many lives both in the developed and developing countries (Ogbonnia et al., 2011). It has been succinctly described as the common metabolic disorder of carbohydrate and fat metabolism, which is due to absolute or relative lack of insulin and is characterized by hyperglycaemia and hyperlipidemia (Sharon and Marvin, 1975; Walter, 1977). Diabetes is a multiple disease state and has been defined as "a state of premature cardiovascular death that is associated with chronic hyperglycemia and also associated with blindness and renal failure" (Fisher and Shaw, 2001). This assertion was to draw attention and to encourage multiple clinical approaches that would altogether help reduce cardiovascular risk factors in diabetic patients (Ogbonnia et al., 2011). Diabetes especially the type 2 model might be postulated to occur primarily due to underlying abnormality of insulin resistance - that is resistance of the body to the biological actions of insulin. The consequences of insulin resistance lead to hyperinsulinaemia and are associated with CRFs - dyslipidaemia including athrogenic lipid profile with increase in low and very-low density lipoprotein-cholesterols (LDL-c and VLDL-c) and reduction in the anti-athrogenic high density lipoprotein-cholesterol (HDL-c). Cardiovascular risk factors have been implicated and even occur at a frequency much higher than expected in some other disease states such as benign prostatic hyperplasia (BPH). Benign prostatic hyperplasia is a neoplastic enlargement of the prostate gland and is common in elderly men (Ejike and Ezeanyika, 2010). Epidemiological studies have demonstrated that many of the risk factors associated with cardiovascular diseases are the same as found in BPH (Dharmananda, 2011), and these risk factors include obesity, hypertension and diabetes. The diabetes connection may be considered very strong and the risk centers on the non-insulin dependent diabetes mellitus (NIDDM) which most often involves excessive insulin levels, a possible direct contributor to the growth of the prostrate (Hammarten and Hogstedt, 2011). The treatment of BPH became a medical issue mainly in 1970s at the same time that the cardiovascular disease therapy came to fore and the incidence of the disease has become higher (Dharmananda, 2011). Herbal or phytomedicines are now being investigated with some recorded successes for the management of cardiovascular risk factors with the accompanied disease states. Herbal remedies with active components understood to be sterols, such as beta-sitosterol has been used as a therapeutic agent for BPH (Bombardelli and Morazzoni, 1997).

2. Cardiovascular risk factors

Cardiovascular risk factors consisting mostly of plasma lipids including triacylglycerol (triglycerides), cholesteryl esters and cholesterol are synthesized by the liver and adipose tissues and may also be absorbed from the diet (Stryer, 1988). They are also efficiently synthesized from carbohydrate diets largely in the intestinal epithelia tissues in addition to the liver (Metzler, 1974), and are transported between various tissues and organs for utilization and storage. These plasma lipids like other lipids are generally insoluble in water and pose a transportation problem in aqueous blood plasma. This problem is overcome by associating the nonpolar lipids comprising triacylglycerol (triglycerides) and cholesteryl esters with amphipatic lipids such as phospholipids, cholesterol and proteins to produce water-miscible lipoproteins (Conn and Stumpf, 1976; Stryer, 1988). A lipoprotein is a particle consisting of core hydrophobic lipids surrounded by a shell of polar lipid and apoprotein and mediates the cycle by transporting lipids from the intestine as chylomicrons – and from the liver as very low density lipoproteins-cholesterol (VLDL-c) - to most tissues for oxidation and to adipose tissue for storage. Lipoproteins are grouped according to increasing densities by centrifugation as follow:

i.   Chylomicrons which incorporate intestinal absorbed triacylglycerol from intestinal absorption of triacylglycerol and other lipids.

ii. Very low density lipoprotein-cholesterol (VLDL-c, or pre – β- Lipoprotein), are derived from the combination of newly synthesized triacylglycerol together with small amounts of phospholipids and cholesterol and apolipoproteins all synthesized in the liver (Stryer, 1988).

iii. Intermediate density lipoprotein (IDL)

iv. Low density lipoprotein-cholesterol (LDL-c) (LDL-c or β-Lipoproteins), representing a final stage in the catabolism of VLDL-c, and

High density lipoproteins-cholesterol (HDL-c, or α-Lipoproteins), involved in cholesterol transport and also in VLDL-c and chylomicron metabolism.

Major groups of lipoproteins have been identified to be physiologically important and are used in clinical diagnosis. The primary role of LDL-c appears to be the transport of esterified cholesterol to tissue while that of the high density lipoproteins-cholesterol (HDL-c) is to carry excess cholesterol away from most tissues to the liver. The size of the lipoprotein particles also varies from a 200 – to 500 –nm diameter for chylomicrons to as little as 5 nm for the smallest HDL particles (Metzler, 1974).

Lipoprotein is made up of triacylglycerol (16%) which is the predominant lipid in chylomicrons and VLDL-c, while phosholipids (30%) and cholesterol (14%) are the predominant lipids of HDL-c and LDL-c respectively and cholesterol esters (36%) (Stryer, 1988). It also contains much smaller fraction of unesterified long chain fatty acids (free fatty acids) which are metabolically the most active of plasma lipids. These constitute what is collectively known as 'Cardiovascular Risk Factors' which are implicated in many disease states as potent or latent causes of death. Lipoproteins may be separated according to their electrophoretic properties into: α-, β-, and pre -β- Lipoproteins (Holme and Peck, 1998).

The protein moiety of a lipoprotein is known as apolipoprotein or apoprotein constituting nearly 70% of HDL-c and as little as 1% of chylomicrons. Some apolipoproteins are integral and can not be removed, whereas others are free to transfer to other lipoprotiens. Seven principal apoprotein, A – 1, A – 2, A – 4, B – 48, B – 100, C and E have been isolated and characterized. They are synthesized and secreted by the liver and the intestine and generally have two principal roles: they solubilize highly hydrophobic lipid and also they contain signals that regulate the movement of particular lipid into and out of specific target cells and tissues.

Lipoprotein	Source/major core lipid	Diameter (nm)	Density (g/mL)	Composition	Main Lipid Components		Mechanism of lipid delivery
				Protein (%)	Lipid (%)	< 0.95	
Chylomicrons	Dietary triacylglycerol Intestine	90-1000	< 0.95	1-2	98-99	< 1.006	Hydrolysis by lipoprotein lipase
Chylomicrons remnants	Dietary cholesterol esters Chylomicrons	45-150	< 1.006	6-8	92-94	0.95-1.006	Receptor-mediated endocytosis by liver
VLDL	Endogenous triacylglycerols Liver (Intestine)	30-90	0.95-1.006	7-10	90-93	1.006-1.019	Hydrolysis by liproprotein lipase
IDL	Endogenous cholesterol esters VLDL	25-35	1.006-1.019	11	89	1.019-1.063	Receptor-mediated endocytosis by liver and conversion to LDL
LDL	Endogenous cholesterol esters VLDL	20-25	1.019-1.063	21	79		Receptor-mediated endocytosis by liver and other tissues
	Endogenous cholesterol esters						Transfer of cholesterol esters to IDL and LDL

Table 1. Composition of the Lipoproteins in plasma of humans.

Each apolipoproteins carry out one or more distinct roles.

i.   The apo B, stabilizes lipoproteins micelles and as the sole protein of LDL-c serves the function of solubilizing cholesterol within LDL-c complex which in turn increases the transport capacity of LDL-c for subsequent deposit on arterial wall (Madhumathi et al., 2006).

ii. They are enzyme cofactors. The apoC-II has specific function of activating the lipoprotein lipase that hydrolyses triacylglycerols of chylomicrons and VLDL. Lack of either C-II or the lipase results in a very high level of triacylglycerol in the blood.

iii. They act as ligands for interaction with lipoprotein receptors in tissues, e.g apoB-100 and apo E for the LDL receptors, apo E for the LDL receptor– related protein (LRP) which has been identified as the remnant receptor, and apo A-1 for the HDL-c receptor. The function of Apo A-IV and apo D, however, are not yet clearly defined, although apo D, is believed to be an important factor in human neurodegenerative disorders.

2.1 Cholesterol

Cholesterol is physiologically very essential for all animal life, and is primarily synthesized from simpler substances within the body. It is an amphipathic waxy steroid of fat that is manufactured in the liver or intestines. It constitutes essentially structural component of membrane required in establishing proper membrane permeability and fluidity and is also a constituent of the outer layer of plasma lipoproteins. Cholesterol is the principal sterol synthesized by animals and transported in the blood plasma of all mammals (Leah, 2009). It is also an important component implicated in the manufacture of bile acids, steroid hormones, and vitamin D (Jain, 2005; Maxifield and Tabas, 2005; Hasimun, 2011). The hydroxyl group on cholesterol interacts with the polar head groups of the membrane phospholipids and sphingolipids, while the bulky steroid and the hydrocarbon chain are embedded in the membrane, alongside the nonpolar fatty acid chain of the other lipids. In this structural form, cholesterol reduces the permeability of the plasma membrane to protons (positive hydrogen ions) and sodium ions.

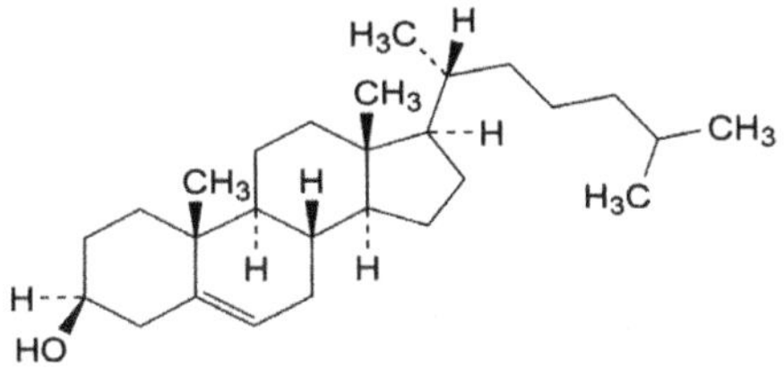

Fig. 1. Chemical structure of cholesterol

Most cholesterol is carried in the blood by low density lipoprotein (LDL), which delivers it directly to cells where it is needed. Both a 74-kDa cholesteryl ester transfer protein and a phospholipid transfer protein are also involved in this process. Cholesterol esterases, which release free cholesterol, may act both on lipoproteins and on pancreatic secretions. The LDL-cholesterol complex binds to LDL receptors on the cell surfaces. These receptors are specific for apolipoprotein B-100 present in the LDL. The occupied LDL-receptor complexes are taken up by endocytosis through coated pits; the apolipoproteins are degraded in lysosomes, while the cholesteryl esters are released and cleaved by a specific lysosomal acid lipase to form free cholesterol.

Animal fats are complex mixtures of triglycerides, with fewer amounts of phospholipids and cholesterol. As a consequence all food containing animal fats contain cholesterol to varying extent. Plasma cholesterol concentration elevation is, therefore ,one of the important CRFs as its transportation within lipoprotein is affected and is strongly associated with progression of atherosclerosis.

2.2 Triacylglycerols

Triacylglycerols (figure 2b see the figure below) serve as biochemical energy reserves in the cell and may be oxidized in the liver to provide energy or deposited as depot fat in characteristic regions of the animal where they act as a long-term food store and insulator (Plummer, 1998). They are the neutral and saponifiable lipids found in most organisms. Triacylglycerols (triglycerides) which are chemically fatty acid esters of the trihydroxy alcohol, glycerol (Figure 2a), are compounds that usually make up the bulk of ingested lipids and are transported to the blood via the lymphatic system in the form of chylomicrons. Triacylglycerols synthesized endogenously as against those obtained from the diet, are carried by VLDL produced primarily by the liver (Styer, 1988). Studies have suggested that triacylglycerol (TG)-rich lipoprotein(TRL) plays an important role in the development of atherosclerosis because both coronary artery   disease and myocardial infarction have been associated with abnormal postprandial lipoprotein pattern (Moreno-Luna et al., 2007)

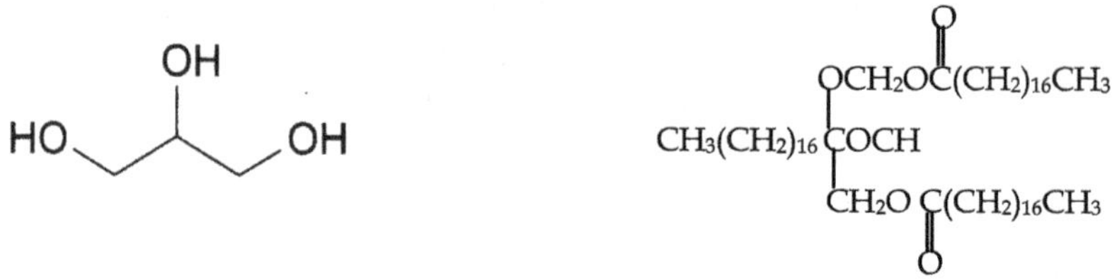

A triacylglycerol (Tristearin)

(a)   (b)

Fig. 2. (a) Chemical structure of cholesterol (b) chemical structure of triacylglycerol

Most of the fatty acids synthesized or ingested by an organism are either transformed into triacylgylcerols and stored for metabolism to give energy or incorporated into phospholipids components of the membrane. Triacylgylcerols have as precursor fatty acyl-CoAs and glycerol-β-phosphate but many enzymatic steps are involved in their biosynthesis in animal tissues. Although the triglycerides have been found to be important predictors of CVD in many studies, no clinical trial data has established that lowering triglycerides in individuals with or without diabetes independently leads to lowering of CVD occurring rates even after changes in HDL-cholesterol are adjusted for. From the foregoing, it is evident that elevated cholesterol, low HDL-c, high TG and high LDL-c are all risk factors for CVD. The pattern of occurrence of these abnormalities in type 2 DM especially has been severally reported in both developed and developing economies (Idogun et al., 2007; Williams et al., 2008).

2.3 Very Low Density Lipoprotein-cholesterol (VLDL-c or preβ- lipoproteins)

VLDL-c is synthesized in the liver and contains primarily triglycerides in their lipid cores for their export and also some cholesterol ester (Botham and Mayes, 2006). As their triglycerides are cleaved by endothelial lipoprotein lipase and transferred to hepatic tissues, the VLDL (very-low-density lipoprotein) particles lose most of their apolipoprotein C and become intermediate-density lipoproteins. VLDL is one of the five major groups of lipoproteins which functions to enable fats and cholesterol to move within the water-based solution of the bloodstream. VLDL-c particles have a diameter of 30-80 nm each and transports endogenous products such as triglycerides, phospholipids, cholesterol, and cholesteryl esters, whereas chylomicrons transport exogenous (dietary) products. It functions as the body's internal transport mechanism for lipids.

2.4 Low Density Lipoprotein-cholesterol (LDL-c)

The primary role of LDL-c appears to be the transport of esterified cholesterol to tissues (Guyton and Hall, 2006). Low density lipoprotein results when triacylglycerols are released from VLDL-c by the action of the same lipase that acts on chylomicrons and the remnants which are rich in cholesterol esters are called intermediate density lipoprotein (IDL). IDL particles have two fates as half of them are taken up by the liver and the other half converted into LDL which is the major carrier of cholesterol in blood (Styer, 1988). LDL-c or β- lipoprotein represent the final stage in the metabolism of VLDL. Originally, LDL-cholesterol was determined by a lengthy, laborious process called ultracentrifugation of serum. A much more rapid test became available based on the following Friedwald equation: Total cholesterol = LDL-cholesterol + HDL-cholesterol + VLDL-cholesterol (VLDL-cholesterol = triglycerides/5). One can rapidly and easily do a lipid profile by enzymatically measuring the important lipids—total cholesterol, HDL- cholesterol, and triglycerides. Dividing triglycerides by five gives the relatively unimportant, but hard to measure, VLDL-cholesterol, which is useful in then calculating the very important LDL cholesterol (Holme and Peck, 1998).

2.5 High Density Lipoprotein-cholesterol (HDL-c or 〈-lipoprotein)

HDL-c is involved in the cholesterol transport and in VLDL and chylomicron metabolism. Unlike LDL which primary role appears to be the carriage of esterified cholesterol to the tissues, HDL functions to carry excess cholesterol away from most tissues to the liver. The apoA-I present in the HDL-c particle binds lipid and also activates lecithin cholesterol acyltransferase (LCAT), which catalyzes formation of cholesteryl esters which migrate into the interior of the HDL-c and are carried to the liver (Metzler, 1974). Recent studies on patients with LCAT deficiency have shown a modest but significant increase in incidence of cardiovascular disease consistent with a beneficial effect of LCAT on atherosclerosis (Rousset et al., 2009) HDL particles compared to other lipoproteins, are assembled outside of cells from lipids and proteins, some of which may be donated from chylomicrons or other lipoprotein particles. HDL has higher protein content than other lipoproteins and is more heterogeneous. The major HDL protein is apolipoprotein A-I, but many HDL particles also contain A-II, and apolipoproteins A-IV, D, and E may also be present. A low plasma level of HDL-cholesterol is associated with a high risk of atherosclerosis.

3. Implicated disease states

3.1 Diabetes

Diabetes mellitus is a major global health problem and is now recognized as one of the leading causes of death in the developing countries, where the high prevalence of the disease could be attributed to improved nutritional status coupled with a gross lack of modern facilities for the early diagnosis of the disease (Uebanso et al., 2007; Ogbonnia et al., 2008[a]). Diabetes mellitus (DM) is a complex disease characterized by abnormal pattern of fuel usage resulting from over production of glucose and its under utilization by other organs (Stryer, 1988). Diabetes has been succinctly described as the common metabolic disorder of carbohydrate and fat metabolism, which is due to absolute or relative lack of insulin and is characterized by hyperglycaemia (Walter, 1977; Shah et al., 2008 and Sharma et al., 2010; Dinesh et al., 2011).

Diabetes mellitus is therefore a multifactorial disease associated with hyperglycemia, (Shah et al., 2008; Sharma et al., 2010); lipoprotein abnormalities, raised basal metabolic rate and high oxidative stress inducing damage to beta cells. The abnormalities in carbohydrates and lipid metabolism in diabetes also result in excessive production of reactive oxygen species (ROS) and defect in ROS scavenging enzymes in addition to oxidative stress. The low level of insulin associated with diabetes has been found to increase the activity of anti-enzyme, fatty acyl Coenzyme A oxidase, which initiates the β-oxidation of the fatty acids, resulting in lipid peroxidation (Shah et al., 2008). Increased lipid peroxidation has also been found to impair membrane function by decreasing membrane fluidity and changing the activity of the membrane-bound enzyme and receptors. The resulting lipid radicals and lipid peroxides are harmful to the cell in the body and are associated with atherosclerosis and brain damage.

Chronic hyperglycemia which occurs in diabetes causes glycation of body proteins which in turn leads to secondary complications affecting eyes, kidneys, nerves and arteries (Mishra and Garg, 2011). These may be delayed, lessened or prevented by maintaining blood glucose values close to normal in modern medicine, though no satisfactory effective therapy is available for total cure of diabetes mellitus.

Diabetes mellitus is also associated with hyperlipidaemia with profound alteration in the concentrations and compositions of plasma lipid. Changes in the concentration of the lipids in diabetes contribute to the development of vascular disease. Excessive levels of blood cholesterol accelerate atherogenesis and lowering high blood cholesterol reduces the incidence of CHD (Grundy, 1986). One of the risk factors for coronary heart disease is elevated total cholesterol (TC), low density lipoprotein-cholesterol (LDL-c) and lowered high density lipoprotein-cholesterol (HDL-c). The development of cardiovascular disease in DM is often predicted by several factors which include central obesity, hypertriglyceridemia and hypertension. Hypertriacylglyceridemia and low high-density liopoproteinaemia are two components of the atherogenic profile seen in DM. Elevated low density lipoprotein-cholesterol (LDL-c) has also been found to be an independent risk factor for the development of cardiovascular disease and is often reported to be the commonest lipid abnormality found in patients with DM (Udawat and Goyal, 2001; Idogun et al., 2007).

3.2 Atherosclerosis

Atherosclerosis or arteriosclerosis is a disease of large and medium size muscular arteries and is characterized by endothelial dysfunction vascular inflammation and build up of lipids, cholesterol, calcium and cellular debris within intima of vessel wall. This build up results in plaque formation, vascular remodeling, acute and chronic luminal obstruction, abnormalities in the blood flow and diminished oxygen supply to the target organ. (Madhumathi et al., 2006). Atherosclerotic disease has been found to be the most common cause of myocardial ischemia. Myocardium is said to be ischaemic when the pumping capability of the heart is impaired as a result of fall in the coronary blood flow which could not meet up with the metabolic need of the heart. In artherosclerotic disease, there is a localised lipid deposits called plaques develop within the arterial walls. In the severe cases of the disease these plaques become calcified and are so large that they physically narrow the lumen of the arteries producing stenosis (Mohrman and Heller, 2006). umerous studies have revealed important risk factors for the development of arthrosclerosis and these include diseases such as diabetes mellitus, arterial hypertension, and also smoking and elevated blood cholesterol

Current concepts in atherosclerosis suggest that oxidation of LDL-c is involved in its pathogenesis. The critical role of oxidized LDL-c in atherogenesis may be due to its rapid uptake by the foam cells lining the arterial intima, which are thought to have macrophage-like properties. When LDL-c is oxidized chemotactic effect is exerted on monocytes and this increase the uptake of LDL-c leading to the formation of arterial plaque. Lipid oxidation can be inhibited by the use of antioxidants such as vit E which inhibit the formation of lesions in hypercholesterolemic rabbits (Chein and Frishman, 2003).

Hypercholesterolemia has also been implicated in the process of atherogenesis and a curvilinear relationship has been documented between increasing cholesterol and increasing incidence of CVD (Brunzell et al., 2008). The role of LDL-c in the development of CVD cannot be overemphasized as there is documented evidence that high levels of LDL-c not only cause atherosclerosis but pharmacological interventions that reduce LDL-c are associated with stabilization and regression of atherosclerosis in proportion to the cholesterol lowering achieved (O'Keefe et al., 2004). Low levels of HDL-c have been consistently reported in cardiovascular diseases (Idogun et al., 2007; Sani-Bello et al., 2007, Singh et al., 2007). Primary treatment of coronary artery disease (and atherosclerosis in general) should include attempts to lower blood lipid by dietary and pharmacological techniques to prevent and possibly reverse further deposit of plaques.

3.3 Benign Prostatic Hyperplasia (BPH)

Benign Prostatic Hyperplasia (BPH) is a neoplastic enlargement of the prostate gland, and is a common problem among aging men (Ejike and Ezeanyika, 2010; Dharmananda, 2011). The etiology of this disease is still poorly understood, but it has been proposed to have two phases:

One of the phases involves no clinical sign but there maybe some microscopic changes while the other manifests as the disorder of urination caused by the obstruction of the urinary tract by an enlarged prostate gland (Dharmananda, 2011).

Epidemiological studies have demonstrated that many of the risk factors associated with cardiovascular diseases apply also as risk factors for BPH. The problems associated with diabetic may be considered very strong as the risk in non-insulin dependent diabetes (NIDDM); which most often connected with insulin resistance may be a possible direct contributor to the growth of BPH (Dharmananda, 2011). NIDDM which arises from either impairment of insulin utilization or dysfunction on the metabolism of carbohydrates, fats and protein or both culminates in hyperlipidemia- hence elevation in plasma cardiovascular risk factor. BPH is therefore associated with metabolic syndrome (Kasturi et al., 2006; Ozden, 2007).

4. Herbal drugs used to control CRF in the disease states

Herbal medicines may be described as medicines prepared either with a single plant part or combinations of different plant parts either fresh,dried or as extract are now recognized as potent therapeutic agents. Plants derived medicines commonly referred to as "phytomedicines" have been effectively employed in the management of variety of pathological conditions and are associated with fewer side effects (Nirmala et al., 2011; Ogbonnia et al, 2011). In recent years, they have been found to be effective both as hypoglycaemic and hypolipidemic agents (Ogbonnia et al., 2008[c]; 2010[b]) and have also been empirically used by many people from various cultures to lower cholesterol levels (Hamed, et al., 2010). Herbal medicines owe their therapeutic activities to the presence in them of secondary organic compounds or natural products constituents called the 'active constituents'.

4.1 Herbal active constituents

Herbal drugs contain natural products or secondary metabolites as the active constituents responsible for their physiological and pharmacological activities. The physiological and pharmacological activities have been found amongst alkaloids, phenolics and flavonoid compounds, glycosides (steroidal and saponins), and terpenoids, and is brought about through one or combination of two or more of the mechanisms that are the same as in the disease state they are being used. The mechanisms of their antidiabetic and antilipidemic activities which contribute to lowering of plasma lipids are the same mechanisms responsible for lowering of cardiovascular risk factors. These include the following: Glycosidase (Glucosidase) inhibition mechanism; alpha-amylase inhibition mechanism; antioxidant activities mechanism; inhibition of hepatic glucose metabolizing enzymes mechanism and inhibition of glycosylation of haemoglobin mechanism. These different mechanisms of activities are briefly discussed below

4.2 Possible mechanism of actions

The different classes of secondary product active constituents present in different herbal medicines may act through one or different mechanisms to bring about lowering or clearing of cardiovascular risk factors in a patient which may be probably the same mechanism through which they act exert their pharmacological action to control the disease state in question. Notably some of these possible mechanisms of actions may include:

4.2.1 Glycosidase (Glucosidase) inhibitor mechanism

One of the earliest features of type II diabetes and also observed in pre-diabetic phase is the loss of early phase secretion of insulin. Early phase insulin secretion is seen after a meal or after oral or intravenous ingestion of glucose and it is responsible for inhibition of hepatic glucose output and its absence results in postprandial hyperglycemia. (Ogbonnia and Anyakora 2009[c]). The α-glucosidase inhibitors category of drugs have been found to decrease postprandial glucose level by interfering with carbohydrate digestion and delaying gastrointestinal absorption of glucose . Slowing down digestion and breakdown of starches may have beneficial effects on insulin resistance and glycaemic index control on people suffering from diabetes. In this group some cryptic or water soluble alkaloids especially polyhydroxy alkaloids, have been identified to be potent glucosidase inhibitor (Kameswara et al., 2001). This as a whole comprises of relatively simple monocyclic pyrrolidine and piperidine alkaloids, necines, amino alcohols which are derivatives bicyclic pyrrolizidine, and are mostly esters of amino alcohols and of aliphatic carboxylic acids.

4.2.2 Inhibition of hepatic glucose metabolizing enzymes mechanism

Synthesis of glucose by the liver and kidney from non carbohydrate precursor such as lactate, glycerol and amino acid constitutes a process known as gluconeogenesis. The liver hydrolytic enzymes glucose-6-phosphatase and fructose-1, 6- diphoshatase have been shown to play a crucial role in gluconeogenesis contributing to hyperglycaemic condition found in diabetes. Herbal drug products may act by binding with the enzymes. Treatment with an herbal drug has been observed to decrease the activities of these liver enzymes significantly with a concomitant decrease in blood sugar level (Lazar, 2006).

4.2.3 Antioxidants effects

Phenolics and polyphenolics are associated with antioxidant properties and have been reported to categorically reduce the oxidation of the LDL-c (Kar, 2007). Flavonoids in hawthorn extract have been found to reduce wall tension in normal and sclerotic blood vessels. These chemicals are also presumed to stimulate beta-2-receptors and thus widen coronary arteries and blood vessels in skeletal muscle . Flavonoids and other antioxidants act to destroy free radicals which are particles that can damage cell membranes, interact with genetic material and possibly develop heart diseases and cancer. They have also been found to decrease two other markers of cardiovascular disease, homocysteine and C-reactive protein. C-reactive protein (CRP) has been reported to be associated with increased risk of cardiovascular disease, myocardial infection (MI) coronary artery disease mortality among individuals with angina pectoris.

Oxidative stress has been reported to increase in diabetic patients and is regarded as common pathway by which many classical cardiovascular disease (CVD) risk factors and postprandial dysmetabolism may initiate and promote atherosclerosis (WHO 1985). Studies have shown that treatment with antioxidant reduces diabetic complications (Negappa et al., 2003). Flavonoids have been shown to scavenge reactive oxygen species (ROS) that are produced under severe stress conditions and protect plant cell and animal cell from oxidative stress and may have important role in human health.

4.2.4 Inhibition of glycosylation of haemoglobin mechanism

It has now become apparent that both fasting and postprandial hyperglycaemia contributes to overall glycaemic burden and therefore total glycosylation of haemoglobin, HbA. Many studies have shown that there is substantial evidence and a very strong correlation between hyperglycaemia and the risk of developing cardiovascular disease and mortality. Postprandial hyperglycemia has been found to occur together with postprandial hyperlipidaemia which is also associated with increased oxidative stress and endothelia dysfunction. However, one could therefore postulate that herbal drug products that are effective in the reduction of postprandial hyperglycaemia may not only play a role in managing type II diabetes but could also offer a tantalizing possibility of reducing cardiovascular risk.

S/no	Plant/Herbal Drugs	Work Done	Reference
1.	Alstonia congensis Engler (Apocynaceae) bark and Xylopia aethiopica (Dunal) A. Rich (Annonaceae) fruits	Evaluation of acute in mice and subchronic toxicity	Ogbonnia et al., 2008[a]
2	Leone Bitters, a Nigerian polyherbal formulation	Antimicrobial evaluation, acute and subchronic toxicity studies	Ogbonnia et al., 2008[a], 2010[a]
3.	Parinari curatellifolia Planch, (Chrysobalanaceae) seeds	Assessing plasma glucose and lipid levels, body weight and acute toxicity following oral administration of an aqueous ethanolic extract.	Ogbonnia et al., 2008[b]
4.	poly-herbal formulation	on alloxan- induced diabetic rats	Ogbonnia et al., 2008[b], 2010[b]
5.	Treculia africana Decne and Bryophyllum pinnatum Lam	Evaluation of Hypoglycaemic and Hypolipidaemic Effects of Aqueous Ethanolic Extracts	Ogbonnia et al., 2008[c]
6.	Stachytarpheta angustifolia	Evaluation of acute and subchronic toxicity in animals and phytochemical profile	Ogbonnia et al., 2009a
7.	Parinari curatellifolia Planch (Chrysobalanaceae) seeds	Evaluation of acute in mice and subchronic toxicity	Ogbonnia et al., 2009[b]
8.	Parinari curatellifolia and Anthoclista vogelli	Diabetes and cardiovascular factors	Ogbonnia et al., 2011
9.	Azadirachta indica	Diabetes Mellitus and hypolipidemic effects	Dinesh et al., 2011
10.	Holarrhena antidysenterica	Diabetes	Ali et al., 2009
11.	Annona muricata Linn Centratherum anthelmintica	Diabetes Diabetes	Shah et al., 2008
12.	Grape seed extract	cholesterol	http://www.nativeremedies.com/article/cholesterol-education-heart-disease.html
13.	Red yeast rice contains a natural form of lovastatin	cholesterol	
14.	Vilis vinifera extract and Oroxylum indicum	cholesterol	D'Mello et al., 2011
15.	Garlic	Cholesterol, antithrombic Cardiovascular diseases	
16.	Hawthorn leaf and flower		Hoareau and DaSilva,1999

17.	Cinnamomic camphoric aetherolleum	Coronary artery disease (CAD)	
18.	Rosmarini folium (Rosemary leaf)		
19.	Pini aetheroleum(pine neddle)		
20.	Eucalypti folium (Eucalyptus leaf)		
21.	Menthae aetheroleum (menthol)		
22.	Bacopa monnieri Linn	Diabetes	Ghosh et al., 2006
23.	Feronia elephantum Corr	Diabetes	Mishra and Garg, 2011
24.	Achilleamellifolium (yarrow) Convallaria majalis (lilly of the valley)Crategeus laevigata (hawthorn) Cynarascolymus (globeantichoke) Gingko biloba (gingko) Vibumum opulus	Cardiovascular diseases	Hoareau and DaSilva, 1999

Table 2. Some researched plants and plant medicines found to have lowering effects on cardiovascular risk factors.

5. Summary

- The danger and the increasing prevalence of heart diseases world over are now of a great concern
- These diseases could be attributed to the cardiovascular risk factors which also have been identified to be the underlying latent or potent causes of death in heart diseases in particular and also in many other disease states
- Cardiovascular risk factors include triacylglycerols (triglycerides), cholesterol, cholesteryl esters, very low density lipoprotein – cholesterol (VLDL-c), low density lipoprotein-cholesterol (LDL-c), and anti-athrogenic HDL which are collectively referred to as plasma lipids
- Cholesterol is a fat-like substance that is present in cell membranes and is a precursor to steroid hormones and bile acids.
- Coronary atherosclerosis is the deposition of cholesterol and fibrin complexes within the lumen of a coronary artery that narrows the lumen, thereby limiting blood flow.
- Coronary heart disease (CHD) is atherosclerosis of one or more coronary arteries that has resulted in symptomatic disease such as angina pectoris, myocardial infarction, or congestive heart failure, or has required coronary artery surgery or coronary angioplasty.
- Lipoproteins are lipid-containing proteins in the blood that transport cholesterol throughout the body.
- Disease states with underlying cardiovascular risk factors include diabetes, atherosclerosis and benign prostatic hyperplasia.

6. References

Ali, K M., Chatterjee K, De D. Bera TK and Ghosh D. 2009. Efficacy of aqueous extract of seed of Holarrhena antidysenterica for the management of diabetes in experimental model rat: A correlative study with antihyperlipidemic activity. International Journal of Applied Research in Natural Products. Vol. 2 no 3: 13-21.

Bombardelli E and Morazzoni, P. 1997. Prunus africana, Phytotherapy Vol.68 no3:205-218.

Botham MK and Mayes AP. 2006. Lipid Transport and Storage. In Murray KM, Granner KD and Rodwell WV Eds. Happers Illustrated Biochemistry. 27th edn. McGraw Hill Singapore: 217-229.

Brunzell JD, Davidson M, Furberg CD, Goldberg RB, Howard BV, Stein J, Witztum JL. 2008. Lipoprotein management in patients with cardiometabolic risk. Consensus statement from the American Diabetes Association and the American college of Cardiology Foundation. Diabetes Care, 31:811-822.

Chein C. P and Frishman H. W. 2003. Lipid disorders. In. Grawford H. Michael Ed. Current Diagnosis and Treatment in Cardiology 2nd edition. International edition. Large medical Books/McGraw Hill. New York. 17

Conn E E and Stumpf PK. 1976. Lipids. In: Outline of Biochemistry. 4th edn. John Wiley& Sons Inc. New York, London Sidney and Toronto pp 57-72

D'Mello PM, Darji KK, Shetgiri PP. 2011. Evaluation of antiobesity activity of various Plant extracts. Pharmacognosy Journal, Vol. 3 no 21:56-59

Dharmananda S, 2011. Herbal therapy for Benign prostatic hyperplasia. Clin. Exp. Pharmacol. Physiol., 33: 808-812.

Dinesh k B, Analava M, Manjunatha M. 2011. Azadirachtolide: An anti-diabetic and hypolipidemic effects from Azadirachta indica leaves Pharmacognosy Communications www.phcogcommn.org Vol. 1 no 1:78- 84

Ejike ECC C and Ezeanyika US L, 2010. Hormonal Induction of Benign Prostatic Hyperplasia in Rats: Effects on Serum Macromolecular Metabolism. International Journal of Current Research. Vol 6: 065-067.

Fisher M, Shaw KM. 2001. Diabetes- a state of premature death. Pract.Diab.Vol.18 no6: 31-37

Ghayour –Mobarhan M, Yaghootkar H, Lanham-New SA, Lamb DJ and Ferns GA 2007. Association between serum CRP concentration with dietary intake in healthy and dyslipidaemic patients. Asia Pac J. Clin Nutr. Vol. 16 no.2 262-268 (http://herbaltreatment.us/index.php/cardiovascular-disease/coronary-artery-disease).Flavonoids

Ghosh T, Maity KT, Sengupta P, Dash KD and Bose A, 2006. Antidiabetic and In Vivo Antioxidant Activity of Ethanolic Extract of Bacopa monnieri Linn. Aerial Parts: A Possible Mechanism of Action. Iranian Journal of Pharmaceutical Research. Vol. 7no.1: 61-68

Grundy, S.M., 1986. Comparison of monounsaturated fatty acid and carbohydrates for lowering plasmacholesterol. N. Eng. J. Med. Vol.314: 745-748.

Guyton C A and Hall E J+. 2006. Lipid Metabolism In: Medical Physiology. 11th International edition Elsevier Inc. Philadelphia, Pennsylvania: 540-851. ISBN 0-8089-2317X

Hamed M Raouf, Hassanein, MA Nahed Ali A Azza and. EL-Nahhas M.Y Toqa 2010. An Experimental Study on the Therapeutic Efficacy of the Combined Administration of Herbal Medicines with Atorvastatin against Hyperlipidemia in Rats Journal of Applied Sciences Research, Vol. 6 no.11: 1730-1744.

Hammarsten J and Hogstedt B. 2001. Hyperinsulinemia as a risk factor for developing benign prostatic hyperplasia, European Eurology, Vol.39 no 2: 151-158

Hasimum P., Sukandar E.., Adnyana I.K., and Tjahjono DH. 2011. A simple method for screening Antihyperlidemic Agents. International Journal of pharmacology. Vol 7, no 1: 74-78 doi:10. 3923/ij p.2011.74.78

Hoareau L and DaSilva J. E. 1999. Medical plants: are emerging health and plant Biotechnology vol 2 no 2: 1-5

Holme J. D and Peck H. 1998. Lipid. In Analytical Biochemistry. 3rd Edn Addison Wesley Longman Ltd. ISBN 058229438-X: pp 403 – 433 – 450.

Idogun ES, Unuigbe EP, Ogunro PS, Akinola OI, Famodu AA. 2007. Assessment of serum lipids in Nigerians with type 2 diabetes mellitus complications. Pak J Med Sci Vol. 23:708-712.

Imafidon K E. 2010. Tissue lipid profile of rats administered aqueous extract of Hibiscus Rosa-Sinensis, Linn. Journal of Basic and Applied Sciences Vol. 6, no. 1: 1-3,

Jain J, L, Jain S and Jain N. 2005. Pyruvate oxidation and citric acid cycle. In: Fundamentals of Biochemistry Reprint S. Chgnd and Company Ltd, New Delhi-India : 481-521.

Kameswara, R.B.; Kesavulu, M.M.; Apparao, C. 2001. Journal of Ethnopharmacology, Vol. 78: 67-71

Kar A. 2007. Nutriceuticals. In: Pharmacognosy and Pharmacobiotechnology.2nd edn. New Age International Publisher, New Delhi: 735-778

Kasturi S, Russell S and McVary KT. 2006. Metabolic syndrome and lower urinary tract symptoms secondary to benign prostatic hyperplasia. Curr Urol Rep., Vol. 7:288-292.

Lazar, F.G.; Saltiel, R.A. 2006. Nature Review: Drug Discovery, Vol.15,no4: 333-342.

Leah Emma 2009. "Cholesterol". Lipidomics Gateway. doi:10.1038/lipidmaps.2009.3. http://www.lipidmaps.org/update/2009/090501/full/lipidmaps.2009.3.html

Lewis R, Gaffin D, Hoefnagels M and Paker B. 2002. Circulatory System Spare Parts. In Life.4th edn., McGraw –Hill Higher Education, a division of the McGraw –Hill Companies, ISBN 0-07-027134-8 pp 680-699

Madhumathi BG, Venkataranganna MV, Gopumadhavan S, Rafiq M and Mitra SK. 2006. Induction and evaluation of atherosclerosis in New Zealand white rabbits. Indian J Exp Biol.Vol.44 : 203-208

Maruthapan, V., Shree K. Sakthi. 2010. Antihyperlipidemic potential of a polyherbal dug (Geriforte) on atherogenic diet induced hyperlipidemia: A Comparison with Ayurslim. International Journal of Chemical and Analytical Science Vol. 1. no 3:37-39

Maxfield FR and Tabas I. 2005 Roles of cholesterol and lipid organization in disease. Nature., 438: 612-621 metabolic syndrome. *Am J Cardiovasc Drugs* 2005, 5(6):379-387.

Metzler E. David 1974. Specific Aspects of Lipid Metabolism. In Biochemistry: The chemical reactions of living cells. 2nd Edition.. Elsevier Academic Press. Vols 1 & 2:1180- 1225

Mishra A and Garg P G, 2011. Antidiabetic activity of fruit pulp of Feronia elephantum Corr Pharmacognosy Journal Vol 3 no 20: 27-32

Mohrman. E. David and Heller Jane Lois. 2006 Cardiovascular disease. In Cardiovascular physiology. 6th edition. McGraw Hill, Boston: 205-221

Moreno-Luna, Rafael, Perez-Jimenez Francisco, Marin Carmen, Perez-Martinez Pablo, Gomez Purification, Jimenez-Gomez Yolanda, Delgado-Lista Javier, Moreno Junan A., Tanaka Toshiko, Orodovas Jose M and Lopez-Miranda J. 2007. Two Independent Apolipoprotein A5 Haplotypes Modulate Postprandial Lipoprotein Metabolism in a Healthy Caucasian Population. Journal of Clinical Endocrinology & Metabolism, diol: 10. 1210/jc.2006-1802, Vol. 92, no. 6: 2280-2285.

Nagappa, A.N.; Thakurdesai, P.A.; Venkat, R.N.; Singh, J. 2003. Antidiabetic activity of Terminalia catappa Linn fruits. Journal of Ethnopharmacology, Vol. 88: 45-50

Nirmala A. Saroja S Gayathri Devi. G. 2011. Antidiabetic Activity of Basella rubra and its Relationship with the Antioxidant Property. British Biotechnology Journal. Vol. 1 no1: 1-9.

Ogbonnia S, Adekunle A A, Bosa M.K, and Enwuru VN. 2008a. Evaluation of acute and subacute toxicity of Alstonia congensis Engler (Apocynaceae) bark and Xylopia aethiopica (Dunal) A. Rich (Annonaceae) fruits mixtures used in the treatment of diabetes. African Journal of Biotechnology. Vol. 7 no.6:701-705

Ogbonnia S, Adekunle A, Olagbende- Dada S, Anyika EN, Enwuru NV, Orolepe M. 2008b. Assessing plasma glucose and lipid levels, body weight and acute toxicity following oral administration of an aqueous ethanolic extract of Parinari curatellifolia Planch, (Chrysobalanaceae) seeds in alloxan-induced diabetes in Rats. African Journal of Biotechnology vol.7 no.8: 3520-3525

Ogbonnia Steve O., Odimegwu Joy I. Enwuru Veronica N. 2008c. Evaluation of Hypoglycaemic and Hypolipidaemic Effects of aqueous ethanolic extracts of Treculia africana Decne and Bryophyllum pinnatum Lam. and their Mixture on Streptozotocin (STZ)-induced diabetic rats. African Journal of Biotechnology Vol.7no 15: 2535-2539 (http://www.umm.edu/altmed/articles/garlic-000245.htm

Ogbonnia SO, Nkemehule FE, Anyika EN. 2009a. Evaluation of acute and subchronic toxicity in animals and phytochemical profile of aqueous ethanolic extract of Stachytarpheta angustifolia (Mill) Vahl (Fam. Verbanaceae) plant. Journal of Biotechnology vol.8 no.9: 3213-2539.

Ogbonnia SO, Olayemi SO, Anyika EN, Enwuru VN, Poluyi O.O. 2009b. Evaluation of acute in mice and subchronic toxicity of hydroethanolic extract of Parinari curatellifolia Planch (Chrysobalanaceae) seeds in rats. Journal of Biotechnology vol.8 no.9: 3245-3251

Ogbonnia SOand Anyakora C 2009c Chemistry and Biology Evaluation of Nigerian Plant with anti-Diabetic Properties. Juliani H.R., Simon J.E and Ho C-T. (Eds.). In African Natural Products: new discoveries and challenges in chemistry and quality American Chemical Society, Washington DC. ISBN 978-0-8412-6987-3

Ogbonnia SO, Mbaka G. O, Igbokwe NH, Anyika E, A lli P, Nwakakwa N. 2010a. Antimicrobial evaluation, acute and subchronic toxicity studies of Leone Bitters, a Nigerian polyherbal formulation in rodents. Agriculture and Biology Journal of North America, Vol. 1 no. 3: 366-376. ISSN Print: 2151-7517, ISSN Online: 2151-7525 Science Huβ, http://www.scihub.org/ABJNA

Ogbonnia SO, Mbaka G. O, Adekunle A, Anyika E. N, Gbolade O. E, Nwakakwa N. 2010[b] Effect of a poly-herbal formulation, Okudiabet, on alloxan-induced diabetic rats. Agriculture and Biology Journal of North America, Vol.1no.2: 139-145. ISSN Print: 2151-7517, ISSN Online: 2151-7525 Science Huβ, http://www.scihub.org/ABJNA

Ogbonnia, S.O.; Mbaka, G.O.; Anyika, E.N.; Ladiju, O.; Igbokwe, H.N.; Emordi, J.E. and Nwakakwa, N. 2011. Evaluation of Anti-diabetics and Cardiovascular Effects of Parinari curetellifolia Seed Extract and Anthoclista vogelli Root Extract Individually and Combined on Postprandial and Alloxan-Induced Diabetic Albino Rats. British Journal of Medicine & Medical Research 1(3): 146-162.

O'Keefe JH, Cordain L, Harris WH, Moe RM, Vogel R., 2004. Optimal lowdensity lipoprotein is 50 to 70 mg/dl: lower is better and physiologically normal. J Am Coll Cardiol Vol.43:2142-2146.

Ozden C, Ozdal OL, Urganioglu G, Kovuncu H, Gokkaya S and Mermis A. 2007. The correlation between metabolic syndrome and prostatic growth in patients with benign prostatic hyperplasia. Eur Urol., Vol. 51:199-206.

Plummer T. D, 1998. Lipids. In: An introduction of practical Biochemistry. 3rd edn. Tata McGraw – Hill Educational Private Limited. New Delhi- India: pp 189-204. ISBN – 13:978-0-07-099487-4, ISBN-10: 0-07-099487-0.

Rousset X, Vaisman B, Amar M, Sethi A A and Remalev AT. 2009. Lecithin: cholesterol acyltranferease...from biochemistry to role in cardiovascular disease. Current Opinion Endocrinology Diabetes Obesity Vol.16 no.2:163-171.

Sani-Bello F, Bakari AG, Anumah FE. 2007. Dyslipidaemia in persons with type 2 diabetes mellitus in Kaduna, Nigeria. Int J Diabetes and Metabolism Vol.15:9-13.

Shah JG, Patel MS, Patel KV and Gandhi TR 2008. Evaluation of Anti-diabetic and Anti-oxidant Activity of Centratherum anthelmintica in STZ-induced Diabetes in Rats. The International Internet Journal of Pharmacology, Vol.6 no1:1-10.

Sharma VK, Kumar S, Patel HJ and Hugar S. 2010. Hypoglycemic activity of Ficus glomerata in alloxan induced diabetic rat. International Journal of Pharmaceutical Sciences Review and Research, Vol. 1 no 2:18-22.

Sharon, G. B., Marvin, R. B. (1975). Synthesis and evaluation of potential hypoglycaemic agents I: carnitine analogs, J Pharm. Sci., 64(12), 1949-1952.

Singh IM, Shishehbor DO. 2007. Ansell BJ: High-density lipoprotein as a therapeutic target: a systematic review. JAMA 298:786-798.

Stryer L. 1988. Biosynthesis of Membrane Lipids and Steroids Hormones. In: Biochemistry.3rd edn. W.H. Freeman and Company, New York, USA: 547-574

Udawat H, Goyal RK. 2001. Lipid lowering effect of simvastatin in patients of type 2 DM. Indian Heart J 53:172-176.

Uebanso T, Arai H, Taketani Y, Fukaya M, Yamamoto H, Mizuno A, Uryu K, Hada T and Takeda E, 2007. Extracts of Momordica charantia Suppress Postprandial Hyperglycemia in Rats. J Nutr Sci Vitaminol, 53, 482 – 488.

Walter, B.J. (1977). An introduction to the principles of disease. W.B. Saunders Company. Philadelphia USA, pp. 374-377.

WHO Expert Committes. In WHO Technical Report Series of Diabetes Mellitus, 1985, 727.

Williams K, Tchernof A, Hunt KJ, Wagenknecht LE, Haffner MS, Sniderman AD. 2008. Diabetes, abdominal adiposity and atherogenic dyslipoproteinaemia in women compared with men. *Diabetes* 57:3289-3296.

7

Morphology and Functional Changes of Intestine, Trophology Status and Systemic Inflammation in Patients with Chronic Heart Failure

G.P. Arutyunov and N.A. Bylova
The Russian State Medical University (RSMU),
Russia

1. Introduction

1.1 Morphological and functional changes of the small intestine in patients with different classes of chronic heart failure

Current understanding prompts to view chronic heart failure (CHF) as a systemic condition. Traditionally, the following organs are considered the target organs of CHF: heart, kidneys, brain. However, low cardiac output and increased activity of the renin-angiotensin-aldosterone system (RAAS), which lead to vasospasm and ischemia, are bound to have effect on functions of other organs, including small intestine, large intestine, and adipose tissue. The increased activity of RAAS is likely to have effect on morphological restructuring of the intestine as well. It can be assumed that accumulation of collagen in the intestinal wall, as well as development of edema and ischemia, decrease the functional activity of the intestinal wall and are a major factor of the malabsorption syndrome, which, in its turn, leads to progressive loss of body mass. This results in progression of certain clinical manifestations in patients with CHF, such as: weakness, fatigue, and progressive decrease of exercise tolerance, which cannot be explained by changes in peripheral circulation alone. The incidence of these complaints is known to increase as the NYHA class of the CHF grows, and it reaches its peak in patients with class IV (Harrington & Anker, 1997).

Loss of body mass means a significantly worse prognosis for the patients with CHF. According to SOLVD study, ≥6 % decrease of body mass in patients with CHF is a potent predictor of negative impact on survival along with other factors such as age, gender, LV ejection fraction, NYHA class (Anker et al., 2003).

Therefore, decrease of body mass should be considered an important sign, equal in significance to such symptoms as dyspnea and edema.

Obviously, a search for new methods to correct the nutritional status in patients with CHF is necessary. The method of nutritional support may be one of these promising options to treat and stop development the malabsorption syndrome, as this method constitutes a system with pathogenesis-based rationale that implies prescription of balanced nutritive mixtures characterized by maximum degree of absorption even in the setting of morphological changes in the intestine.

1.2 Materials and methods

This was an open-label prospective study approved by the Ethics Committee of the Russian State Medical University. All of the patients participating in this study had signed the informed consent.

The study included 110 patients with New York Heart Association (NYHA) class I-IV ischemic CHF, with history of CHF for more than 24 months. Age of the patients was 45 to 65 years, mean age was 58.7±5.3 years. All of the patients were allocated to different groups based on the severity of their CHF. The control group included 38 patients (24 male and 14 female), 45 to 65 years old (mean age 60.6±2.6), in which no signs of CHF were found after testing. The patient populations had comparable basic parameters at baseline.

All of the patients with the signs of CHF received standard basic therapy, which included ACE inhibitors, β-blockers, loop diuretics or thiazide diuretics, cardiac glycosides, nitrates, aspirin, and aldosterone antagonists. Patients in the control group received therapy for their main condition.

Patients were investigated using the following sets of tests:

- Endoscopy with biopsy of the small intestine (the samples were taken 10 cm below the plica duodenojejunalis). Preparation and analysis of microscopic specimens were performed in the Pathology Department of the Bakulev Scientific Center of Cardiovascular Surgery.
- Assessment of functional activity of the small intestine (measurement of excretion of fat in feces, biochemical measurement of total protein and protein fractions in feces via nitrogen content, measurement of carbohydrate absorption in the small intestine using the D-xylose test).

Statistical analyses of the results were performed using standard statistical formulas with Microsoft Excel 7.0 and BIOSTAT software. Arithmetic means of values in the sample population (M) and standard deviations (σ) were determined. The significance of differences between groups was determined using Student test at $p < 0.05$. Relationship between parameters was assessed by calculating the correlation coefficient (r) with the level of errorless prognosis at 95 % ($p<0.05$).

1.3 Results

1.3.1 Morphological changes of the small intestine in patients with NYHA class I-IV CHF

The photographs of microscopic specimens (Fig. 1) demonstrate the pattern of the mucosa of the small intestine typical for patients with NYHA class IV CHF (a) and healthy individuals (b). Collagen fibers are stained pink.

These photographs demonstrate that in patients with NYHA class III-IV CHF the collagen fibers stained pink take up a significant area of the small intestine mucosa, while in patients without signs of CHF only solitary collagen fibers are present.

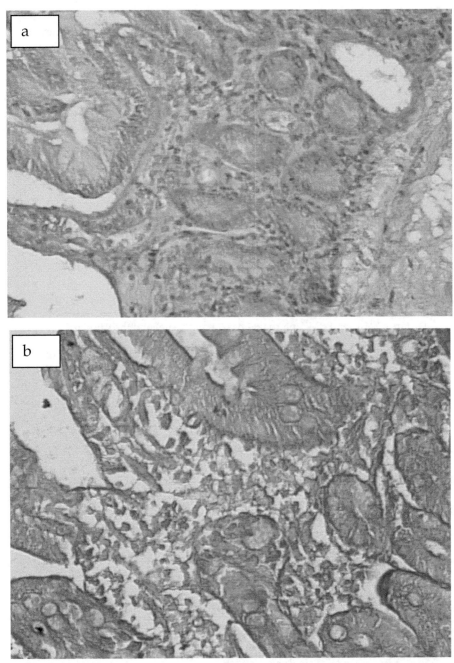

Fig. 1. The microscopic sample of the mucosa of the small intestine from a patient with
NYHA class IV CHF (a) and a patient without signs of CHF (b). Van Gieson's stain,
magnification x 400.

Collagen deposition level in patients with NYHA classes III and IV was significantly different from values measured in patients with NYHA classes I or II and in patients without signs of CHF. Comparison of collagen relative density between patients without CHF and with NYHA class I or II CHF did not reveal significant differences. However, a clear trend towards increase of collagen level in the latter was noted. Also, the difference in the amount of collagen between CHF patients with NYHA classes III and IV was not significant.

When assessing the microscopic specimens of the small intestine, high amount of collagen was observed to mechanically push enterocytes away from a capillary vessel. This increases the intestine-blood barrier and may have an impact on nutrient absorption.

The measured data are presented in Table 1.

Groups	Distance between EBM and a capillary vessel, μm	Significance of difference between groups
1. No CHF	8.4±0.7	p1-2 >0.05; p1-3>0.05; p1-4<0.05; p1-5<0.05
2. NYHA class I	10.1±1.2	p2-3>0.05; p2-4>0.05; p2-5>0.05
3. NYHA class II	11.3±1.1	p3-4<0.05; p3-5<0.05
4. NYHA class III	18.6±1.4	p4-5>0.05
5. NYHA class IV	19.1±1.2	

Table 1. Distance between EBM (enterocyte basal membrane) and the capillary wall

Even primary assessment of microscopic photographs revealed atrophy of villi of the small intestine mucosa in patients with NYHA class III-IV CHF. Fig. 2 shows pattern of the mucosa in a patient with NYHA class IV CHF (a) compared to a patient from the control group (b).

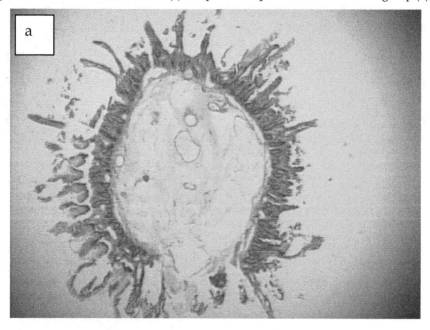

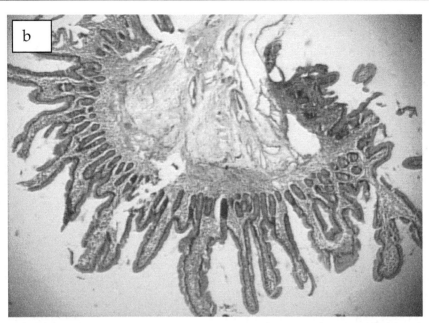

Fig. 2. Villi of the small intestine mucosa in a patient with NYHA class IV CHF (a) and a patient without CHF (b).Magnification x100. Hematoxylin-eosin stain.

Quantitative values describing changes in the villi of the small intestine in patients with different classes of CHF are shown in the Table 2.

Groups	Mean length of a villus, μm	Mean width of a villus, μm	Significance of difference between groups
No CHF	372±9.9	98±4.4	p1-2>0.05; p1-3>0.05; p1-4<0.05; p1-5<0.05
Class I CHF	369±7.4	94±3.5	p2-3>0.05; p2-4>0.05; p2-5>0.05
Class II CHF	374±6.9	91±6.1	p3-4<0.05; p3-5<0.05
Class III CHF	254±5.5	65±3.1	p4-5>0.05
Class IV CHF	223±6.1	59±3.0	

Table 2. Length and width of mucosal villi in the small intestine of patients with CHF.

To conclude, analysis of the small intestine mucosa biopsy samples demonstrated significant morphological changes, which worsen with the severity of CHF. Increase of intestine-blood barrier and decrease of the absorbing area of the villi determined further study of nutrient absorption, which, supposedly, should have decreased significantly in patients with CHF.

1.3.2 Functional changes of the small intestine in patients with NYHA class I-IV CHF

Analysis of protein absorption parameters revealed the following pattern: in patients with NYHA class I CHF, losses of total nitrogen were virtually below the upper limit of normal range, reaching 7.1±0.2 % of daily consumption. No significant differences were found between the patients of the control group (5.9±0.21 %) and classes I or II (p>0.05). With NYHA class IV CHF, the loss of protein was significantly higher – 18.6±1.3 %; this was on average 3.1 times higher than in the group of patients without CHF (p<0.05). In the group of patients with NYHA class III, the loss of protein was 16.7±1.8 %. Comparison of the protein loss levels in CHF patients with NYHA class III and IV vs. the protein loss levels in patients with NYHA class I and II showed a significant difference (p>0.05).

Levels of total fat loss were most pronounced in CHF patients with NYHA class III and IV (22.4±2.1 % and 24.1±2.12 % of the daily consumption, respectively) and exceeded the levels in patients without CHF (5.5±0.86 %) 4-fold on average. For NYHA classes I and II, fat loss levels were at the upper limit of normal (6.1±1.1 and 7.2±0.9 % of daily consumption, respectively) and were not significantly different from the values in the group of patients without CHF (p>0.05).

Analysis of D-xylose test results demonstrated a dependency similar to the one observed for absorption of proteins and fats. In patients with NYHA class IV CHF, the 5-hour excretion of D-xylose was 0.89±0.05 g. This was 1.4 times lower than the values for the control group. For NYHA class III CHF, D-xylose excretion was 0.96±0.03 g. This was also significantly different from normal values. Patients with NYHA class I and II did not show significant differences compared to the control group.

To conclude, patients with CHF experience deterioration of absorption for all basic nutrients, and the absorption reduction demonstrates dependence upon the severity of the CHF.

1.4 Attempts for correction

Taking into consideration the pronounced changes of the small intestine in patients with severe CHF that lead to development of malabsorption syndrome and protein-energy insufficiency, such patients demand specific correction of their nutritional status. Naturally, raw nutrients will hardly be utilized in the intestine that underwent these changes. A possibility to use specifically treated nutrients in the form of standard mixes for oral feeding was the objective that we assessed in the second phase of this study.

This part was an open-label, randomized, prospective, 24-week study.

Patients with NYHA class III and IV CHF were screened for this study. Total number of subjects was 74 (46 males, 28 females).

Randomization was performed using a random number method, with even numbers corresponding to the standard-of-care group (Group 1), and odd numbers corresponding to the nutritional support group (Group 2). The number of patients assigned to Group 1 was 36. Group 2 included 38 patients.

Figure 3 shows the study design.

Subjects in Group 1 (n=36) received standard basic therapy and their usual nutrition within the standard diet for cardiovascular patients.

Subjects in Group 2 (n=38), in addition to the basic therapy and standard diet, received a balanced nutritive mix, comprising 25 % of daily calories.

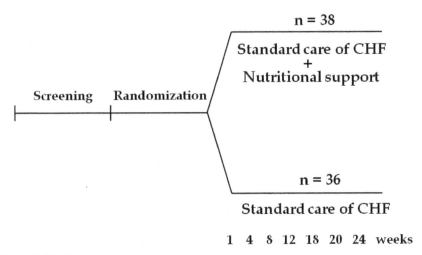

Fig. 3. Study Design.

The absolute majority of the patients were male and had history of ischemic origin of their disease. Their mean age was over 60 years. Mean NYHA class within these groups was 3.5 and 3.4, respectively. The resulting groups were identical in structure by gender, age and other clinical characteristics, warranting their comparability. The following tests were performed during this study: 6-minute test, echocardiography (LVEF), diet review, measurement of body mass and BMI, estimation of body fat mass and lean body mass, total protein, albumin, absolute lymphocyte count, hand dynamometry, assessment of absorption for proteins, fats, and carbohydrates, morphometric study of small intestine mucosa biopsy specimens, count of hospitalizations due to CHF progression.

Estimations of energy and nutrient demands were performed for all subjects before therapeutic diet and nutritional support were prescribed.

Subjects in Group 2 had 25 % of their energy demands (daily energy consumption) covered using balanced nutritive mixes, and the remaining 75 % were covered using the standard diet. All patients maintained dietary diaries, which allowed us to control the amount of energy they have received with their usual diet.

The balanced nutritive mixes used for nutritive support were Peptamen (Nestle, Switzerland), Berlamin Modular (Berlin-Chemie, Germany), Unipit and Nutrien-standard (Nutritek, Russia).

Assessment of nutritional support efficacy included change of 6-minute test parameters over time, change of LBM over time, and number of hospitalizations due to CHF progression compared between the experimental group and the control group.

During 24-week observation, a total of 11 patients died in 2 groups: 4 males and 2 females in Group 1 (standard-of-care), and 3 males and 2 females in Group 2 (oral nutritional support). Total number of hospitalization events throughout 24 weeks was 54 and 42 in Group 1 and Group 2, respectively. Table 3 shows causes of death and hospitalization.

Cause	Hospitalization		Death	
	Group 1	Group 2	Group 1	Group 2
CHF progression	36 (66,7%)	28 (66,7%)	4 (66,7%)	3 (60%)
Recurrent MI	6 (11,1%)	7 (16,7%)	1 (16,7%)	2 (40%)
Pneumonias	10 (18,5%)	6 (14,3%)	1 (16,7%)	0
Other	2 (0,4%)	3 (0,7%)	0	0
Total	54	42	6	5

Table 3. Causes of death and hospitalization for Groups 1 and 2.

Three patients chose to withdraw from study: 2 of them were from the standard-of-care group, and another one from the nutritional support group (the reason was moving to another city). Compliance was assessed using patient diaries, where their adherence to basic therapy and to nutritional support was recorded. Compliance below 80 % was reported for 2 subjects in Group 1 and 2 subjects in Group 2 (these subjects were excluded from the final analysis). As a result, in the standard-of-care group 26 patients completed the study, and in the nutritional support group 30 patients completed the study.

1.4.1 Changes of 6-minute test parameters over time

The trend for growth of the parameters in Group 2 was noticeable starting from Week 2. The curves of 6-minute test for the 2 groups diverged significantly starting from Week 8. After 24 weeks, the exercise tolerance in patients receiving standard nutrition decreased significantly (p=0.025). The baseline values for 6-minute test in this group were 85 to 243 m, mean 203.4±41.6 m. After 24 weeks, the mean distance walked in 6 minutes decreased by 19 % (164.7±48.1 m).

Six patients with NYHA class III CHF experienced substantial deterioration of their health – worsening of dyspnea, weakness, edema, i. e. their condition progressed to NYHA class IV.

In the group of patients receiving the nutritional support, the baseline for the 6-minute test was 182.2±45.6 m (range 34 m to 221 m), and Week 24 mean was 231.3±41.1 m (75 m to 295 m), i. e. a statistically significant (p=0.015) increase in exercise tolerance was observed. In this group, progression of NYHA class III to class IV was recorded for 2 patients only.

To conclude, in patients receiving the standard diet, Week 24 exercise tolerance decreased significantly, whereas in patients receiving nutritional support, significant increase of the exercise tolerance was observed. Statistical significance for the difference between the groups was p=0.021.

1.4.2 Change of hand dynamometry measurements over time

After 24 weeks of monitoring, no significant differences were found for dynamometry variables when comparing pre-treatment and post-treatment values; however, there was a trend towards increase for these variables in the nutritional support group (mean increase 0.2 kg, p=0.084). In the standard-of-care group, the variables decreased, with mean change of 0.4 kg; this change was not statistically significant (p=0.09).

1.4.3 Change of LBM over time

For most of the patients receiving nutritional support, a significant increase of LBM was shown (mean change 5.8±1.2 kg or 8.9 %, p=0.038). For 2 patients, a progressive decrease of LBM was recorded on treatment (the LBM decreased by 2.1 kg and 3.4 kg). In the standard nutrition group, 23 patients experienced statistically significant decrease of their LBM (mean decrease 3.6±0.7 kg or 4.9 %, p=0.036). The LBM did not change significantly in 2 patients, and an increase of LBM (+1.7 kg) was reported for 1 patient.

To conclude, long-term nutritional support leads to statistically significant increase of LBM, while in the standard nutrition group the LBM continues to decrease progressively. The differences between groups were statistically significant (p=0.04).

1.4.4 Changes of laboratory variables over time (absolute lymphocyte count and serum albumin)

In the nutritional support group, a statistically significant increase of nutritional status was demonstrated: the absolute lymphocyte count increased from 1590 to 1710 x109 (+12.5 %, p=0.04), and the albumin level increased from 25.1 to 29.4 g/L (+17.1 %, p=0.045). In the standard-of-care group, no significant changes were observed after 24 weeks of monitoring for the lymphocyte count and albumin. The differences between groups were statistically significant (p=0.04).

To conclude, the nutritional support demonstrated a favorable effect for all basic nutritional status variables.

1.4.5 Other variables

For the effect of nutritional support on protein, fat and carbohydrate absorption variables see Table 4.

Absorption variables	Group 1		Group 2	
	Baseline	Week 24	Baseline	Week 24
Total protein loss, % of daily consumption	18.1±0.3	17.9±0.2	17.9±0.2	15.48±0.9
Total fat loss, % of daily consumption	22.5±0.6	21.6±0.4	23.4±0.4	20.7±1.3
D-xylose excretion with urine, g/5 h	0.81±0.05	0.85±0.04	0.82±0.04	0.83±0.04

Table 4. Absorption of nutrients in patients with NYHA class III-IV CHF, pre-treatment and post-treatment.

No statistically significant changes were demonstrated in either group for morphometric variables during the treatment period of 24 weeks.

1.5 Conclusion

The study of the small intestine condition revealed marked changes of structure and functional activity of the intestine in all patients with CHF. The degree of the small intestine impairment directly depends on the severity of the CHF. This suggests direct impact of heart failure on gastrointestinal restructuring.

We consider the oral nutrition system involving prescription of balanced nutritional mixes to be one of the promising options to treat cardiac cachexia, as it has a pathogenesis-based rationale. This study was an attempt to evaluate the efficacy of the nutritional support during CHF progression.

2. Morphological and functional changes of the large intestine in patients with different classes of chronic heart failure

2.1 Introduction

Current understanding acknowledges the role of the following factors in the pathogenesis of CHF: neuroendocrine imbalance with excessive production of neurohormones, impairment of various target organs (cardiac muscle, kidneys, skeletal muscles, small intestine). However, many authors observed increased level of pro-inflammatory cytokines in CHF patients that cannot be explained by neuroendocrine activation. A number of authors reported a correlation between cytokine levels and blood plasma concentration of the endotoxin (lipopolysaccharide of gram-negative bacteria).

In an attempt to find the origin of the endotoxin, various bacteria were considered, particularly the bacteria of upper and lower respiratory tract, H. pylori, microorganisms of urinary tract and intestine. The strongest changes were found in the flora of the large intestine, where increase of the total number of microorganisms was observed, predominantly gram-negative. However, there were no reports of detailed analysis of the intestinal flora composition, and the parietal mucin layer flora was not taken into account.

The data on flora changes suggested potential methods of correction, particularly the selective decontamination method. However, according to literature reports, a course of selective decontamination reduces the number of microorganisms in the large intestine in the phase of antibacterial treatment only, while as early as 6 weeks after their discontinuation characteristics of the flora return to baseline. This shows lack of efficacy of the selective decontamination alone in CHF patients with high NYHA classes.

From our perspective, there are two possible approaches to correct the endotoxemia that leads to systemic inflammation: (1) development of methods that act on the intestinal wall by decreasing its permeability to the endotoxin, and (2) treatment that has direct effect on the intestinal flora towards normalization of both numbers and the composition of the flora.

2.2 Materials and methods

Laboratory tests.

Quantitative assay of endotoxin level using Kinetic-QCL test №50-650 U "Bioscience Cambrex Wallkersville", USA.

Quantitative assay of IL-6 (IL-6 Human ELISA Kit (1 x 96 Well Plate), Cytokine company, Russia), TNF-alpha (TNF alpha Human ELISA Kit (1 x 96 Well Plate), Cytokine company, Russia), CRP (C Reactive Protein Human ELISA Kit - 1 x 96 Well Plate, Abcam, USA) plasma levels using solid phase ELISA.

2.3 Assessment of the microbial landscape, large intestine wall structure, endotoxin levels, and pro-inflammatory cytokines in CHF patients with different NYHA classes

To study these variables, three consecutive groups were enrolled: Group 1: 65 patients with NYHA class III-IV CHF; Group 2: 60 patients with NYHA class I-II CHF; Group 3: 56 patients, control group (patients with ischemic heart disease and arterial hypertension without signs of CHF).

2.3.1 Changes in lumen flora of the large intestine in CHF patients with different NYHA classes and in the control group

Comparison of the first and the second study groups revealed statistically significant differences ($p<0.05$) for the following variables: total number of enterobacteria was 10^9 colony-forming units (CFU)/g in Group 1 vs. 10^7 CFU/g in Group 2. Enterobacteria pool growth was predominantly formed by *E. coli* (10^7 CFU/g in NYHA I-II group vs. 10^9 CFU/g in NYHA III-IV group, $p<0.0001$), various *Klebsiella sp.* (10^5 CFU/g in NYHA I-II group vs. 10^7 CFU/g in NYHA III-IV group, $p<0.005$), and citrate-assimilating enterobacteria (10^6 CFU/g in NYHA I-II group vs. 10^8 CFU/g in NYHA III-IV group, $p<0.005$). Differences in concentrations of *Citrobacters, Enterococci* and *Candida* yeasts were also statistically significant.

Comparison of the results for Group 1 (NYHA class III-IV) and control group subjects showed differences similar to the comparison of Group 1 versus Group 2, with the exception of differences in Clostridia populations (lecithinase- and hydrogen sulfide-positive strains): 10^7 CFU/g in CHF patients with NYHA III-IV vs. 10^5 CFU/g in the control group ($p<0.05$).

Comparison of Group 2 (NYHA I-II CHF) versus control group demonstrated minimal changes in the gut microbiome. Statistically significant differences were shown for *Bacteroides* only (10^9 CFU/g in NYHA class I-II patients vs. 10^{10} CFU/g in the control group, $p<0.05$). In CHF patients with NYHA class III-IV the levels of *Bacteroides* were not significantly different from results reported for the control group; therefore, from our perspective, these data can be ignored in practice.

Statistically significant differences were demonstrated for *Clostridia* (hydrogen sulfide-positive, lecithinase-positive): 10^5 CFU/g in the control group vs. 10^7 CFU/g in CHF patients with NYHA class III-IV, as well as for *Enterococci* and *Candida* yeasts ($p<0.05$). No statistically significant differences between groups were demonstrated for other microorganisms.

Conclusion: the higher is NYHA class of CHF, the stronger are the changes in the large intestine flora due to growth of gram-negative species.

2.4 Changes of the parietal mucin layer flora in CHF patients with NYHA class I-IV

The microorganisms located in the parietal mucin layer have the most significant impact on the host. Therefore, our objective was to study the changes in parietal mucin layer flora in CHF patients with NYHA class I-IV.Taking into account the minimal changes in lumen flora between NYHA class I-II patients and the control group, and considering technical difficulties associated with parietal flora studies, we decided to skip investigation of parietal mucin layer flora in the large intestine for the control group.We decided to approximate the results from biopsies of CHF patients with NYHA class I-II as normal.

Biopsy studies showed changes similar to those reported for feces. A statistically significant changes of the enterobacteria population in CHF patients with NYHA class III-IV was demonstrated (10^8 CFU/g vs. 10^5 CFU/g in patients with NYHA classes III-IV and I-II, respectively; p<0.0001).These changes were due to growth of *E. coli* (10^8 CFU/g vs. 10^5 CFU/g in NYHA III-IV vs. NYHA I-II, respectively; p<0.0001), *Klebsiella* (10^8 CFU/g vs. 10^5 CFU/g in NYHA III-IV vs. NYHA I-II, respectively; p<0.005), and citrate-assimilating enterobacteria (10^8 CFU/g vs. 10^5 CFU/g in NYHA III-IV vs. NYHA I-II, respectively; p<0.005).No statistically significant differences were found in the biopsy specimens for *Clostridia, Enterococci,* as well as for *Candida* yeasts. However, statistically significant differences were demonstrated for the population of *Bifidobacteria*: 10^3 CFU/g vs. 10^6 CFU/g in NYHA III-IV vs. NYHA I-II, respectively (p<0.05).

Conclusion: the parietal mucin layer flora changes corresponded to the changes of the lumen flora: the higher is NYHA class, the greater is the population of gram-negative microorganisms. No changes in the population levels of gram-positive flora was demonstrated for lumen flora, while in the parietal mucin layer a decrease of *Bifidobacteria* population was reported.

2.5 Changes in the structure of the intestinal wall in CHF patients with NYHA class I-IV

Changes found in the microbial landscape of both lumen flora and parietal mucin layer flora prompted us to study the large intestine wall structure in CHF patients with NYHA class I-IV.

In Group 2, no changes were observed in the biopsy specimens of large intestine mucosa. In Group 1, hyperemic vessels and focal dense lymphoid-cellular infiltrates were reported in the lamina propria of the large intestine mucosa (Fig. 4). This pattern is consistent with marked chronic inflammation.

To confirm the lymphoid nature of the infiltrates, OLA reaction (common lymphocytic antigen) was performed (Fig. 5).

A strong positive infiltrate (derivates of white blood cell line) was observed in the lamina propria of the large intestine mucosa. Particularly, intraepithelial lymphocytes were seen clearly. CD8+ staining (Fig. 6) revealed intraepithelial CD8+-positive T-lymphocytes in the superficial layer of the large intestine mucosa.

Ki67 reaction revealed positive cells of gland epithelium (Fig. 7) in the proliferation phase. At the same time, there were solitary cells positive for Muc5 reaction (i. e. containing mucin 5) in the superficial epithelium of the large intestine mucosa.

Histopathology also revealed a large number of siderophages (Fig. 8), suggesting chronic congestion in the large intestine vessels. We considered these changes to be a sign of the chronic heart failure.

Conclusion: the CHF patients with NYHA class III-IV showed signs of marked chronic inflammation in the large intestine mucosa, along with tissue edema and venous congestion. The severity of these changes increased with higher NYHA class and the severity of CHF decompensation symptoms.

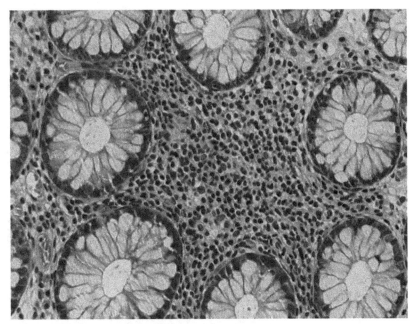

Fig. 4. Biopsy sample of the large intestine mucosa. Hematoxylin-eosin stain.

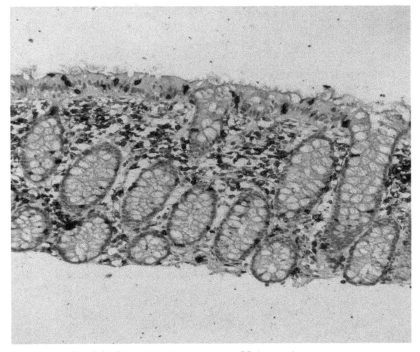

Fig. 5. Biopsy sample of the large intestine mucosa. OLA reaction.

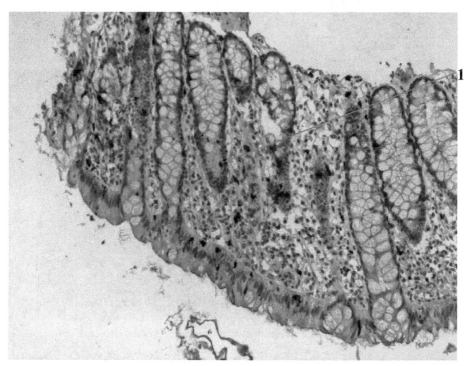

Fig. 6. Biopsy sample of the large intestine mucosa, CD8+ lymphocyte stain. 1 – CD8+ lymphocytes.

2.6 Endotoxin level assessment

Plasma levels of the endotoxin were 1.2±0.03 EU/L in NYHA class III-IV subjects and 0.46±0.01 EU/L in NYHA class I-II subjects (EU – endotoxin units). The level of the endotoxin in the control group subjects was 0.35±0.02 EU/L. Notably, plasma endotoxin levels directly correlated with the changes in population numbers of the large intestine gram-negative flora.

The CHF patients with NYHA class III-IV had levels of IL-6 at 11.5±0.3 U/L, TNF-alpha at 6.6±0.4 U/L, and CRP at 8±0.65 mg/ml. The CHF patients with NYHA class I-II had levels of IL-6 at 4.6±0.3 U/L, TNF-alpha at 3.7±0.4 U/L, and CRP at 5.5±0.29 mg/ml. The levels of these pro-inflammatory cytokines in the control group were within normal limits: : IL-6 was 2 U/L, TNF-alpha was 1.5 U/L, and CRP was 2.9 mg/ml. The identified changes prompted us to suggest two approaches to correction of these conditions:

1. Targeting the large intestine wall using different diuretic regimens, including agents with tissue activity.
2. Selective decontamination in combination with probiotics.

2.7 Use of different diuretic regimens

Figure 9 shows the study design.

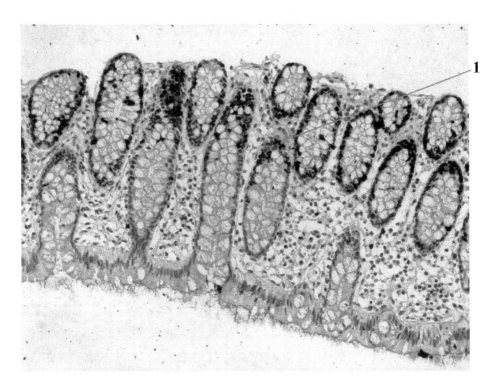

Fig. 7. Biopsy sample of the large intestine mucosa, Ki67 reaction.

1 – proliferating epithelial cells of a gland.

The study drugs were prescribed for the first 5 days after the screening visit. After that, the study drug was discontinued and patients remained on the standard-of-care therapy for the 30 days of follow-up (until compensation of their clinical status).

The following tests were performed in this study:

- body mass and the volume of excreted fluid,
- results of 6-minute test,
- Clinical Status Assessment Scale score (points),
- plasma levels of the endotoxin,
- feces flora composition and enzyme activity of the microorganisms,
- results of colonoscopy with cecum biopsy and further histopathology and histochemistry of the obtained samples.

These tests were performed on Day 1, Day 6 and Day 30 of the study.

After the study treatment period, all patients were switched to the supportive care regimen and received the standard-of-care therapy; this phase lasted for 30 days.

One patient died while on study (CHF decompensation was the cause of death).

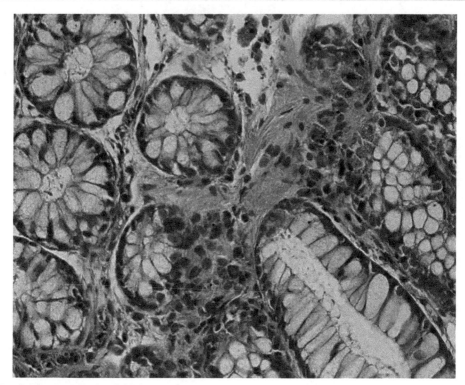

Fig. 8. Biopsy sample of the large intestine mucosa. Hematoxylin-eosin stain. 1 – siderophage.

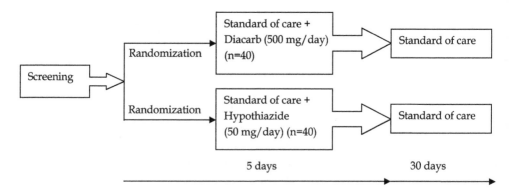

Fig. 9. Study design for the assessment of efficacy of Diacarb (acetazolamide) and Hypothiazide (hydrochlorothiazide) in comprehensive therapy of CHF patients with NYHA III-IV.

Data from 79 subjects who completed the study was therefore used for the analysis of study results.

During the study, 15 adverse reactions were reported, but none of these caused discontinuation of the study treatment.

No statistically significant differences between groups were demonstrated for the main variables.

2.8 Changes of body mass and volume of excreted urine over time

To determine efficacy of each study diuretic regimen, changes of the body mass and the volume of excreted urine were evaluated throughout the study. After the first five days, a decrease of body mass to 83±0.5 kg and 83.1±0.36 kg was demonstrated in both Group 1 and Group 2, respectively. The decrease was statistically significant against the baseline body mass of 87 kg, but the difference between groups was not statistically significant (p=0.872).

The volume of excreted urine in the study groups was the highest on the first day of treatment, comprising 2.51±0.1 L and 2.5±0.25 L for Group 1 and Group 2, respectively. This effect decreased proportionally during the following five days in both groups. Notably, no statistically significant difference was detected between groups both in terms of body mass change (p=0.99) and in terms of the volume of excreted urine.

2.9 Changes of endotoxin levels over time

Substantial decrease of endotoxin levels on the follow-up Day 21 (1.2±0.02 EU/L to 0.2±0.01 EU/L) was demonstrated in all groups. However, in the Diacarb group, this process was substantially faster: as early as on Day 5, the endotoxin levels were at 0.4±0.02 EU/L, whereas in the thiazide diuretic group the levels were at 0.78±0.01 EU/L (p=0.012). Notably, while the diuretic effects in the Hypothiazide and Diacarb groups were almost identical, the latter group demonstrated faster decrease of the endotoxin level.

This is probably due to tissue pH change caused by Diacarb, which facilitates fast dehydration of the large intestine wall and decreases its permeability for the endotoxin. To support this hypothesis, we performed histopathology and histochemistry studies using the biopsy samples from the large intestine at Day 1 and Day 5. To exclude the role of the large intestine flora, we also monitored its composition throughout the study.

2.10 Assessment of diuretic regimen effects on structural changes in the large intestine wall over time

Assessment of the histological and histochemical patterns in the large intestine mucosa during Diacarb or Hypothiazide treatment demonstrated the following changes.In the thiazide group (Fig. 10 and Fig. 11), there were signs of reduced mucosal edema on treatment (Day 6); however, a rise of local inflammatory reaction was also evident (lymphoplasmocytic infiltration, increased number of segmented WBCs, predominantly eosinophils).This may be a relative effect caused by reduction of edema and shortening of intercellular distances rather than an absolute growth of the inflammatory infiltration.

A decrease of edema on Day 6 was also seen in the Diacarb group (Fig. 12, Fig. 13), but, in addition to that, the level of local inflammation decreased (the infiltration by lymphoid cells is consistent with low-intensity chronic inflammation).

Most probably, the difference between Diacarb and Hypothiazide in their effects on large intestine wall edema causes different permeability of the wall for the endotoxin, which results in different kinetics of blood endotoxin level reduction in the CHF patients with NYHA class III-IV. These findings may result from changes in pH of the intestinal wall, better microcirculation, and consequent decrease of infiltration. Another possibility is that Diacarb, a carbonic anhydrase inhibitor, blocks alpha-carbonic anhydrase of gram-negative bacteria, depressing their pathogenic effect on the intestinal wall.

2.11 Assessment of effects of diuretic regimens on changes of flora over time

No statistically significant changes in concentration of gram-negative bacteria both in feces and in biopsy material were demonstrated, regardless of the treatment regimen.

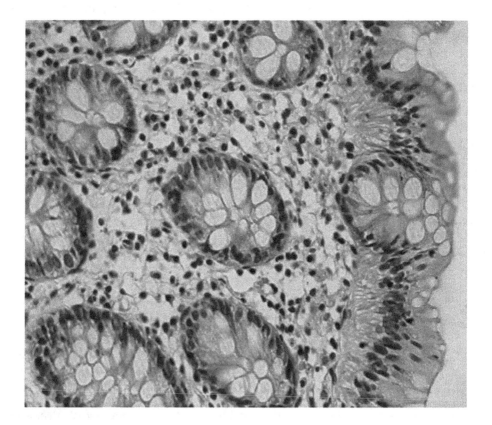

Fig. 10. Magnification x 400 (good), hematoxylin and eosin stain.Before treatment, "fuzzy" lymphoid-cellular infiltration and solitary eosinophils were noted in the *lamina propria* of the large intestine mucosa.

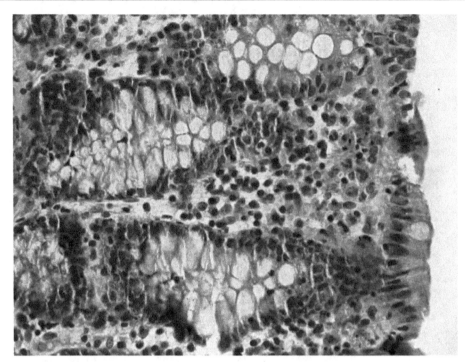

Fig. 11. Magnification x 400 (good), hematoxylin and eosin stain.Day 6 of the treatment period.Lymphoplasmocytic infiltration increases. The population of segmented WBCs, particularly eosinophils, increases significantly.

These results demonstrate that plasma endotoxin levels in CHF patients with NYHA class III-IV are affected not only by the gram-negative flora population in the intestine, but also by the severity of edema, and therefore by the degree of decompensation of patient's clinical status.The endotoxin levels in this case are probably affected by the increase of the intestinal wall permeability for the endotoxin caused by the edema.

As patient's status improves towards compensation, the endotoxin levels decrease to normal values. This process is faster with the use of Diacarb compared to the use of Hypothiazide. However, this is not accountable to their diuretic effects, because there were no statistically significant differences in the changes of body mass and the volume of excreted urine between Diacarb and Hypothiazide.It is likely that Diacarb improves microcirculation by changing tissue pH, and causes not only improvement of renal urine filtration, but also faster shrinking of tissues, particularly shrinking of the intestinal wall, which decreases its permeability for the endotoxin.

Differences in the inflammatory infiltrate intensity between Hypothiazide and Diacarb groups were discovered (in addition to decreased edema, Diacarb reduces the inflammation in the large intestine mucosa). This effect is probably accountable to improved microcirculation in the intestinal wall in the Diacarb group, as well as carbonic anhydrase inhibition produced by Diacarb leading to block of alpha-carbonic anhydrase of gram-negative bacteria, which reduces their pathogenic effect on the intestinal wall.

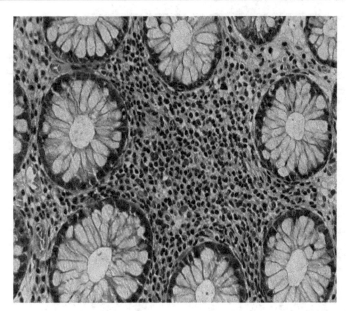

Fig. 12. Magnification x 400 (good), hematoxylin and eosin stain.Before treatment, there were hyperemic vessels and focal dense lymphoid-cellular infiltration in the *lamina propria* of the large intestine. This pattern is typical for strong chronic inflammation.

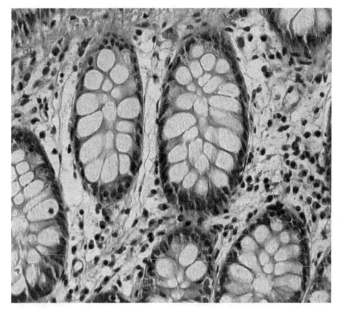

Fig. 13. Magnification x 400 (good), hematoxylin and eosin stain. Day 6 of the treatment period."Fuzzy" lymphoid-cellular infiltration is seen in the *lamina propria* of the large intestine mucosa, which is consistent with the pattern of weak chronic inflammation.

Conclusion: administration of Diacarb facilitates faster decrease of plasma endotoxin levels, which allows for faster compensation of patient's clinical status.

2.12 Use of selective decontamination alone vs. selective decontamination in combination with probiotics in comprehensive therapy of NYHA class III-IV CHF

All patients included in this phase of the study received standard-of-care therapy, including:

- ACE inhibitors/ angiotensin receptor blockers (mean daily dose of 10 mg/160 mg);
- beta-blockers (prescribed from Day 5 after the start of the therapy, dose titration from the minimum therapeutic dose, mean daily dose was 50 mg of metoprolol per day);
- digoxin 0.00025 g per day (in case of atrial fibrillation with tachycardia or LVEF below 25 %);
- aspirin 125 mg/day (secondary prophylaxis method);
- Cordarone 200 mg/day (in case of ventricular disturbances with risk of high Lown grades);
- loop diuretics (Lasix) with mean daily dose of 70 mg/day.

The following drugs were chosen for the study:

- antibacterial fluoroquinolone: ciprofloxacin with daily dose of 1000 mg;
- probiotic: Primadophilus Bifidus, 1 capsule per day.

At the study start, all patients received a 5-day selective decontamination with oral ciprofloxacin 1000 mg/day.After that, patients were randomized into two groups:

- Group 1 (n=45) received standard-of-care;
- Group 2 (n=45) received the probiotic – Primadophilus Bifidus, 1 capsule per day for 14 days.

After the completion of probiotic treatment, both groups received standard-of-care.

The following study variables were evaluated on Day 1, Day 5, and Day 21:

- results of 6-minute test,
- Clinical Status Assessment Scale score (points),
- plasma levels of the endotoxin,
- feces flora composition and enzyme activity of the microorganisms.

In this phase, 2 deaths occurred in the group receiving selective decontamination alone.In the Primadophilus Bifidus group, one patient experienced adverse effects leading to patient's decision to discontinue the drug.

Data from 87 subjects who completed the study was therefore used for the analysis of study results.

Ten cases of adverse reactions were reported during the study. Only one of these cases caused the patient to stop the drug.

The resulting groups had comparable basic characteristics.

2.13 Changes of the large intestine flora over time with the use of selective decontamination alone or selective decontamination combined with the probiotic

By Day 5 of the study, a statistically significant decrease was demonstrated in Group 1 for total population of both gram-negative microorganisms (baseline value was $10^{12\pm0.1}$ CFU/g, the value after the selective decontamination was $10^{6\pm0.4}$ CFU/g; p=0.000) and gram-positive microorganisms (baseline value was $10^{6\pm0.56}$ CFU/g, the value after the selective decontamination was $10^{4\pm0.32}$ CFU/g; p=0.000)However, on Day 21 study visit, gram-negative and gram-positive populations returned to their baseline levels ($10^{11.9}$ CFU/g and $10^{6.1}$ CFU/g, respectively; p=0.000). These results support literature reports of low efficacy of the selective decontamination used alone.

In the group where probiotics were prescribed after the course of selective decontamination, Day 5 populations decreased similarly to Group 1, both for gram-negative (baseline $10^{12.05\pm0.6}$ CFU/g, post-decontamination $10^{6.3\pm0.4}$ CFU/g; p=0.000) and gram-positive (baseline $10^{5.2\pm0.5}$ CFU/g, post-decontamination $10^{4.2\pm0.2}$ CFU/g; p=0.000) microorganisms.However, after Primadophilus Bifidus administration for 14 days, gram-positive flora population grew to $10^{8.02\pm0.1}$ CFU/g, and an insignificant growth of gram-negative flora to $10^{7.27\pm0.1}$ CFU/g was demonstrated, which is consistent with normal values for gram-negative population in the large intestine.

Conclusion: administration of probiotics after a course of selective decontamination normalizes large intestine flora levels, whereas decontamination alone leads to reduction of microbial populations for a short term only.

2.14 Changes of the endotoxin level over time

In Group 1, Day 5 endotoxin levels decreased from baseline significantly (baseline: 1.2±0.9 EU/L, Day 5: 0.55±0.06 EU/L; p=0.000), which corresponded to the reduction of gram-negative population in the large intestine. However, at Day 21, as the gram-negative population in the large intestine grew, the plasma endotoxin levels returned to their baseline values (1.18±0.05 EU/L); on Day 30, the endotoxin concentration remained high (1.21±0.045 EU/L).

In Group 2, after the selective decontamination was completed and the gram-negative population in the large intestine reduced, the plasma endotoxin levels also declined (baseline: 1.24±0.01 EU/L, Day 5: 0.67±0.03 EU/L, p=0.000). A trend towards decline of plasma endotoxin levels and achievement of normal values was demonstrated subsequently (Day 21: 0.56±0.02 EU/L, Day 30: 0.26±0.08 EU/L). These results can be explained by the reduction of the gram-negative populations in the large intestine due to administration of the selective decontamination followed by probiotic.

2.15 Assessment of changes in plasma pro-inflammatory cytokine levels over time

With the use of the selective decontamination alone, the decrease of the following variables on Day 5 was demonstrated: IL-6 to 4.1±0.03 U/L (baseline 4.9±0.01 U/L), TNF-alpha to 5±0.09 U/L (baseline 5.7±0.04 U/L), and CRP to 4 mg/ml (baseline 8.6 mg/ml).However, as early as on Day 12, these cytokine variables were shown to return to their baseline levels, which persisted till Day 30. This demonstrates poor efficacy of the selective decontamination alone for the system inflammation marker endpoints.

When the selective decontamination was used in combination with the probiotic, decrease in the population of enterobacteria in the large intestine and decrease of plasma endotoxin levels were reported.However, while levels of the pro-inflammatory cytokines decreased by Day 5 (CRP: 4.2 ± 0.1 mg/ml on Day 5 vs. baseline 7.82 ± 0.05 mg/L; IL-6: 3.9 ± 0.05 U/L on Day 5 vs. baseline 5 ± 0.01 U/L; TNF-alpha: 5.01 ± 0.02 U/L on Day 5 vs. baseline 5.8 ± 0.02 U/L), but on Day 21 they already rebounded above the baseline levels, and on Day 30 there was a trend towards further growth of their levels.

This is probably accountable to the decrease of gram-negative flora population in the large intestine due to the antibacterial treatment, and consequent decline of plasma levels of the endotoxin.Normal population numbers of the gram-negative flora are further maintained by the administration of the probiotic. However, the probiotic contains gram-positive microorganisms, which bind to the Toll-like receptors, initiating the synthesis of pro-inflammatory cytokines in the large intestine enterocytes, leading to further exacerbation of the systemic inflammation.

These results demonstrate lack of efficacy for the selective decontamination used alone.When the selective decontamination was combined with the probiotic, normalization of the intestinal flora and plasma endotoxin levels was reported. However, a significant growth of the pro-inflammatory cytokine levels occurs with this regimen, which affects patient's status and is likely to require additional correction.

These data demonstrated that comprehensive therapy for CHF combined with the selective decontamination alone (i. e. without probiotic) caused to a short-term decline of gram-negative flora population, while the population numbers of gram-positive flora remained almost unaffected. A short-term decline in plasma levels of the endotoxin and pro-inflammatory cytokines was also reported. However, as early as one week after the discontinuation of the antibacterial treatment, gram-negative flora population numbers returned to their baseline levels, accompanied by the increase in plasma levels of the endotoxin and the pro-inflammatory cytokines. A potential explanation for this pattern is that CHF patients with NYHA class III-IV develop significant restructuring of their large intestine walls, providing favorable conditions for domination of gram-negative flora.Isolated use of the selective decontamination, neither supported by any agents that repair large intestine wall structure, nor combined by any probiotics, fails to provide stable, long-term changes in the large intestine flora.

However, administration of probiotics added to the antibacterial treatment demonstrated persistent effect: normalization of gram-negative flora levels and plasma endotoxin levels. Notably, with the use of the probiotic, blood CRP levels increased, which is probably accountable to the presence of gram-positive flora in the probiotic, prompting the host to produce more antibodies. Unfortunately, the CRP levels were not followed for a longer period of time, and the time needed for the CRP to reach normal levels remained unknown.It can only be assumed that this period should not take too much time, because the subjects were exposed to the probiotic for 2 weeks only. However, if a long-term, persistent growth of the CRP levels in blood do occur, decompensated CHF patients with NYHA class III-IV might benefit from administration of statins.

3. Clinical significance of adipose tissue changes over time in patients with chronic heart failure of ischemic origin. Treatment options

3.1 Introduction

Syndrome of cardiac cachexia is one of the most severe complications of chronic heart failure. Among the latest advancements in the field of immunology is the concept of cytokine activation system and its role in the pathogenesis of chronic heart failure and development of cardiac cachexia. Currently, two main classes of cytokines are known to participate in the development of heart failure:vasoconstrictive cytokines (endothelin-1 and big endothelin) and vasodepressive cytokines (TNF-α, IL-1, IL-6, IL-8). Patients with signs of cardiac cachexia are known to have higher levels of inflammation markers than patients with normal body mass (Francis, 1998; Monteiro, 2007). Notably, adipose tissue is one of the sources of cytokines.In addition to leptin and adiponectin, adipose tissue was demonstrated to participate in production of TNF-α and IL-6 (Moses, 2004; Nagaya, 2001; Springer, 2010).

We assumed that one of the methods to decrease the activities of pro-inflammatory cytokines could be the increase of dry body mass (body muscle mass, body fat mass) (Dostalova et al., 2003). Therefore, one of the options to correct the levels of inflammatory markers in this category of patients could be nutritional support.

From our perspective, there are two possible approaches to correct the systemic inflammation:development of methods that can increase the mass of the adipose tissue and methods that have direct effect on the synthesis of pro-inflammatory cytokines.

3.2 Assessment of body composition, levels of leptin, adiponectin, and pro-inflammatory cytokines in patients with different NYHA classes of CHF

To study these variables, three consecutive groups were enrolled in the first part of the study: Group 1 included chronic heart failure patients with NYHA class I-II, Group 2 included chronic heart failure patients with NYHA class III-IV (subgroup A: without cachexia; subgroup B: with cachexia), Group 3 was a control group.Patient screening was performed in the population of patients with history of CHF of ischemic origin with NYHA class I-IV for more than 6 months, older than 40 years of age, admitted to a general internal medicine department or a cardiology department (n=197).The control group included outpatients of the Consultation and Diagnostics Polyclinic (n=52).

Clinical characteristics of the patients:

Age:these three groups were comparable in terms of patients' age.

From the results of analysis of associated clinical conditions, diabetes mellitus was reported in 57.1 % of CHF patients with NYHA class III-IV with cachexia and in 48.6 % without cachexia, as well as in 14 % of patients with NYHA class I-II.

Analysis of concomitant medications: CHF patients with NYHA class III-IV with/without cachexia were on ACE inhibitors or ARB in 64.2 %/63.8 %, on beta-adrenoblockers in 82.1 %/80 %, on digoxin in 75 %/76.1 %, on diuretics in 35.7 %/34.3 %, and on Cordarone in 28.6 %/19.5 % of cases, respectively.For NYHA class I-II patients, the corresponding variables were: on ACE inhibitors/ARB 51.6 %, on beta-adrenoblockers 59.4 %, on digoxin 9.3 %, on diuretics 45.3 %, on Cordarone 3.1 %.

3.3 Comparison of methods used to evaluate body composition in patients with CHF of different NYHA class and the control group patients

Two methods were used to study body composition: caliper measurement and bioimpedance analysis.comparison of these methods in all three groups did not reveal any statistically significant differences between the values obtained using caliper measurements and bioimpedance analyzer.However, the method of caliper measurements is subjective and is not suitable for patients with decompensated heart failure (i. e. with severe edema syndrome).Moreover, unlike caliper measurements, bioimpedance analyzer of body composition allows to estimate not only the body fat mass, but also total fluid content, which is important for the assessment of the body composition in patients with decompensated chronic heart failure.

Comparison of Group 1 vs. Group 2 revealed statistically significant differences in the adipose tissue mass, which was 29.7±2.2 kg in Group 1 and 22.2±2.1 kg in Group 2 (p<0.001), as well as in the lean body mass, which was 54.8±6.9 kg in Group 1 and 59.7±6.1 kg (p<0.001) in Group 2. This was associated with changes in total fluid content, which was 38.2±3.1 kg in Group 1 vs. 48.8±3.3 kg in patients with NYHA class III-IV (p<0.001).BMI did not differ significantly between groups.

Comparison of the study results between Group 2 (NYHA III-IV) and the control group revealed changes similar to those between Group 1 and Group 2.

Comparison of Group 1 (NYHA I-II) vs. the control group revealed statistically significant differences in the body fat mass, which was 29.7±2.2 kg in Group 1 vs. 32.6±2.4 kg in Group 3 (p<0.001), and statistically significant differences in total fluid content, which was 38.2±3.1 kg in Group 1 vs. 25.6±2.9 kg in Group 3 (p<0.001).

In patients with cachexia, a significantly lower LBM of 55.2±4.9 kg and body fat mass of 15.65±1.8 kg were reported. Notably, the total fluid content levels in these patients was greater than levels of this variable in patients without cachexia, but the differences of this variable were not statistically significant.

Conclusion: the higher is NYHA class of CHF, the stronger are changes of body composition; with higher NYHA class, adipose tissue mass declines, total fluid content grows.These changes were stronger in patients with cachexia.

3.4 Levels of leptin, adiponectin, and pro-inflammatory cytokines in patients with different NYHA classes and in the control group

The patients with NYHA III-IV were found to have adiponectin levels at 18.6±4.9 µg/mL, leptin levels at 43.8±8.3 ng/mL, IL-6 levels at 11.7±0.3 U/L, TNF-α levels at 6.6±0.2 U/L, CRP levels at 8.8±0.4 mg/ml. These values were significantly higher than values reported for patients with NYHA class I-II and for patients in the control group, who had their levels of adipokines and pro-inflammatory cytokines within normal range.

Comparison of patients with NYHA class III-IV with and without cachexia demonstrated the following differences: leptin levels were significantly higher in patients without cachexia (47.9±4.2 ng/mL), while levels of adiponectin, IL-6, TNF-α, and CRP were significantly higher in patients with cachexia.

Conclusion: the higher is NYHA class of CHF, the stronger is the intensity of chronic inflammation. While this may be an effect of growing intoxication in patients with advanced stages of CHF, this could also be associated with the role of the adipose tissue in production of pro-inflammatory cytokines and biologic agents that stimulate cytokine production. Higher classes of NYHA are associated with lower adipose tissue mass, which leads to increase of adiponectin plasma levels.However, the levels of leptin in patients with NYHA class III-IV are also high, which may be accountable to big dimensions of adipocytes. Patients with cachexia have significantly lower levels of leptin when compared to patients without cachexia; this is probably associated with shrinking of the lipid droplet in the adipocyte.

3.5 Evaluation of visceral and subcutaneous tissue structure in patients with different CHF classes

To study this variable, autopsies of deceased patients (with NYHA class I-IV chronic heart failure diagnosed before their death) were performed. Patients were allocated into two groups: Group 1: before death, patients were diagnosed with NYHA I-II chronic heart failure; Group 2: before death, patients were diagnosed with NYHA III-IV chronic heart failure. Patients of Group 2 were divided in two subgroups: patients with cachexia and patients without cachexia. All patients were admitted to GKB no. 4 (City Clinical Hospital no. 4) before death. For NYHA I-II patients, the main reasons for hospitalization were: unstable angina, acute myocardial infarction, hypertensive crisis, heart rhythm disorder, cerebrovascular accident; for NYHA III-IV patients, the main reasons for hospitalization were: decompensation of CHF, acute/recurrent myocardial infarction, heart rhythm disorder, cerebrovascular accident.The postmortem assessment included measurement of the subcutaneous fat, measurement of the omentum mass, morphometric study of the subcutaneous fat, omental fat and pericardial fat.

Of 118 subjects total, 50 subjects were in the first group, 56 subjects were in the second group, and 12 subjects belonged to the third group. These three groups were comparable in terms of patients' age. The main cause of death for NYHA I-II patients was the acute myocardial infarction (46.0 %), and for NYHA II-III patients (both with cachexia and without cachexia) the main cause of death was post-infarction cardiosclerosis (58.3 %, 48.2 %, respectively). The most frequent complication leading to death in patients with NYHA class I-II CHF was acute heart failure; in patients with NYHA class III-IV the most frequent complication leading to death was CHF decompensation. Pneumonia incidence in patients with NYHA class III-IV was higher (22 %) than in NYHA I-II patients (4 %). Multiple complications were reported for 22.0 % patients with NYHA I-II, 46.4 % patients with NYHA III-IV without cachexia, and 100 % of patients with NYHA III-IV with cachexia.

During autopsy, the following investigations were performed: measurement of subcutaneous fat thickness 2 cm below the navel, measurement of omentum weight; autopsy samples of subcutaneous fat, omental fat, and pericardial fat at the apex of the heart were collected.

There were no statistically significant differences between patients with NYHA I-II and NYHA III-IV without cachexia in the thickness of subcutaneous fat: it was 5.3±1.7 cm and 5.1±2.2, respectively (p=0.6).In CHF patients with NYHA III-IV with cachexia, the difference in thickness of subcutaneous fat (2.4±1.1 cm) was statistically different from NYHA III-IV patients without cachexia (p<0.001).

In CHF patients with NYHA class III-IV, omentum weight was significantly lower than in patients with NYHA I-II (387±134 g vs. 521±142 g, respectively; p<0.001).In CHF patients with NYHA classes III and IV, the omentum weight was 164±87 g, which is significantly lower than in patients without cachexia (p<0.001).

The morphometric analysis of the samples showed the following changes.In the subcutaneous fat, lymphocytic infiltration was the strongest in patients with NYHA class III-IV with cachexia (average 12.4±4.7 %); in patients with NYHA class I-II this variable was 3.8±2.2 % (comparison: p<0.001), and in NYHA III-IV patients without cachexia it was 4.3±2.4 % (comparison: p<0.001).No significant differences in the proportion of fibrous tissue in the subcutaneous fat was found between the groups.The percentage of fibrous tissue was 3.8±1.9 % in NYHA class I-II patients, 4.1±2.3 % in NYHA class III-IV patients without cachexia, and 4.6±2.6 % in NYHA class III-IV patients with cachexia (p1-2=0.469, p1-3=0.229, p2-3=0.506). See Fig. 14, 15, 16.

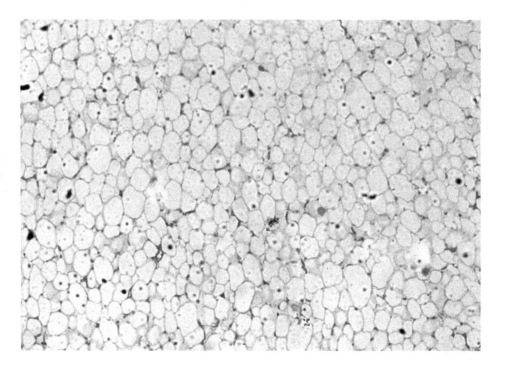

Fig. 14. Subcutaneous fat in a CHF patient with NYHA class I. Romanowsky-Giemsa stain.

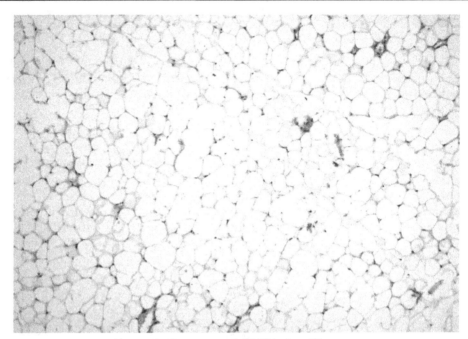

Fig. 15. Subcutaneous fat in a CHF patient with NYHA class III.

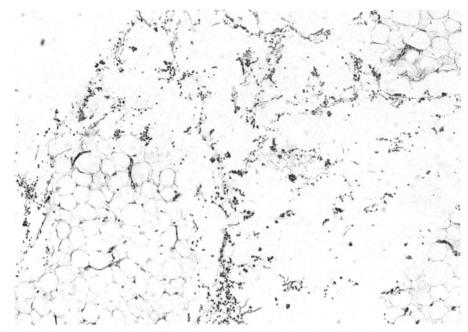

Fig. 16. Subcutaneous fat in a CHF patient with NYHA class IV with cachexia.
Romanowsky-Giemsa stain.

Analysis of the visceral fat (omentum, pericardial fat) showed the strongest lymphocytic infiltration in subjects with NYHA class III-IV, both with cachexia and without cachexia. This variable was 53.4±7.8 % in the omentum and 49.7±8.4 % in the pericardium in patients with cachexia, and 42.1±6.7 % in the omentum and 42.6±8.8 % in the pericardium in patients without cachexia (compare to patients with NYHA I-II, who had the lymphocytic infiltration of 5.1±2.3 % in the omentum (p1<0.001, p2<0.001) and 4.9±2.6 % in the pericardium (p1<0.001, p2<0.001)).The amount of fibrous tissue in NYHA class III-IV patients without cachexia was higher than in the patients with NYHA class I-II: 15.2±4.9 % vs. 3.1±1.2 % in the omental adipose tissue (p<0.001), 14.8±5.4 % vs. 3.2±0.9 % in the adipose tissue of the pericardium (p<0.001), respectively.In NYHA III-IV patients with cachexia, the amount of fibrous tissue was significantly higher than in NYHA III-IV patients without cachexia: 24.8±3.7 % in the omentum (p<0.001) and 24.3±3.2 % in the pericardium (p<0.001).See figures 17-22.

Mean diameter of adipocytes was measured, with the following results:In CHF patients with NYHA class I-II, the diameter of adipocytes was 38.6±12.2 µm in the subcutaneous fat samples, 44.2±16.1 µm in the omentum, 42.3±11.4 µm in the pericardial fat. In CHF patients with NYHA class III-IV without cachexia, the diameter of adipocytes was 42.7±14.2 µm in the subcutaneous fat samples (p=0.116), 56.4±13.9 µm in the omentum (p<0.001), 52.2±11.3 µm in the pericardial fat (p<0.001). In NYHA class III-IV patients with cachexia, the diameter of adipocytes was 28.2±11.5 µm in the subcutaneous fat samples (p=0.01), 32.8±14.3 µm in the omentum (p=0.028), 30.3±12.4 µm in the pericardial fat (p<0.001).

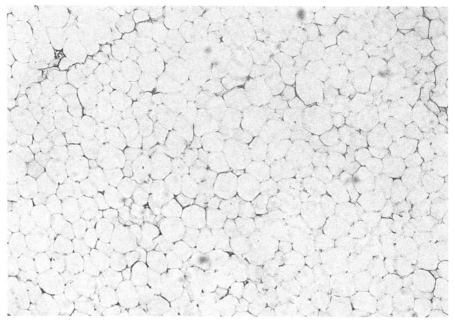

Fig. 17. Visceral adipose tissue (pericardial fat) in a CHF patient with NYHA class I. Romanowsky-Giemsa stain.

Fig. 18. Visceral adipose tissue (omentum) in a CHF patient with NYHA class I. Romanowsky-Giemsa stain.

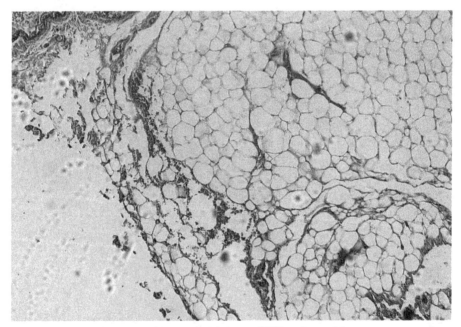

Fig. 19. Visceral adipose tissue (pericardial fat) in a CHF patient with NYHA class III.Romanowsky-Giemsa stain.

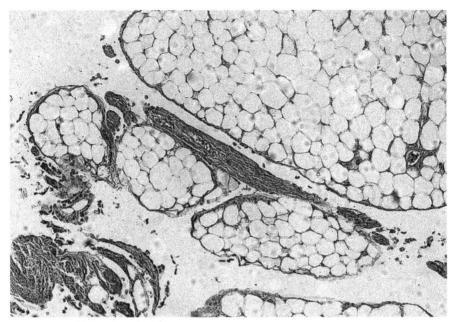

Fig. 20. Visceral adipose tissue (omentum) in a NYHA class III patient without cachexia. Van Gieson's stain.

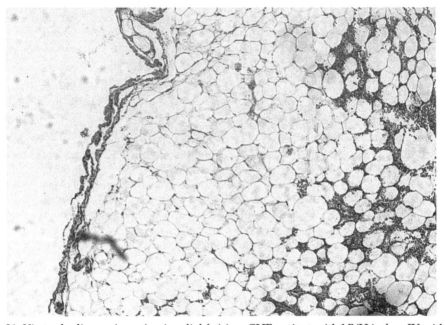

Fig. 21. Visceral adipose tissue (pericardial fat) in a CHF patient with NYHA class IV with cachexia.Romanowsky-Giemsa stain.

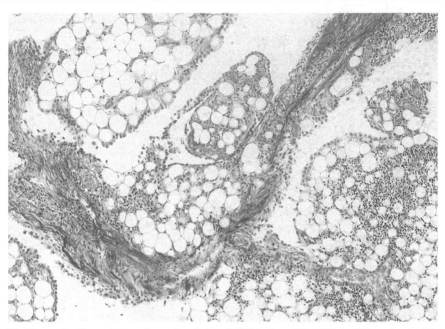

Fig. 22. Visceral adipose tissue (omentum) in a NYHA class IV patient with cachexia. Van Gieson's stain.

Therefore, the higher is NYHA class, the lower are the subcutaneous fat and the omentum weight. The higher is NYHA class, the more intensive is the chronic inflammation, manifested by the lymphocytic infiltration and the content of fibrous tissue, especially in the visceral fat.These changes are stronger in NYHA III-IV patients with cachexia.

In patients with NYHA III-IV and cachexia, a decrease in the content of adipose tissue was demonstrated to be the result of adipocyte shrinking, as well as substitution of the adipose tissue by fibrous tissue.

Currently, there is no solution for the problem of how to increase the body muscle mass and body fat mass in patients with cachexia, particularly with cardiac cachexia. Unfortunately, all attempts to use anabolic steroids in this patient population have been unsuccessful.We assumed that using nutritional support in this patient population would allow to change the nutritional status in addition to reducing the malabsorption syndrome. Moreover, nutritional mixes that have both local and systemic anti-inflammatory effect are currently available. Administration of these mixes might help fighting the inflammation observed in the large intestine of the CHF patients with higher classes of NYHA, as well as reducing their blood levels of pro-inflammatory cytokines.

3.6 Comparison of efficacy of Modulen vs. Peptamen added to standard-of-care therapy in CHF patients with NYHA III-IV

Screening was performed in a consecutive population of patients hospitalized to general internal medicine or cardiology departments (n=144).

Morphology and Functional Changes of Intestine, Trophology Status and Systemic Inflammation in Patients with
Chronic Heart Failure

161

Inclusion and exclusion criteria are shown in Table 5.

Inclusion criteria	Exclusion criteria
• CHF of ischemic origin • CHF history for more than 12 months • Age > 40 years old • Patient's consent to participation in the study	• Acute or chronic infectious diseases • Cancer within last 5 years • Severe impairment of liver or kidneys (AST, ALT > 3 x upper limit of normal, creatinine > 250 µmol/L) • Mental disorders • Primary or secondary immunodeficiency conditions • Alcohol or substance dependence • Any conditions that can cause cachexia (at investigator's discretion) • Lack of tolerance to enteral nutrition regimen • Unable to sign the informed consent • Unable to follow the study procedures

Table 5. Inclusion and exclusion criteria.

Chronic heart failure patients with NYHA class III-IV were randomized into three groups, 40 subjects in each:

- Patients in Group 1 received Modulen (balanced nutritional mix for enteral tube feeding or oral feeding) in addition to standard-of-care therapy.
- Patients in Group 2 received Peptamen (balanced nutritional mix for enteral tube feeding or oral feeding) in addition to standard-of-care therapy.
- Patients in Group 3 received the standard-of-care therapy only, as well as the necessary amount of nutrients in a standard diet designed for cardiology patients.

All patients received standard-of-care therapy, which included:

• ACE inhibitors/ angiotensin receptor antagonists (mean daily dose of 10 mg/160 mg);
• beta-blockers (prescribed from Day 5 after the start of the therapy, dose titration from the minimum therapeutic dose, mean daily dose was 12.5 mg of carvedilol per day);
• digoxin 0.00025 g per day (in case of atrial fibrillation with tachycardia or sinus rhythm with LVEF below 25 %);
• aspirin 125 mg/day (secondary prophylaxis method);
• loop diuretics (Lasix) with mean daily dose of 60 mg/day.

The following procedures were performed for every patient:medical history; physical examination, including measurement of weight, height, waist circumference, hip circumference, wrist circumference, arm circumference; casual BP; heart rate; fasting chemistry lab blood samples; 6-minute test; echocardiography for the measurement of the ejection fraction; caliper measurements; bioimpedance analysis of body composition to measure the lean body mass (LBM), body fat mass (BFM), total water content (TW); Clinical Status Assessment Score.

Group 1 patients received nutritional mix Modulen (100-130 g of dry mix), which accounted for 25 % of their daily energy demands, in addition to their basic diet.Group 2 patients received nutritional mix Peptamen (100-130 g of dry mix), which accounted for 25 % of their daily energy demands, in addition to their basic diet.Group 3 patients received their standard therapy only, as well as the necessary amount of nutrients within a standard diet, based on pre-calculated energy demands.All patients maintained their dietary diaries, which were used to adjust the diet on an individual basis.

The energy demands were calculated using Harris-Benedict formula with adjustment for body mass deficit, taking into account body temperature and activity of a patient.

Energy demands:

$$AEC = EOO*AF*TF*BMD \qquad (1)$$

where:AEC — actual energy consumption (kcal/day);

EOO — basal metabolic rate, calculated using Harris-Benedict equations:

EOO (men) = 66 + (13.7*body mass, kg) + (5*height, cm) - (6.8*age)

EOO (women) = 655 + (9.6*body mass, kg) + (1.8*height, cm) - (4.7*age)

AF — activity factor (bed rest: 1.1, movement within room: 1.2, no limitations: 1.3), TF — temperature factor (36–37.0°C: 1.0, 37.1–38.0°C: 1.1, 38.1–39.0°C: 1.2), BMD — body mass deficit (10–20 %: 1.1, 20–30 %: 1.2, >30 %: 1.3).

This study enrolled 120 patients.Males: 18 subjects (45 %) in Group 1, 19 subjects (47.5 %) in Group 2, and 21 subjects (52.5 %) in Group 3.Females: 22 subjects (55 %) in Group 1, 21 subjects (52.5 %) in Group 2, and 19 subjects (47.5 %) in Group 3.

Total duration of CHF history was 15.3±4.3 months, 15.7±4.1 months, and 15.6±4.4 months for Group 1, Group 2, and Group 3, respectively.These characteristics were not significantly different between study groups.

Compensated type 2 diabetes mellitus was reported in 52.5 %, 55 %, and 42.5 % of subjects in Group 1, Group 2, and Group 3, respectively.

Charlson index was > 5 in all groups.

As demonstrated above, there were no statistically significant differences between groups in gender, age, and co-morbidity rates.

In all three groups, decreases of weight and LBM were demonstrated on Day 21 of the treatment period:in Group 1, Day 21 body weight was 56.4±2.6 kg (baseline 66.9±3.5 kg); in Group 2, Day 21 body weight was 56.4±2.1 kg (baseline 66.2±2.9 kg); in Group 3, Day 21 body weight was 55.4±1.7 kg (baseline 67.0±2.9 kg); in Group 1, Day 21 LBM was 40.9±1.7 kg (baseline LBM 47.2±1.9 kg); in Group 2, Day 21 LBM was 42.0±2.0 kg (baseline LBM 47.3±2.0 kg); in Group 3, Day 21 LBM was 41.2±1.9 kg (baseline LBM 46.9±1.8 kg).However, on Day 224, the body weight in Group 1 increased to 62.6±2.7 kg, but was significantly lower than in Group 2 (66.8±2.4 kg) and Group 3 (68.7±1.9 kg).The LBM also increased on Day 224, but it was lower than baseline LBM in Group 1 (44.4±1.6 kg), whereas it reached the baseline in Group 2 (47.4±2.2 kg) and significantly exceeded the baseline in Group 3 (48.1±1.9 kg).

In Group 2 and Group 3, a statistically significant decrease of total fluid content on Day 21 was demonstrated: 34.6±1.8 kg in Group 2 (baseline 47.3±2.1 kg) and 34.4±1.7 in Group 3 (baseline 47.1±1.7 kg).On Day 224, the total fluid content increased in both of these groups: 47.2±2.0 kg and 48.3±1.9, respectively.In Group 1, the total fluid content also decreased by Day 21 (34.3±1.9 kg) compared to baseline (46.8±2.0 kg), but there was no significant increase of the total fluid content on Day 224 (39.3±1.9 kg), unlike in other two groups.

On Day 224, the body fat mass increased significantly in Group 1 to 18.6±1.11 kg (baseline 16,8±1.13 kg), while no significant change in the body fat mass was reported for Group 2 and Group 3:16.8±1.13 kg (baseline 16.5±1.16 kg) in Group 2 and 16.6±1.33 kg (baseline 16.5±1.19 kg) in Group 3.

On Day 21, the BMI decreased from baseline in all groups:21.2±0.60 kg/m^2 in Group 1 (baseline 24.1±0.93 kg/m^2); 21.4±0.59 kg/m^2 in Group 2 (baseline 24.1±0.86 kg/m^2); and 21.5±0.64 kg/m^2 in Group 3 (baseline 24.3±1.01 kg/m^2).On Day 224, the BMI returned to baseline and was 23.7±0.62 kg/m^2 in Group 1, 23.7±0.58 kg/m^2 in Group 2, and 24.5±0.60 kg/m^2 in Group 3.

The body mass increased in all three study groups, but in patients on Modulen this was accountable to increase of muscle and fat mass, and not to increase of total fluid content.This suggests that administration of Modulen improves the nutritional status profile.

Assessment of NT-proBNP, adiponectin, leptin, CRP, IL-6, TNF-α during administration of Modulen and Peptamen added to standard-of-care therapy in CHF patients with NYHA class III-IV.

The level of NT-proBNP in all groups was over 3000 pg/mL.

Reduction of chronic inflammation intensity was demonstrated in patients receiving Modulen:on Day 224, there was a decrease in levels of CRP (4.7±0.4 mg/ml vs. baseline 8.9±0.7 mg/mL), IL-6 (5.2±0.4 U/L vs. baseline 11.8±0.8 U/L), TNF-α (3.4±0.2 U/L vs. baseline 6.8±0.4 U/L).Levels of adiponectin also declined in patients on Modulen: 15.8±1.5 μg/mL vs. baseline 24.4±1.5 μg/mL. No significant changes were demonstrated in Group 2 and Group 3.

There were no significant changes of leptin levels in any of the groups.

Assessment of hospitalization events showed the following results.In Group 1, during treatment with Modulen, 32 hospitalization events were reported per year: 22 hospitalizations were due to CHF decompensations, in 12 of these cases congestive pneumonia was also present; 2 events were due to myocardial infarctions; 5 events were for hypertensive crisis, with 2 of them progressing to CVA; 3 events were due to fibrillation paroxysms. Per-patient hospitalization rate was 0.55±0.01 event/person.There were 5 deaths over one year of observation in Group 1:2 deaths were caused by CHF decompensation, 2 deaths were caused by CVA, 1 death was caused by AMI.

In Group 1, during treatment with Peptamen, 38 hospitalization events were reported over one year of observation:of these, 27 hospitalization events were due to CHF decompensations, with 15 cases accompanied by congestive pneumonia; 3 events were due to acute myocardial infarctions; 7 events were due to hypertensive crisis, 1 of them progressed to CVA; 4 events were due to fibrillation paroxysms. Per-patient hospitalization rate was 0.95±0.02 event/person.There were 8 deaths over one year of observation in Group 2:5 deaths were caused by CHF decompensation, 2 deaths were caused by AMI, 1 death was caused by CVA.

In Group 3, 48 hospitalizations were reported over one year of observation: 41 events were due to CHF decompensations, in 22 of which congestive pneumonia was also present; 2 events were due to acute myocardial infarctions; 4 events were for hypertensive crisis, with 2 cases progressing to CVA; 1 event was due to a fibrillation paroxysm.Per-patient hospitalization rate was 1.2±0.03 event/person.There were 12 deaths over one year of observation in Group 3:8 deaths were caused by CHF decompensation, 2 deaths were caused by AMI, 2 deaths were caused by CVA.

4. Conclusion

Rates of hospitalization events and deaths over one year were lower in subjects receiving Modulen compared to Peptamen and standard-of-care therapy.

5. References

Anker S.D., Negassa A, Coats AJ et al. (2003). Prognostic importance of weight loss in chronic heart failure and the effect of treatment with angiotensin-converting-enzyme inhibitors: an observational study. *Lancet,*Vol.361, No.9363, (March 2003), pp.1077-1083, ISSN0140-6736

Dostalova I., Kavalkova P., Papezova H., Domluvilova D., Zikan V., Haluzik M. (2010).Association of macrophage inhibitory cytokine-1 with nutritional status, body composition and bone mineral density in patients with anorexia nervosa: the influence of partial realimentation.*Nutrition & Metabolism,*Vol.7, (April 2010), pp.34, ISSN 1743-7075

Francis G.S. (1998). Changing the remodeling process in heart failure: basic mechanism and laboratory results. *Current opinion in cardiology,* Vol.13, No.3, (May 1998), pp.156-161, ISSN 0268-4705

Harrington D., Anker S.D. (1997).Skeletal muscle function and its relation to exercise tolerance in CHF.*Journal of the American College of Cardiology,* Vol.30, No.7, (December 1997), pp.1758-1764, ISSN 0735-1097

Monteiro M.P., Ribeiro A.H., Nunes A.F. (2007).Increase in grelin levels after weight loss in obese zucker rats is prevented by gastric banding. *Obesity Surgery,*Vol.17, No.12, (November 2007), pp.1599-1607, ISSN 0960-8923

Moses A.W.G., Slater C., Preston T., Barber M.D., Fearon K.C.H. (2004). Reduced total energy expenditure and physical activity in cachectic patients with pancreatic cancer can be modulated by an energy and protein dense oral supplement enriched with n-3 fatty acids. *British Journal of Cancer,*Vol.90, No.5, (March 2004), pp.996-1002, ISSN 0007-0920

Nagaya N., Uematsu M., Kojima M. (2001). Elevated Circulating Level of Ghrelin in Cachexia Associated With Chronic Heart Failure. *Circulation,*Vol.104, No.17, (October 2001), pp. 2034-2038, ISSN 0009-7322

Springer J., Adams V., Anker S. D. (2010).Myostatin Regulator of Muscle Wasting in Heart Failure and Treatment Target for Cardiac Cachexia.*Circulation,*Vol.121, No.3, (January 2010), pp. 354-356, ISSN 0009-7322

8

Role of Echocardiography in Research into Neglected Cardiovascular Diseases in Sub-Saharan Africa

Ana Olga Mocumbi
National Health Institute & University Eduardo Mondlane,
Mozambique

1. Introduction

Echocardiography is a non-invasive imaging technique that has been important in improving the quality and reliability of cardiovascular diagnosis, but access to it remains limited in most developing countries in Africa due to the costs of the technique and the lack of highly specialized personnel to perform it. Training in echocardiography is part of the postgraduate residency training requirements in cardiology in most African countries, despite the absence of an accreditation process such as that designed in Europe and United States of America (Ogah et al., 2006). While the use of transthoracic echocardiography has been spreading slowly around the continent, transesophageal echocardiography is still limited to few centers.

Barriers to obtaining ultrasound services in Sub-Saharan Africa include distance, time, cost of transfers and ultrasound charges (Shah et al., 2008). However, compared to other diagnostic imaging modalities echocardiography is safe, portable and inexpensive, uses simple power supply, and requires minimal maintenance. These characteristics make it the most suitable imaging technique for low-resource areas of Sub-Saharan Africa, where the introduction of smaller and battery-powered ultrasound machines is being used to reach out for people living in remote areas that traditionally did not have access to specialized cardiovascular diagnosis and care.

While witnessing an increasing awareness of the epidemic of cardiovascular disease, encompassing conditions such as hypertension, acute coronary syndrome, stroke and chronic heart failure, Sub-Saharan Africa still has a high burden of several infectious-related cardiovascular diseases and specific conditions such as cardiomyopathies. These neglected cardiovascular diseases include amongst others rheumatic heart disease (RHD) and endomyocardial fibrosis (EMF), both representing a considerable source of burden to the communities and playing a major role in determining premature mortality around the continent. Having recognized the potential of echocardiography as a research tool, African scientists have been using this technique to describe the epidemiology and profile of neglected cardiovascular conditions, as well as to bring new insights into the main causes of heart failure in both pediatric and adult populations (Mocumbi et al., 2008; Sani et al., 2007; Jaiyesimi & Antia, 1981a, b; Marijon et al., 2007; Adesanya 1979).

RHD and EMF have been the subject of community- and hospital-based research using echocardiography. This has resulted in an increase in the number of publications from Africa in indexed medical journals during the last decade. However, the increase is far from the desirable as the number of epidemiological and clinical studies using echocardiography augmented from 6 to 15 for RHD and from 2 to 4 for EMF (Figure 1).

In this chapter we review the recent use of transthoracic echocardiography worldwide for advancing knowledge about the pathogenesis and natural history of RHD and EMF, focusing on the modalities most readily available in low-resource settings, namely bidimensional, M-mode, pulsed and continuous Doppler. Finally, we discuss the specific role of echocardiography in fostering research into these two endemic diseases in Africa, and present the current challenges and opportunities of the use of this technique in Sub-Saharan Africa.

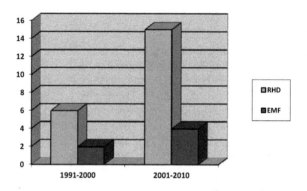

Fig. 1. Number of publications in indexed journals that reported hospital or community-based epidemiological and clinical studies using echocardiographic diagnosis for Rheumatic Heart Disease (RHD) and Endomyocardial Fibrosis (EMF) in the last two decades in Africa.

2. Endomyocardial fibrosis

EMF is a restrictive cardiomyopathy of unknown etiology characterised by progressive fibrous thickening of the ventricular endocardium, leading to restrictive physiology associated with atrioventricular valve dysfunction. Most of our knowledge of this condition comes from hospital-based studies in endemic areas of Uganda, Cote d'Ivoire, Nigeria, India and Brazil. Data on its exact epidemiology are scarce, but variations in geographical and ethnic distribution have been reported, stimulating the search for both environmental factors and genetic factors.

EMF is thought to be the commonest restrictive cardiomyopathy worldwide (Somers, 1990), affecting mainly children and adolescents of low-income communities from tropical regions of Africa, Asia and South America. Established and advanced disease can be easily diagnosed by clinical examination in endemic areas, but the finding of relatively asymptomatic individuals who present important echocardiographic abnormalities is not rare (Mocumbi et al., 2008; Salemi et al., 2005). The characterisation of early stages of the disease has not been systematically done, leading to major gaps in our knowledge of its pathogenesis and natural history.

The use of echocardiography for diagnosis of EMF, started almost half a century ago, has contributed to characterization of the disease and better understanding of its pathophysiology, resulting in improvements in management and prognosis. Several authors from different parts of the world have described the clinical and echocardiographic findings in EMF (Acquatella et al., 1979; Gonzalez-Lavin et al., 1982; Vijayaraghavan et al., 1983; Okereke et al., 1991; Rashwan et al.,1995), and more recently there have been attempts to use this technique for understanding its epidemiology (Mocumbi et al., 2008) as well define prognostic criteria prior to surgery (Mady et al., 2004).

2.1 Echocardiographic features

The hallmark of established EMF is the presence of thickened endocardium, ventricular obliteration and dilated atria. The typical image of restrictive cardiomyopathy is that of inversion of the size of heart cavities with small obliterated ventricles and dilated atria (Hassan et al., 2005; Berensztein et al., 2000). The wide spectrum of distribution and severity of the fibrotic lesions, as well as the changes in heart shape and distortion mandate a careful and comprehensive echocardiographic evaluation of each patient, using the usual and less conventional views.

The most characteristic echocardiographic features of EMF are large endocardial plaques, patchy endocardial thickening, obliteration of ventricular apices or valve recesses, ventricular and atrial thrombi, ventricular cavity volume reduction, enlarged atrium, restricted mobility of the atrioventricular valve leaflets, fusion of the papillary muscles to the wall and abnormalities of the ventricular regional wall motion (Okereke et al., 1991; Mady et al., 2005; Hassan et al., 2005; Berensztein et al., 2000). Less specific echocardiographic abnormalities include diffuse atrioventricular valve leaflet thickening, enhanced echodensity of the moderator band or trabeculae, abnormal movement of the interventricular septum and/or posterior LV wall, and presence of thickened left ventricular "false tendon" (Mocumbi et al., 2008). Moderate to massive pericardial effusion is a frequent finding in both left and right forms of EMF (George et al., 1982; Lowenthal & Teeger, 2000). Occasionally, endocardial calcification may be seen in the ventricles (Lowenthal & Teeger, 2000; Morrone et al., 1996; Trigo et al., 2010).

The pattern of distribution of the morphological and hemodynamic abnormalities allows the classification of EMF in different forms according to exclusive or predominant distribution of structural lesions in one or both sides of the heart. Hence the description of right, left and bilateral EMF.

2.1.1 Endocardial thickening

Thickening of the endocardium is the most characteristic feature of established EMF (Ojereke et al., 1991; Connor et al., 1967). It may consist of large plaques affecting one or both ventricles, as well as patchy endocardial thickening evenly distributed in the ventricular walls or affecting exclusively the interventricular septum. These abnormalities can be assessed by both bidimensional and M-mode. The most striking and constant features are increased amplitude echos at the right ventricular trabecular region, left ventricular apex and the region of the posterior mitral valve leaflet (Vijayaraghavan et al., 1983).

2.1.2 Ventricular thrombosis

Spontaneous contrast and ventricular thrombi are frequently seen in normally contracting ventricles in early stages of EMF, as part of the initial process that leads to endocardial fibrosis (Berensztein et al., 2000). The presence of ventricular thrombi, calcified or not, is a major determinant of management and prognosis.

2.1.3 Ventricular obliteration

This characteristic abnormality of EMF consists in partial or complete exclusion of a portion of the ventricle from the circulation (Figure 2). In right EMF the trabecular portion of the ventricle is separated from the remaining cavity by a large fibrotic endocardial plaque, underneath which there is myocardium of apparently normal texture (Trigo et al., 2010). Left ventricular obliteration affects both the apex and the recesses of the posterior mitral valve leaflet excluding these parts from the ventricular cavity (Berensztein et al., 2000). It is thought that obliteration by thrombi and subsequent scarring fibrosis are the mechanisms involved (Connor et al., 1967), both leading to reduction of the diastolic properties of the ventricles. Also, thrombi may involve the sub-valvar apparatus, leading to scarring and fusion of leaflets to the ventricular wall, therefore resulting in leaflet movement restriction and severe atrioventricular valve dysfunction.

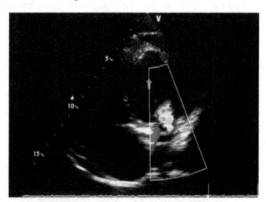

Fig. 2. Left-sided EMF with obliteration and endocardial thickening at the ventricular apex. The atypical mitral regurgitation jet is frequent in moderate disease.

With progression of the disease to more advanced stages cavity retraction occurs with further reduction of the effective ventricular cavity volume, seemingly due to progressive organization and fibrosis of the mural thrombi and adjacent endocardium. Particularly in the right ventricle, this process is associated with pulling of the wall by the retracted tricuspid valve apparatus, resulting in the distinctive finding of advanced right-sided EMF called "apical notch" (Figure 3). The apical notch gives the heart a shape that resembles the map of Africa, hence the designation "Heart of Africa" (Davies, 1960). On the left side the ventricular apex is never retracted; it becomes thicker leading to considerable reduction of the longitudinal diameter of the ventricle, resulting in a spherical ventricular shape.

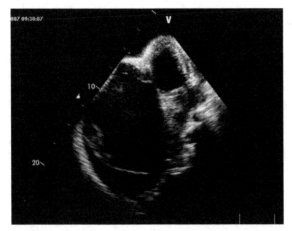

Fig. 3. Transthoracic image obtained during field research using a portable ultrasound machine showing retraction of the trabecular portion of the right ventricle with reduction of cavity size and aneurysmal right atrium in which a thrombus can be seen.

2.1.4 Diffuse leaflet thickening

Diffuse thickening of the atrioventricular valve leaflets occurs in some patients with EMF. This pattern helps differentiating left-sided EMF with predominant valvular lesion from chronic rheumatic disease of the mitral valve in endemic areas for both diseases. In chronic rheumatic mitral regurgitation leaflet thickening is usually restricted to or exaggerated at the tip of the valve, extends to the chordae, and is never associated to obliteration of the contralateral ventricle (Saraiva et al., 1999; Metras et al., 1983).

2.1.5 Septal motion abnormalities

The restricted movement of the fibrotic left ventricular apex and its obliteration are accompanied by compensatory contractile mechanism that results in exaggerated and distinctive motion of the basal portion of the left ventricle, the so-called Merlon sign (Vijayaraghavan et al., 1983; Berensztein et al., 2000). On M-mode the interventricular septum has a rapid anterior movement in early diastole (Acquatella et al., 1979) assuming an M-shaped movement. In some patients the septal motion may be reversed (paradoxical septal movement).

2.1.6 Restrictive filling pattern

A tall E wave with E/A ratio greater than 2, deceleration time less than 120ms and isovolumic relaxation time inferior to 160ms are the criteria used to define the presence of ventricular restrictive filling pattern. This evaluation is usually compromised by the presence of severe mitral regurgitation. The brisk early diastolic filling with poor filling in the remainder of diastole, the absence of respiratory changes, the presence of normal pericardium and the usual association to pericardial effusion, enable distinction from constrictive pericarditis.

2.1.7 Atrioventricular valve regurgitation

Mild mitral regurgitation is found in initial stages of left EMF. The jet is atypical and seems to start inside the ventricular cavity (figure 2). In severe left EMF thickening and scarring of the valve leaflets and the mitral valve apparatus lead to severe mitral regurgitation that is usually eccentric, due mainly to restricted movement of the posterior leaflet. The regurgitation has a high velocity jet directed to the posterior wall of the left atrium, reaching the pulmonary veins in most cases (Figure 4).

The tricuspid valve apparatus is distorted in EMF with restricted movement of the leaflets in early phases of the disease. In severe right EMF there is massive tricuspid annulus dilatation and non-turbulent low velocity regurgitant jet, witnessing the absence of pressure gradient between the two right cavities. In these cases the right filling pressures are very high, leading to severe dilatation of the cava system and reflux from the right atrium towards the supra-hepatic veins, a phenomenon easily accessed using pulsed and color Doppler.

2.1.8 Atrial dilatation

Both the restriction to ventricular filling and the atrioventricular valve regurgitation result in increase in atrial pressure, leading to progressive atrial dilatation. The consequence is further increase in atrioventricular valve annulus dilatation perpetuating the cycle and being responsible for the frequent finding of aneurysmal atria (Hassan et al., 2005; Berensztein et al., 2000). Annular dilatation, leaflet retraction and fibrosis of the sub-valvar apparatus lead to non-coaptation and free tricuspid valve regurgitation (Okereke et al., 1991), this later seen as a non-turbulent low velocity jet on color Doppler.

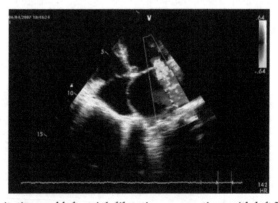

Fig. 4. Mitral regurgitation and left atrial dilatation on a patient with left EMF evaluated using portable ultrasound machine during a community-based study.

2.1.9 Semilunar valve abnormalities

The pulmonary valve is usually spared from structural abnormalities but there is often pulmonary regurgitation that allows estimation of the mean and diastolic pulmonary pressures. In severe cases due to the lack of pressure gradient between the atrium, the ventricle and the pulmonary artery, there is often diastolic opening of the pulmonary valve. The aortic valve is almost always normal, but in few cases there may be thickening of the cusps.

2.1.10 Abnormalities of the left side of the heart

Early left-sided EMF is characterized by thickening of the mitral leaflets, presence of apical thrombus, and/or obliteration of the apex or the recess between the posterior leaflet and the posterior wall. Thrombi may be found in the sub-valvar apparatus involving the free edges of both papillary muscles or in the apex. There is moderate left atrial dilatation but the valve remains non-regurgitant. The flow across the mitral valve reveals early diastolic filling followed by restriction pattern.

In the established left-sided EMF endocardial thickening is prominent in interventricular septum, the apex and posterior wall behind the recess of the posterior mitral leaflet, the ventricular cavity assumes a spherical shape and there is increased contractility at its basal portion. The left ventricular ejection fraction is usually not calculated due to the presence of mitral regurgitation and left ventricular distortion. The heart distortion and change in the position of the heart in the chest explains the fact that contractility is often graded using a visual scale. In patients without severe distortion of the left ventricular shape and no mitral regurgitation, the LV end-systolic and end-diastolic volumes and ejection fraction can be determined from the apical 4-chamber view according to the modified Simpson's rule or the Teicholz method (Feigenbaum, 1994).

Although in rare patients the mitral valve may be stenotic, most patients present an eccentric mitral regurgitation with signs of passive pulmonary hypertension. The left atrium maximal linear dimensions at the end of left ventricular systole are increased in all plans and, in severe cases the cavity may be aneurysmal. However, there is rarely left atrial thrombus.

Regarding the mitral valve there is leaflet thickening and shortage, leading to non-coaptation and severe mitral regurgitation. The posterior mitral valve leaflet appears to be tethered down to the left ventricular posterior wall, with reduced mobility during diastole. In severe cases the leaflet, its chordae and papillary muscle are completely adherent to the wall leading to massive regurgitation.

2.1.11 Abnormalities of the right side of the heart

The initial lesions on the right side consist of thickening of the moderator band. In the longitudinal view of the right ventricle and short axis of the left ventricle at the level of the aorta a stretched moderator band is seen, while in 4 chambers-view the ventricular cavity is separated into two cameras. There may be thickening of the tricuspid leaflets and the analysis of the tricuspid inflow by pulsed Doppler reveals abnormal compliance.

Right ventricular trabecular cavity obliteration is thought to start by separation of the trabecular chamber of the right ventricle from the rest of the cavity, as seen in 4-chambers view (Figure 5). It is usually accompanied by mild to moderate tricuspid regurgitation caused by restriction to the movement of the anterior and septal leaflets of the tricuspid valve. The leaflets may present attachments to the wall leading to an echocardiographic picture that may mimic "Ebstein Malformation" (Vaidyanathan et al., 2009), namely with dilatation of the tricuspid annulus, tricuspid regurgitation with jet originating from the level of non-cooptation of the leaflets, which is dislocated to the trabecular portion of the ventricle. The right ventricular systolic function, evaluated through a visual semi-quantitative scale using two-dimensional guided M-mode in several incidences (four-chambers, parasternal long axis, parasternal short axis and sub-costal views), is globally normal, but may be reduced when there are large endocardial plaques and cavity retraction.

Advanced right EMF is defined by retraction of the ventricular cavity due to elimination of the trabecular portion of the cavity, resulting in the pathognomonic finding of an "apical notch". The right ventricular outflow tract is dilated and hyperdynamic to compensate the loss of the trabecular portion, and the interventricular septal motion may be reversed.

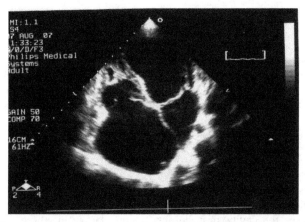

Fig. 5. Right EMF seen in 4-chambers view showing separation of the cavity in two portions, a feature that is characteristic prior to complete obliteration of the trabecular cavity.

Severe tricuspid regurgitation with no turbulence is characteristically associated to restriction of leaflet movements caused by involvement of the papillary muscles in the fibrotic process and to dilatation of the annulus that results from severe right atrial dilatation. At this stage most patients have spontaneous contrast inside the right atrium extending to the inflow tract of RV and also to the inferior vena cava and dilated supra-hepatic veins. Multiple thrombi may be found some moving freely and others attached to the atrial wall. The dilated inferior vena cava and supra-hepatic veins, usually with dynamic echos indicating stasis, do not show the normal respiratory changes, indicating increased systemic venous pressure. Pericardial, pleural and peritoneal effusions are also frequently present in patients in heart failure, best seen in subcostal view.

The colour Doppler is used for semi-quantitative estimation of tricuspid regurgitation severity, taking into account the width and depth of regurgitant jet inside the atrium seen from different views (four-chambers, short-axis and sub-costal). One criteria used to define severe tricuspid regurgitation is the lack of aliasing of the jet and its large width at origin, especially when there is non-coaptation of the tricuspid valve leaflets. The aneurismal right atrium results in heart distortion and compression of the left cavities making it difficult to evaluate the presence of mitral dysfunction. Abundant pericardial effusion and compression of left cavities compromise an adequate evaluation of the left ventricular function.

The lateral and supero-inferior dimensions of the right atrium are always increased and an aneurysmal atrium is usually found. The high pressure inside the atrial cavity pushes the interatrial septum towards the left side opening the *foramen ovale* in many occasions, and allowing a certain degree of right –to-left shunt that causes mild cyanosis. Compression of the left cavities by the severely dilated atrium and tense right ventricle at the level of the admission chamber may impede adequate ventricular filling as well as mask mitral regurgitation. On M-mode these findings are associated with interventricular paradoxical septal motion and small left ventricular cavity.

2.2 Pathological correlation

Surgery can be used to assess the accuracy of transthoracic echocardiography in determining the severity of EMF. This has been achieved by performing standardized transthoracic echocardiography on EMF patients prior to surgery, followed by detailed intra-operative examination of the abnormalities and histopathological evaluation of tissue obtained from excised biopsies (Mocumbi et al., 2010). In this series of patients from Mozambique the echocardiographic description coincided with the intraoperative findings in more than 80% of patients, the concordance being absolute for the most important pathological lesions of EMF, namely fusion of the posterior papillary muscle and leaflet to the wall, left ventricular apical fibrosis, thickening of the atrioventricular leaflets, right ventricular obliteration, right ventricular retraction and ventricular thrombi. This suggested that transthoracic echocardiography can be used in isolation for diagnosis and surgical management of chronic EMF in low-resource endemic areas.

2.3 Challenges and opportunities

Echocardiography can make a confident non-invasive diagnosis of EMF (Vijayaraghavan et al., 1983; Mocumbi et al., 2010), has been useful in determining patients who can benefit from surgery and allows evaluation of the response to treatment. Access to hand-carried echocardiography battery-operated systems has allowed for the first time the design and implementation of epidemiological research in a remote area in Mozambique. In this community, known to have a high attack rate of the disease from previous hospital-based data (Ferreira et al., 2002), 1063 individuals of all ages were randomly selected and submitted to transthoracic echocardiography using a standardized protocol (Mocumbi et al., 2008). A prevalence of 19.8% was found, with the majority of the individuals being asymptomatic and having mild or moderate disease.

For such disease with so many gaps in knowledge there is need to build regional or continental registries starting with phenotypic characterization of individuals in early stages of EMF through echocardiography, using standardized criteria that can be validated on follow-up studies in several endemic areas. This may contribute to uncover aspects related to its natural history, and constitute cohorts to test differences in genetic and to biological profile between healthy individuals and those affected by the disease in endemic areas. Follow-up of individuals with well-established echocardiographic phenotype may also be important to identify predictors of outcome using different disease management strategies.

3. Rheumatic heart disease

RHD is the most important form of acquired cardiovascular disease in children and adolescents in Africa. It is the only chronic sequelae of rheumatic fever (RF), a systemic disease that results from group A streptococcal infections.

Rheumatic Heart Disease (RHD) is still a major concern in Africa (World Health Organization, 2007) despite the dramatic declines in the incidence and prevalence of this condition that have occurred over the last 150 years in the developed world (Gordis, 1985). It is a disease traditionally associated with poverty and overcrowding, and this decline was achieved through improvement in living conditions and widespread use of penicillin for the treatment of streptococcal pharyngitis. The unacceptably high rates of RF/RHD in Sub-Saharan Africa lead to considerable use of health-care resources and a major impact on the patients, their families and the society as a whole.

Although RHD is still a neglected disease, there has been a new surge on research on this condition. This has been centered in developing countries and those populations within middle- and high-income countries where high burdens of disease still exist. Echocardiography is considered the adequate tool for identifying early stages of heart valve disease (Carapetis & Zuhlke, 2011).

3.1 Echocardiographic diagnosis

Echocardiography is an essential tool in diagnosis and management of RF and RHD. Several structural and hemodynamic abnormalities are important for classifying valve lesions, both in the acute and chronic phases of the disease. Even before the advent of colour Doppler flow imaging several studies had already highlighted the utility of echocardiography for the diagnosis of rheumatic carditis, and emphasized its value in defining the mechanisms of valve disease and heart failure associated with severe attacks of carditis (Vansan et al., 1996; Narula et al., 1999). Colour flow Doppler imaging was then considered a useful method of identifying subclinical mitral and aortic valvar disease at all stages of rheumatic fever when carditis cannot be otherwise detected (Folger et al., 1992). Regarding chronic rheumatic heart disease, echocardiography may be used to track the progression of valve abnormalities and to help determine the time for surgical intervention.

3.1.1 Acute carditis

In acute rheumatic disease Doppler-echocardiography identifies and quantifies valve abnormalities, ventricular dysfunction and pericardial effusion (Narula et al., 1999; Folger et al., 1992). The valve most commonly affected is the mitral, followed by the aortic valve (Folger et al., 1992). In the African context, severe pure rheumatic mitral regurgitation is as prevalent as pure stenosis but has an entirely different time course, surgical anatomy, and relation to disease activity, suggesting a separate pathophysiologic mechanism (Marcus et al., 1994).

The usual features of acute rheumatic valvulitis are annular dilatation, elongation of the chordae to the anterior leaflet, and postero-laterally directed mitral regurgitation jet (Vansan et al., 1996; Narula et al., 1999; Folger et al., 1992). Nodular thickening of valve leaflets also occurs (Vansan et al., 1996), and may represent echocardiographic equivalents of rheumatic verrucae seen universally at autopsy in patients who died of acute rheumatic fever (Baggenstoos & Titus., 1968) and noted macroscopically at surgery in a substantial proportion of patients subjected to valve surgery during the acute phase (Kinsley et al., 1981). When acute carditis courses with chordal thickening (Vijayalakshmi et al., 2008), it suggests acute rheumatic fever recurrence in patients with established rheumatic heart valve disease. Mild mitral regurgitation present during the acute phase usually resolves weeks to months after. In contrast, patients with moderate-to-severe carditis have persistent mitral and/or aortic regurgitation.

Valve insufficiency due to endocarditis, rather than myocardial dysfunction caused by myocarditis, is the dominant cause of heart failure in acute rheumatic fever, related to ventricular dilatation and/or restriction of leaflet mobility (Vansan et al., 1996). This has been supported by demonstration of the absence of cTnI elevations during rheumatic fever (Kamblock et al., 2003; Essop et al., 1993). The left ventricle is dilated with preserved or increased fractional shortening in most cases, but variable degree of ventricular dysfunction is not rare in the African setting probably due to the high prevalence of predisposing factors such as anemia.

3.1.2 Chronic rheumatic heart disease

Isolated mitral regurgitation or combined mitral and aortic regurgitation are the most common abnormalities found in chronic RHD (Vansan et al., 1996; Folger et al., 1992; Marcus et al., 1994). Several morphological abnormalities have been considered features of chronic mitral RHD namely (a) valve and/or chordal thickening; (b) restrictive leaflet motion due to chordal thickening, shortening or fusion, commissural fusion and leaflet calcification or thickening; and (c) chordal elongation, rupture or prolapse (Marijon et al., 2007; Paar et al., 2010; Namboodiri et al., 2009; Wilkins et al., 1988). In mitral regurgitation the posterior mitral leaflet is shortened and immobile because its submitral complex is also thickened, fused and shortened, resulting in a gap or non-coaptation of the two leaflets in many patients (Okubo et al., 1984). Mitral stenosis occurs when the leaflets of the affected valves become diffusely thickened, with fusion of the commissures and chordae tendineae, as well as increased echodensity of the mitral valve that may signify calcification. However, valvular calcification is rare in juvenile rheumatic heart disease, frequently seen in Africa (Yuko-Jowi et al., 2005). Left atrial thrombus is a common finding in mitral stenosis.

There are few studies of characterization of aortic valve abnormalities in rheumatic heart disease. Rheumatic aortic valve disease is usually diagnosed in combination with mitral disease, and after exclusion of congenital disease, mainly bicuspid aortic valve. Echocardiographic diagnosis has been based on morphological changes such as the presence of thickened leaflets, rolled leaflet edges, coaptation defect, deformed leaflets, commissural fusion, leaflet retraction, abnormal leaflet mobility, systolic doming of leaflet, hyperechogenicity of leaflet edges and prolapse are used (Marijon et al., 2007; Paar et al., 2010). For community studies a more accurate case-definition and assessment of severity is needed since follow up of patients with RHD shows that those with no or mild aortic valve disease at the time of mitral valve intervention rarely develop severe aortic valve disease, and seldom require aortic valve surgery over the long-term follow up, while the presence of mild aortic stenosis at baseline is predictive of relatively more rapid progression in the minority of cases (Namboodiri et al., 2009).

Two-dimensional echocardiographic criteria of organic rheumatic tricuspid valve disease include thickened leaflets with restriction in motion, diastolic doming, and encroachment of the leaflet tips on the wall of the ventricular inlet (Guyer et al., 1984; Meira et al., 2006). Since pulmonary hypertension is predominant in mitral valve disease, there is commonly annulus dilatation that results from right cavities dilatation and leads to tricuspid regurgitation. This must be differentiated from organic valve disease, which has usually morphological changes similar to that described above for the mitral valve.

3.1.3 Major valvular abnormalities

3.1.3.1 Restrictive or excessive leaflet motion

Restrictive leaflet motion is evident in most patients with established RHD requiring surgery MR (Chavaud et al., 2001), nearly one third of patients with acute RF (Vijayalakshmi et al., 2008; Marcus et al., 1989) and all those with rheumatic mitral stenosis (Wilkins et al., 1988; Naito et al., 1980; Prasad & Radhakrishnan, 1992; Van der Bel-Kahn & Becker, 1986). It is caused by chordal shortening, thickening and fusion, commissural fusion, and leaflet calcification and thickening (Chavaud et al., 2001; Van der Bel-Kahn & Becker, 1986; Carpentier, 1983). The terms used to characterize the abnormal and restricted mobility of the mitral leaflets include elbow, dog-leg and hockey-stick deformity (Paar et al., 2010; Webb et al., 2009; Steer et al., 2009; Reeves et al., 2011; Carapetis et al., 2008) (Figure 6).

Chordal elongation and rupture of the primary chords are the mechanisms responsible for mitral valve prolapse in RHD. These changes must be carefully looked for as they influence the surgical management (Chavaud et al., 2001; Marcus et al., 1989; Carpentier, 1983).

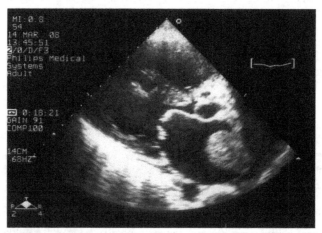

Fig. 6. Long axis parasternal view of a patient with mitral stenosis due to RHD showing thickening of the mitral and aortic valves, as well as restricted motion of the mitral leaflets. Notice a large left atrial thrombus.

3.1.3.2 Valve thickening

The rheumatic valve is fibrotic and firm, with thickening and fusion of leaflets and commissures (Van der Bel-Kahn & Becker, 1986), mostly seen in stenotic valves. Thickening of the mitral valve, especially the anterior mitral leaflet, appears to be a consistent feature of RHD (Figure 6), which can be adequately assessed in the parasternal long axial view where the anterior mitral valve because the ultrasound beam is perpendicular to the leaflet. Regarding the aortic valve both the parasternal and subcostal views allow adequate evaluation. Valve thickness of both mitral and aortic valves increases with age, based on an autopsy study (Sahsakul et al., 1988). However, in populations where RHD is prevalent there are very few additional conditions that are associated with increased thickness of the mitral valve in the age groups affected by RHVD, except for endemic areas for both RHD and EMF (Mocumbi et al., 2008).

3.2 Recent advances and research needs

The knowledge gap regarding epidemiology, pathogenesis and natural history of RF/RHD in Africa is related to several factors. First, group A streptococcal infections that precede RHD are subclinical, and most of the clinical cases are of a minor nature compared with other diseases afflicting children in this setting. Secondly, RF/RHD is not notifiable in most African countries and its impact is underestimated. Thirdly, many children are not brought to medical care when they complain of sore throat or a skin lesion. Finally, the diagnosis of rheumatic fever/carditis, requires clinical sophistication that exceeds the expertise available at many local hospitals that are manned by nurses or trained health care workers.

The echocardiographic diagnosis of RHD is not standardized and there are few studies looking systematically at criteria for diagnosing valve disease using modern echocardiographic tools. However, due to the persisting burden of the disease in some areas of the world echocardiography has been used in community studies in Mozambique and Cambodia (Marijon et al., 2007), Tonga (Carapetis et al., 2008), Nicaragua (Paar et al., 2010), Fiji (Steer et al., 2009; Reeves et al., 2011), Kenya (Anabwani et al., 1996), India (Thakur et al., 1996; Bhaya et al., 2010), Pakistan (Sadiq et al., 2009; Rizvi et al., 2004) and China (Zhimin 2006). These studies applied different inclusion and diagnostic criteria, raising the issue about the need for standardization of the definition of rheumatic heart valve disease by echocardiography.

Patients from African series present severe abnormalities at early ages (Sliwa et al., 2010; Marijon et al., 2008). Because rheumatic heart valve disease has an initial latent stage that can be detected by appropriate tests (among which echocardiography), has adequate affordable therapy, and may have its prognosis improved by interventions at an early stage, it should be the target of screening as a tool of preventive medicine.

3.2.1 Developing guidelines for echocardiographic screening

Early detection of "subclinical" rheumatic valve disease by echocardiography is vital, as it presents an opportunity for case detection at a time when prophylactic penicillin – to prevent recurrent episodes – can stop progression to important valve disease. This is very important in Africa, where most new patients admitted to hospitals have already advanced and complicated rheumatic valvular lesions (Sliwa et al., 2010), often resulting in heart failure and/or arrhythmia that cannot be adequately managed due to unavailability of open heart surgery. A current challenge for African scientists is therefore to make echocardiographic screening reliable, affordable and feasible in low-resource settings, using diagnostic criteria that are clear, simple, robust and reproducible. This would allow their incorporation in protocols for performing, reading and interpreting echocardiograms, in order to avoid over- and under-diagnosis.

Researchers from Africa have been involved in continental efforts to assess the epidemiology of RHD using echocardiography. This has started with the "**A**wareness, **S**urveillance, **A**dvocacy and **P**revention Strategy" lounged by the Pan African Society of Cardiology in 2005, which aims at reducing the burden of RF/RHD in the continent (Mayosi et al., 2006). More recently African researchers have been taking part in a global initiative aiming at standardization of echocardiographic screening that is led by the World Heart Federation (World Heart Federation, 2011).

3.2.2 Disseminating echocardiographic screening

The use of highly trained specialists for large scale echocardiographic screening of RHD in endemic areas of Africa is not practical (Figure 7) but the diffusion of ultrasound technology to nontraditional users has been rapid and far-reaching in the last years (Shah et al., 2008). Experiences for dissemination of echocardiography to non-traditional users in Rwanda and Tanzania have been designed aiming at the evaluation of pericardial effusion, rheumatic heart disease, congestive heart failure and estimation of global left ventricular function (Shah et al., 2008; Adler et al., 2008). The impact of this technology diffusion is being quantified, but early results show that ultrasound is a teachable skill, leads to accuracy of diagnosis, helps in management of common cardiovascular conditions, and improves professional satisfaction of local health providers (Shah et al., 2009). The role of task-shifting inside the health systems to allow non-cardiologists to perform echocardiographic screening for RHD must therefore be studied. However, there is need to carefully choose the health providers to be trained and implement measures of quality assessment and sustainability.

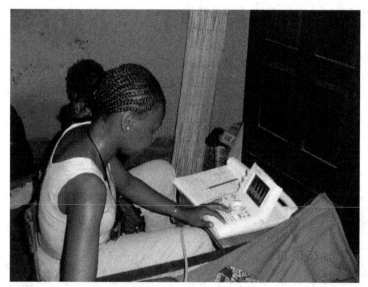

Fig. 7. Photograph of a researcher performing echocardiography in an Africa rural setting.

3.2.3 Definition of curricula and selection of ultrasound machines

Considering the unique pattern of cardiovascular disease in Africa, there is need for designing *curricula* and training materials tailored to the local needs, taking into consideration the differential diagnosis with conditions such as cardiomyopathy, which are also highly prevalent in the continent. In the particular conditions of health care provision in Africa the choice of the ultrasound machines is also of paramount importance. Machine specificities that are suitable for the African environment include durability, portability, battery-operated machines and high two-dimensional image quality. In portable machines a storage bag with room for gel, towels, probe covers and cleaning supplies is recommended (Shah et al., 2008).

4. Conclusions

There has been an increase in scientific publications from African researchers and institutions with the dissemination of echocardiography. Echocardiographic-driven research into neglected diseases such as endomyocardial fibrosis and rheumatic heart disease have contributed to uncover epidemiology and clinical profile of these conditions in the continent, confirming the role for this imaging technique in fostering research and improving quality of care in cardiovascular diseases in resource-deprived areas of Africa. Echocardiography may also help to quantify the health impact of certain neglected cardiovascular diseases in Africa, as well as assist in design and implementation of programs for surveillance, prevention and control of such conditions.

5. References

Anabwani GM, Bonhoeffer P. (1996). Prevalence of heart disease in school children in rural Kenya using colour-flow echocardiography. *East African Medical Journal*;73(4):215-217.

Acquatella H, Puigbo JJ, Suarez C, Mendoza J. (1979). Sudden early diastolic anterior movement of the septum in endomyocardial fibrosis. *Circulation*;59(4):847-848

Adesanya CO. (1979). M-mode echocardiography in the diagnosis of mitral stenosis. *Niger Med J*;9:533-537

Adler D, Mgalula K, Price D, Taylor O. (2008). Introduction of a portable ultrasound unit into the health services of the Lugufu refugee camp, Kigoma District, Tanzania. *Int J Emerg Med*;i:261-266

Baggenstoos AH, Titus JL. (1968). Rheumatic and collagen disorders of the heart. In: Gould SE, ed. Pathology of Heart and Blood Vessels. 3rd ed. Springield, III: Charles C Thomas Publisher;649-722

Berensztein CS, Pinero G, Marcotegui M, Brunoldi R, Blanco MV, Lerman J. (2000) Usefulness of echocardiography and Doppler echocardiographiy in endomyocardial fibrosis. *J Am Soc Echocardiog*; 13(3):226-30

Bhaya M, Panwar S, Beniwal R, Panwar RB. (2010) High prevalence of rheumatic heart disease detected by echocardiography in school children. *Echocardiography*; 27(4):448-453.

Carapetis J, Zuhlke L. (2011)Global research priorities in rheumatic fever and rheumatic heart disease. Annals of Pediatric *Cardiology*;4(1): 4-12.

Carapetis JR, Hardy M, Fakakovikaetau T, Taib R, Wilkinson L, Penny DJ, Steer AC. (2008) Evaluation of a screening protocol using auscultation and portable echocardiography to detect asymptomatic rheumatic heart disease in Tongan schoolchildren. *Nature Clinical Practice Cardiovascular Medicine*;5(7):411-417.

Carpentier A. (1983) Cardiac valve surgery - the "French correction". *J Thorac Cardiovasc Surg.*;86(3):323-337.

Chauvaud S, Fuzellier JF, Berrebi A, Deloche A, Fabiani JN, Carpentier A. (2001) Long-term (29 years) results of reconstructive surgery in rheumatic mitral valve insufficiency. *Circulation*;104(12 Suppl 1):I12-15;

Connor DH, Somers K, Hutt NSR, Manion WC, D'Arbela PGD. (1967) Endomyocardial fibrosis in Uganda (Davies'disease). Part I. *Am Heart J.*;74(5):687-709.

Davies, JNP. (1960) Some considerations regarding obscure diseases affecting the mural endocardium. *Am Heart J*;19(4):600-630

Essop MR, Wisenbaugh T, Sareli P. (1993) Evidence against a myocardial factor as the cause of left ventricular dilation in active rheumatic carditis. *J Am Coll Cardiol*;22:826-829

Feigenbaum, H. (1994) Echocardiographic evaluation of cardiac chambers, In: *Echocardiography*. 5th ed. Lippincott Williams & Wilkins. pp 134-180, ISBN 0-8121-1692-5 Philadelphia

Ferreira B, Matsika-Claquin MD, Hausse-Mocumbi AO, Sidi D, Paquet C. (2002) Origine geographique des cas de fibrose endomyocardique traitées a l'Hôpital Central de Maputo, entre 1987 et 1999 *Bull Soc Pathol Exot*, 95(4): 274-9.

Folger GM Jr, Hajar R, Robida A, Hajar HA. (1992) Occurrence of valvar heart disease in acute rheumatic fever without evident carditis: colour-flow Doppler identification. *Br Heart J*;67:434-439

George BO, Gaba FE, Talabi AI.(1982) M-mode echocardiographic features of endomyocardial fibrosis. *Br Heart J*.48(3):222-8.

Gonzalez-Lavin L, Friedman JP, Hecker SP, McFadden PM. Endomyocardial fibrosis: Diagnosis and treatment. Am Heart J 1982;105(4):699-705.

Gordis L. (1985) The virtual disappearance of rheumatic fever in the United States: lessons in the rise and fall of disease: T. Duckett Jones Memorial Lecture. *Circulation*;72:1155-62

Guyer De, Gillam LD, Foale RA, Clark MC, Dinsmore R, Palacios I, Block P, King ME, Weyman AE. (1984) Comparison of the echocardiographic and hemodynamic diagnosis of rheumatic tricuspid stenosis. *J Am Coll Cardiol* ;3(50):1135-44

Hassan W, Fawzy ME, Helaly SA, Hegazy H, Malik S. Pitfalls in Diagnosis and Clinical, Echocardiographic, and Hemodynamic Findings in Endomyocardial Fibrosis: a 25-year experience. Chest 2005;128:3985-92

Jaiyesimi F, Antia AU. (1981a) Congenital Heart Disease in Nigeria: a ten-year experience at UCH, Ibadan. *Ann Trop Paediatr*; 1;77-85

Jaiyesimi F, Antia AU. (1981b) Childhood rheumatic heart disease in Nigeria. *Trop Geogr Med*;33:8-13

Kamblock J, Payot L, Iung B, Costes P, Gillet T, Goanvic C, Lionet P, Pagis B, Pasche J, Roy C, Vahanian A, Papouin G. (2003) Does rheumatic myocarditis really exists?

Systematic study with echocardiography and cardiac troponin I blood levels. *Eur Heart J*;24:855-862

Kinsley RH, Girwood RW, Milner S.(1981) Surgical treatment during the acute phase of rheumatic carditis. In: Nyhus LM, ed *Surgery Annual*. East Norwalk, Conn: Appleton-Century-Crofts;13:299-323

Lowenthal MN, Teeger S. (2000) Endomyocardial fibrosis with pericardial effusion and endocardial calcification. *Isr Med Assoc J*.;2(3):249.

Mady C, Salemi VMC, Ianni BM, Arteaga E, Fernandes F, Ramires FJA. (2004) Quantitative Assessment of Left Ventricular Regional Wall Motion in Endomyocardial Fibrosis. *Arq Bras Cardiol*;84(3):241-244

Marcus RH, Sareli P, Pocock WA, Barlow JB. (1994) The spectrum of severe rheumatic mitral valve disease in a developing country: correlations among clinical presentation, survival pathological findings and hemodynamic sequelae. *Ann Intern Med*;120930;177-83

Marcus RH, Sareli P, Pocock WA, Meyer TE, Magalhaes MP, Grieve T, Antunes MJ, Barlow JB. (1989) Functional anatomy of severe mitral regurgitation in active rheumatic carditis. *Am J Cardiol*;63(9):577-584

Marijon E, Iung B, Mocumbi AO, Kamblock J, Thanh CV, Gamra H, Esteves C, Palacios IF, Vahanian A. (2008) What are the differences in presentation of candidates for mitral percutaneous commissurotomy across the world and do they influence the results of the procedure? *Arch Cardiovasc Dis*;101(10):611-7.

Marijon E, Ou P, Celermajer DS, Ferreira B, Mocumbi AO, Jani D, Paquet C, Jacob S, Sidi D, Jouven X. (2007) Prevalence of rheumatic heart disease detected by echocardiographic screening. *N Engl J Med*;357(5):470-476.

Mayosi B, Robertson K, Volmink J, Adebo W, Akinyore K, Amoah A, Bannerman C, Biesman-Simons S, Carapetis J, Cilliers A, Commerford P, Croasdale A, Damasceno A, Dean J, Dean M, de Souza R, Filipe A, Hugo-Hamman C, Jurgens-Clur SA, Kombila-Koumba P, Kotzenberg C, Lawrenson J, Manga P, Matenga J, Mathivha T, Mntla P, Mocumbi A, Mokone T, Ogola E, Omokhodion S, Palweni C, Pearce A, Salo A, Thomas B, Walker K, Wiysonge C, Zaher S. (2006) The Drakensberg declaration on the control of rheumatic fever and rheumatic heart disease in Africa. *S Afr Med J*; 96:246.

Meira Z, Goulart E, Mota C. (2006) Comparative Study of Clinical and Doppler Echocardiographic Evaluations of the Progression of Valve Diseases in Children and Adolescents with Rheumatic Fever. *Arq Bras Cardiol*;86 (1):32-8

Metras D, Ouezzin-Coulibaly A, Ouattara K, Bertrand E, Chauvet J. (1983) Endomyocardial fibrosis masquerading as rheumatic mitral incompetence. A report of six surgical cases. *J Thorac Cardiovasc Surg*;86(5):753-6.

Mocumbi AO, Carrilho C, Sarathchandra P, Ferreira MB, Yacoub MH, Burke M. (2010) Echocardiography accurately assesses the pathological abnormalities of chronic endomyocardial fibrosis. *Int J Cardiovasc Imaging*

Mocumbi AO, Ferreira MB, Sidi D, Yacoub MH. (2008) A population study of Endomyocardial Fibrosis in a rural area of Mozambique. *N Eng J Med*; 369:43-9.

Morrone LF, Moreira AE, Lopez M, Kajita LJ, Poterio DI, Arie S. (1996) Endomiocardiofibrose com Calcificação endocárdica maciça biventricular. *Arq Bras Cardiol*;67(2):103-5.

Naito M, Morganroth J, Mardelli TJ, Chen CC, Dreifus LS. (1980) Rheumatic mitral stenosis: cross-sectional echocardiographic analysis. *Am Heart J*;100(1): p. 34-40;

Namboodiri N, Remash K, Tharakan JA, Shajeem O, Nair K, Titus T, Ajitkumar VK, Sivasankaran S, Krishnamoorthy KM, Harikrishnan SP, Harikrishnan MS, Bijulal S. (2009) Natural history of aortic valve disease following intervention for rheumatic mitral valve disease. *J Heart Valve Dis*;18(1):61-7.

Narula J, Chandrasekar Y, Rahimtoola S. (1999) Diagnosis of active carditis: the echos of change. *Circulation*;100:1576-1581

Ogah OS, Adebanjo AT, Otukoya AS, Jagusa TJ. (2006) Echocardiography in Nigeria: use, problems, reproducibility and potentials. *Cardiovascular Ultrasound*; 4: 13 doi:10.1186/1476-7120-4-13

Okereke OUJ, Chikwendu VC, Ihenacho HNC, Ikeh VO. (1991) Non-invasive diagnosis of endomyocardial fibrosis in Nigeria using two-dimensional echocardiography. *Tropical Cardiology*;17(67):97-103

Okubo S, Nagata S, Masuda Y, Kawazoe K, Atobe M, Manabe H. (1984) Clinical features of rheumatic heart disease in Bangladesh. *Jpn Circ J*;48(12):1345-9

Paar JA, Berrios NM, Rose JD, Caceres M, Pena R, Perez W, Chen-Mok M, Jolles E, Dale JB. (2010) Prevalence of rheumatic heart disease in children and young adults in Nicaragua. *Am J Cardiol*.;2010: 105(12):1809-1814.

Prasad k, Radhakrishnan S. (1992) Echocardiographic variables affecting surgical outcome in patients undergoing closed mitral commissurotomy. *Int J Cardiol*;37(2): p. 237-42;

Rashwan MA, Ayman M, Ashour S, Hassanin MM, Zeina AA. (1995) Endomyocardial fibrosis in Egypt: an illustrated review. *Br Heart J*;73:284-9.

Reeves BM, Kado J, Brook M. (2011) High prevalence of rheumatic heart disease in Fiji detected by echocardiography screening. *Journal of Paediatrics and Child Health*: 47(7):473-8

Rizvi SF, Khan MA, Kundi A, Marsh DR, Samad A, Pasha O. (2004) Status of rheumatic heart disease in rural Pakistan. *Heart*;90:394-399

Sadiq M, Islam K, Abid R, Latif F, Rehman AU, Waheed A, Azhar M, Khan JS. (2009) Prevalence of rheumatic heart disease in school children of urban Lahore. *Heart*;95(5):353-357.

Shah S, Noble VE, Umulisa I, Dushimiyimana JMV, Bukhman G, Mukherjee J, Rich M, Epino H. (2008) Development of an ultrasound training curriculum in a limited resource international setting: successes and challenges of ultrasound training in rural Rwanda. *Int J Emerg Med*; 1:193-196

Shah SP, Epino H, Bukhman G, Umulisa I, Dushimiyimana JMV, Reichman A, Noble VE. (2009) Impact of the introduction of ultrasound services in a limited resource setting: rural Rwanda 2008. *BMC International Health and Human Rights*, 9:4

Sahsakul Y, Edwards WD, Naessens JM, Tajik AJ. (1988)Age-related changes in aortic and mitral valve thickness: implications for two-dimensional echocardiography based on an autopsy study of 200 normal human hearts. *Am J Cardiol*;62: 424-430

Salemi VMC, Rochitte CE, Barbosa MM, Mady C. (2005) Clinical and echocardiographic dissociation in a patient with right ventricular endomyocardial fibrosis. *Heart*;91(11):1399

Sani M, Mukhtar-Yola M, Karaye K, Karaye KM. Spectrum of congenital heart disease in a tropical environment: an echocardiographic study. Journal of the National Medical Association 2007;99(6):665-9

Saraiva LR, Carneiro RW, Arruda MB, Brindeiro Filho D, Lira V. (1999) Mitral valve disease with rheumatic appearance in the presence of left ventricular endomyocardial fibrosis. *Arq Bras Cardiol.*;72(3):327-32.

Sliwa K, Carrington M, Mayosi BM, Zigiriadis E, Mvungi R, Stewart S. (2010) Incidence and characteristics of newly diagnosed rheumatic heart disease in urban African adults: insights from the heart of Soweto study. *Eur Heart J*;31(6):719-27.

Somers K. (1990) Restrictive Cardiomyopathies. In Pediatric Cardiology. International Congress Series 906. Pongpanich B, Sueblinvong V, Vongprateep C (eds). Excerpta Medica, Amsterdam.

Steer AC, Kado J, Wilson N, Tuiketei T, Batzloff M, Waqatakirewa L, Mulholland EK, Carapetis JR. (2009) High prevalence of rheumatic heart disease by clinical and echocardiographic screening among children in Fiji. *Journal of Heart Valve Disease*;18(3):327-335; discussion 336.

Thakur JS, Negi PC, Ahluwalia SK, Vaidya NK. (1996) Epidemiological survey of rheumatic heart disease among school children in the Shimla Hills of northern India: prevalence and risk factors. *Journal of Epidemiology & Community Health*;50(1):62-67.

Trigo J, Camacho A, Gago P, Candeias R, Santos W, Marques N, Matos P, Brandão V, Gomes V. (2010) Fibrose endomiocárdica com calcificação maçica do ventrículo esquerdo. *Rev Port Cardiol*;29(0):445-449

Vaidyanathan K, Agarwai R, Sahayaraj A, Sankar M, Cherian KM. (2009) Endomyocardial fibrosis mimicking Ebstein's anomaly. *Tex Heart Inst J*;36(3):250-1

Van der Bel-Kahn J, Becker AE.(198) The surgical pathology of rheumatic and floppy mitral valves. Distinctive morphologic features upon gross examination. *Am J Surg Path*;10(4):282-292

Vansan R, Shrisvastava S, Vijayakumar M, Narang R, Lister B, Narula J. (1996) Echocardiographic evaluation of patients with acute rheumatic fever and rheumatic carditis. *Circulation*;94:73-82

Vijayalakshmi IB, Vishnuprabhu RO, Chitra N, Rajasri R, Anuradha TV. (2008) The efficacy of echocardiographic criterions for the diagnosis of carditis in acute rheumatic fever. *Cardiol Young*;18(6):586-92.

Vijayaraghavan G, Davies J, Sadanandan S, Spry CJF, Gibson DG, Goodwin JF. (1983) Echocardiographic features of tropical endomyocardial disease in South India. *Br Heart J*;50:450-9

WHO Report of the Regional Committee of Africa 2005. (2005) Available at: http://www.afro.who.int/rc55/documents/afr_rc55_12_cardiovascular.pdf.

Wilkins G, Weyman A Abascal V, Block P, Palacios I. (1988) Percutaneous ballon dilatation of the mitral valve: an analysis of echocardiographic variables related to outcome and the mechanisms of dilatation. *Br Heart J*;60:299-308.

www.world-heart-federation.org

Yuko-Jowi C, Bakari M. (2005) Echocardiographic patterns of juvenile rheumatic heart disease at Kenyatta National Hospital, Nairobi. *East Afr Med J*;82(10):514-9

Zhimin W, Yubao Z, Lei S, Xianliang Z, Wei Z, Li S, Hao W, Jianjun L, Detrano R, Rutai H. (2006) Prevalence of chronic rheumatic heart disease in Chinese adults. *Int J Cardiol*;107(3):356-359.

9

Evaluation and Treatment of Hypotension in Premature Infants

Shoichi Ezaki and Masanori Tamura
Division of Neonatal Medicine, Center for Maternal,
Fetal and Neonatal Medicine, Saitama Medical Center,
Saitama Medical University,
Japan

1. Introduction

Sixteen to 98% of extremely preterm infants are treated for hypotension within the first week of life. The enormous variation in this estimate is due to a lack of reliable evidence. While selecting a vasoactive agent, it is necessary to consider the goals of the therapy. To achieve those goals, the clinician must assess the mechanisms of action of the potential therapies. This chapter details the unique characteristics of the neonatal cardiovascular system and defines hypotension in preterm infants. It provides indications for treatment and appropriate therapies for individual cases.

2. Characteristic pathophysiology of hypotension in preterm infants

Blood pressure increases with advancing gestational and postnatal age, which is a developmentally regulated phenomenon (Noori and Seli, 2005). Since cardiac output (CO) and systemic vascular resistance (SVR) both contribute to blood pressure, elevation in blood pressure during development may be the result of increased CO, increased SVR, or both (Fig.1)

2.1 Hypovolemia

In preterm infants, absolute hypovolemia is the most frequent cause of hypotension. Peripheral vasodilation with or without myocardial failure is the most frequent primary etiological factor (Seli and Evans J, 2001). Absolute hypovolemia is defined as a loss of volume from the intravascular compartment; alternatively, relative hypovolemia is defined as vasodilatation with an inadequate volume to fill the expanded intravascular compartment. In both situations, the result is inadequate filling pressure (also known as preload) in the heart. If severe enough, hypovolemia can reduce CO, resulting in inadequate tissue perfusion and oxygenation (Fig 1).

In cases of absolute hypovolemia, the body releases corticosteroids, adrenaline, and noradrenaline, which cause vascular contraction in order to maintain blood pressure and filling pressure and cause increased heart rate and contractility to maintain systemic blood flow (SBF). However, in sick or immature infants, this response may be limited (Ng et al., 2001; Evans N, 2003). In addition, volume administration for the treatment of hypotension in sick infants has been reported to have a dopaminergic effect (Seli and Evans J, 2001).

In preterm infants with acute blood loss (e.g., intraventricular hemorrhage [IVH]) or excessive transepidermal water losses (e.g., gestational age ≤ 25 weeks), absolute hypovolemia should be considered the primary cause of hypotension.

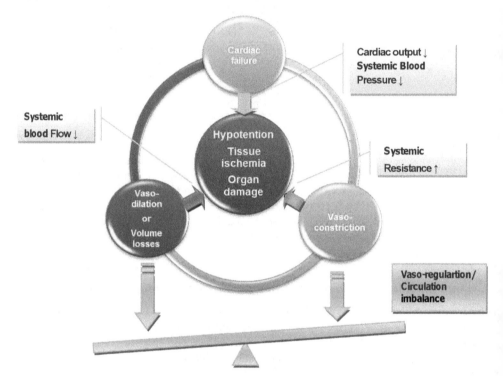

Fig. 1. Mechanism of preterm hypotension

2.2 Myocardial dysfunction

Myocardial contraction and relaxation depend on the regulation of cytosolic calcium concentration and the responsivity of myofilaments to changes in calcium content. Preterm infants, term infants, and adults all have the membrane systems that control cell calcium flux and the sarcomeres that make up the myofibrils. However, the components of each system undergo qualitative and quantitative changes during development. During in the prenatal and newborn periods, myocytes change in size and shape. There are also changes in the number of contractile elements and the nuclear-to-cellular volume ratio.

Cardiac contraction is an energy-dependent process that requires ATP, calcium, and an ATPase located at the myosin head. The processes of contraction and relaxation in immature myocardium as well as calcium homeostasis are different from those in mature myocardium. Specifically, immature myocytes do not rely as heavily on the release and re-uptake of calcium from the sarcoplasmic reticulum; instead, they depend more on extracellular calcium concentration. As such, the immature myocardium of the fetus and newborn depends on L-type calcium channels as a calcium source for contraction. Furthermore, immature myocytes have greater cell surface area-to-volume ratios, which may compensate for their underdeveloped T-tubule systems. The alterations in myocardial structure and function with maturation and the developmental changes in cardiovascular function provide the cellular and molecular bases for differences in myocardial contractility among preterm newborns, term newborns, and older infants (Rowland and Gutgesell, 1995; Noori and Seli, 2005).

Therefore, preterm infants with hypotension have a limited ability to increase CO in response to inotropes or changes in volume (Teitel and Sidi, 1985). Furthermore, they have an elevated sensitivity to increased afterload (Van Hare et al., 1990), which commonly leads to decreased CO (Belik and Light, 1989).

2.3 Abnormal peripheral vasoregulation

Immediately after birth, there is a sudden increase in SVR. This can have a deleterious effect on CO and potentially compromise organ blood flow. After the initial transition period, vasodilation predominates rather than vasoconstriction. Indeed, the complex regulation of vascular smooth muscle tone involves a delicate balance between vasodilators and vasoconstrictors (Fig. 1 and Fig. 2).

hANP: human atrial natriuretic peptide, NO: Nitric oxide, GTP: guanosine triphosphate, cGMP: cyclic guanosine monophosphate

The endogenous vasodilating factors include NO, eicosanoids, hAMP, and endothelin. The endogenous vasoconstrictive factors include catecholamines, vasopressin, and angiotensin II. The balance of these factors determines the blood vessel equilibrium and the tendency toward vasodilation or vasoconstriction (Fig.2). In Figure 2, the vasoconstriction pathway is shown in red, and the vasodilatation pathway is shown in blue. Phosphorylation of myosin is the critical step in vascular smooth muscle contraction. Vasoconstrictors, such as angiotensin II, vasopressin and norepinephrine, activate second messengers to increase cytosolic calcium concentration, which in turn activates myosin light chain kinase. Vasodilators, such as human atrial natriuretic peptide (hANP) and nitric oxide (NO), activate myosin phosphatase, which dephosphorylates myosin to cause vasorelaxation. The plasma membrane is shown at its resting potential (plus signs). cGMP denotes cyclic guanosine monophosphate (Landry and Oliver, 2001). In addition, potassium channels in the smooth muscle cell membrane have recently been implicated in the pathogenesis of vasodilatory shock (Liedel et al., 2002).

Under normal physiologic conditions, CO remains essentially unchanged throughout infancy. Therefore, the increased blood pressure with advancing gestational and postnatal age is primarily the result of increased SVR. Maturation of vascular smooth muscle, changes in the expression of vascular angiotensin II receptor subtypes, and maturation of the central autonomic and peripheral nervous systems play significant roles in increasing vascular tone and SVR. There are 2 major subtypes of angiotensin II receptors. AT1R, which is expressed in mature tissues and the umbilical artery, mediates smooth muscle contraction and regulates fluid and electrolyte balance. AT2R, which is expressed in fetal and newborn tissues, has an unknown function. The developmentally regulated transition from expression of AT2R to AT1R begins following the first 2 weeks of life and is complete by month 3 (Noori and Seli, 2005; Engle, 2001). The vasodilating factor NO increases under conditions of oxidative stress and sepsis. Because preterm infants are prone to these conditions (Ezaki et al., 2009a), their NO levels can easily increase. Together, these physiological characteristics of preterm infants make them susceptible to vasoregulatory dysfunction.

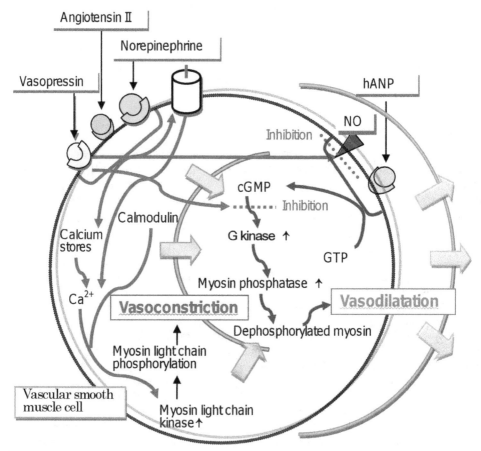

Fig. 2. Regulation of vascular smooth muscle tone

3. The significance of hypotension requiring treatment in preterm infants

3.1 Clinical outcomes

Hypotension is a common complication among preterm infants. Importantly, there is an association between systemic hypotension and neonatal morbidities, including IVH and neurodevelopmental disorders (Watkins et al., 1989; Goldstein et al., 1995). Unfortunately, common conditions among preterm infants, such as sepsis, renal failure, and neonatal asphyxia, can lead to the development of clinical hypotension and confer a poor prognosis.

3.2 Relationship between systemic blood flow and blood pressure

The most important goal in treating hypotension is to prevent cellular and tissue damage resulting from hypovolemia. Seli et al. and Greisen et al. have reported important considerations for the treatment of hypotension (Seli, 2006; Greisen, 2005). If effective treatment is not promptly initiated, the blood pressure may decrease further to the "ischemic threshold, which is said to be about 30 mmHg," resulting in tissue ischemia and permanent organ damage. For example, a loss of cerebral blood flow (CBF) triggers abnormal cerebral function and, finally, tissue ischemia (Fig. 3). Furthermore, high blood pressure is also deleterious. Although, exact value is not noted in existing reports, when blood pressure exceeds "intraventricular hemorrhage (IVH) threshold", risk of IVH increases (Fig. 3).

Loss of vascular autoregulation has not been formally proven as a cause of increased morbidity and mortality in preterm infants (McLean et al., 2008). However, it has consequences that negatively affect prognosis. For instance, loss of autoregulation often triggers IVH. In addition, the amount of blood shunted through the patent ductus arteriosus (PDA), present in preterm infants, can become unstable. Furthermore, the patient is likely to develop necrotizing enterocolitis (NEC) due to compromised blood flow to gastrointestinal tract. Finally, once the patient enters the ischemic stage, there is an increased incidence of periventricular leukomalacia (PVL) and severe renal failure. As such, although the exact reference blood pressure values that cause failure of autoregulation and CBF remain unclear, it is important that hypotension be treated properly.

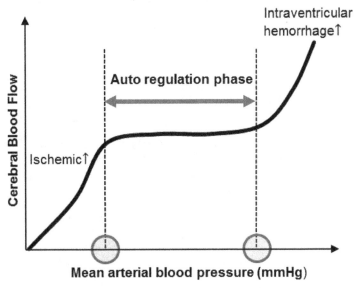

Fig. 3. Proposed relationship between blood flow and mean blood pressure in the cerebral circulation of the preterm infant

4. Definitions of normotension and hypotension in the preterm infant

Most preterm infants admitted to the neonatal intensive care unit (NICU) have medical conditions, such as respiratory disorders, electrolyte abnormalities, or neonatal asphyxia. In addition, because there is a wide range of ages and body weights, it is difficult to define hypotension as a single value in preterm infants. A neonate is considered to be hypotensive if the mean blood pressure is below the fifth or tenth percentile of the normative data according to gestational and postnatal age and weight (Cunningham et al., 1999). Another definition of hypotension is a mean blood pressure less than or equal to the patient's gestational age in weeks. Although this definition is a useful tool, it is only valid during the first 48 hours of life (Nuntnarumit et al., 1999). However, due to its simplicity, this value is a good indicator for neonatologists to suspect hypotension.

4.1.1 Definition of preterm hypotension and its relationship to low systemic perfusion

Figure 3 indicates blood pressure values that are thought result from a failure of autoregulation. Although they would be an ideal definition of hypotension, no consensus has yet been reached. Of preterm infants with a gestational age of 23–26 weeks, >90% have a mean blood pressure >30 mmHg (Nuntnarumit et al., 1999). Recent studies suggest that it may be as high as 28–30 mmHg, even among extremely low birth-weight infants (Munro et al., 2004).

4.1.2 Permissive hypotension

A recent study in very preterm neonates suggested that blood pressure below the clinically-accepted lower limit during the first postnatal days may not require intervention, as long as adequate tissue perfusion is maintained (Dempsey et al., 2009). This study suggested that although treatment must be initiated promptly, overzealous treatment may worsen the prognosis. Therefore, a diagnosis of hypotension must be based on clinical and laboratory findings.

4.2 Clinical signs

Many conditions may trigger hypotension in preterm infants (Table 1). The need for tests and treatments to prevent decreased tissue perfusion is examined.

Vasoregulation imbalance
Hemorrhage: Placental hemorrhage, abruption placenta prevail, feto-maternal hemorrhage, birth trauma-subaponeurotic bleed, massive pulmonary hemorrhage.
Other: Twin-to-twin transfusion, third-space losses, asphyxia, sepsis and septic shock, disseminated intravascular coagulopathy, NEC
Cardiogenic shock
Asphyxia, electrolyte abnormality, cardiac disease: arrhythmias, congenital heart disease, PDA, cardiomyopathy, myocarditis, air leak syndromes
Endocrine
Adrenal hemorrhage, adrenal insufficiency
Drug induced
Anesthetic drugs, sedative drugs

Table 1. Causes of hypotension in preterm infants

4.3 Hemodynamic monitoring in preterm infants

An ideal method for monitoring blood pressure would be simple, reliable, non-invasive, and painless and would provide continuous measurement. However, such an ideal method has not yet been developed. As such, the only reasonable approach to obtaining meaningful hemodynamic data in preterm infants is the use of complex, multi-channel, real-time monitoring towers combined with streamlined data-acquisition systems and observation of clinical symptoms.

4.3.1 Conventional assessment

Direct invasive measurements (via umbilical or peripheral artery catheterization) allow for constant monitoring of blood pressure in hypotensive preterm infants. Although this method is controversial, in our experience, blood pressure values obtained through intra-arterial catheterization are more accurate than non-intermittent blood pressure measurements taken during times of vasoconstriction. In addition, once intermittent blood pressure measurements become necessary, the patient's condition is often already severe, making the insertion of an arterial catheter impossible. It is important to note the risks of an indwelling catheter, including thrombus formation, hemorrhage, and infection.

In neonates admitted to the NICU, heart rate is continuously, accurately, and routinely monitored. However, factors such as anemia, drugs affecting the cardiovascular system, and infection can also affect heart rate. Therefore, heart rate monitoring has a limited role in the diagnosis of circulatory compromise.

Similarly, SpO2 measurements are performed routinely on neonates admitted to the NICU. This measures arterial oxygenation as an indicator of the arterial circulation. However, in contrast to adults, neonates have unique clinical complications. Clinical oximeters cannot detect carbon monoxide hemoglobin, methemoglobin, fetal hemoglobin, or other hemoglobin variations. Therefore, blood tests are needed for the accurate assessment a neonate's oxygenation status (Shiao and Ou, 2007). Nevertheless, SpO2 monitors are also useful for estimating the extent of the peripheral circulation on the basis of oxygenation waveforms.

Conventional monitoring of neonatal hemodynamics was restricted to intermittent evaluation of indirect clinical and laboratory indices of perfusion, such as peripheral-to-core temperature difference, skin color, urine output, capillary refill time, acid-base balance, and serum lactate levels. There are limited data available on capillary refill time in preterm infants. In the first 24 hours, the use of a capillary refill time of $\geq$ 3 seconds had a 55% sensitivity and 81% specificity for detecting low superior vena cava (SVC) flow (Osborn et al., 2004). In addition, abnormalities in skin color, urine output, base excess, and serum lactate often arise in other conditions of poor tissue oxygenation. For example, anemia can cause skin color abnormalities; kidney disease can cause abnormal urine output; dehydration and late metabolic acidosis can exacerbate BE and cause abnormal lactate levels. Hence, these measurements are not specific to hypotension and must be assessed in combination with other test findings.

4.3.2 Echocardiography

Echocardiographic examination may provide useful information regarding CO, contractility, pulmonary hemodynamics, and PDA shunting in hypotensive preterm infants. Recently, functional echocardiography has been increasingly used to assess CO, myocardial function, and organ blood flow in neonates requiring intensive care (Kluckow et al., 2007).

4.3.2.1 Systolic performance

Left ventricular systolic performance can be assessed by measuring the shortening factor (SF) and ejection fraction. Normal neonatal values for the SF are 28–40% (El-Khuffash and McNamara, 2011). A normal neonatal value for the ejection fraction is approximately 55% (Evans N and Kluckow, 1996).

4.3.2.2 Cardiac output

Normal left and right ventricular output ranges from 170 to 320 mL · kg-1 · min-1. Low left and right ventricular output is defined as < 150 mL · kg-1 · min-1 (normal values range from 170 to 320 mL · kg-1 · min-1) (Evans N and Kluckow, 1996). Superior Vena Cava Flow (SVC flow) in preterm infants is 50–110 mL · kg-1 · min-1. Low SVC flow is defined as below 30 mL · kg-1 · min-1 at the first 5 hours post-natally or below 46 mL · kg-1 · min-1 at the first 48 hours postnatally (Kluckow, 2005). Approximately 35% of preterm infants of < 30 weeks gestational age encounter a period of SVC flow below 40 mL · kg-1 · min-1 during the first 12 hours postnatally. After this point, SVC flow typically improves (Kluckow and Evans N, 2000).

4.3.2.3 Assessment of hypovolemia

The left ventricular end-diastolic diameter (LVEDD) is used to assess hypovolemia. LVEDD is measured at the point of maximal ventricular filling. Normally, the mean LVEDD increases from 11 mm at 23–25 weeks, 12 mm at 26–28 weeks, and 13 mm at 29–31 weeks to 14 mm at 32–33 weeks (Skelton et al., 1998). However, the utility of LVEDD as an indicator of hypovolemia in infants has not been systematically examined. In addition to LVEDD, other factors can affect left ventricular load in the transitional circulation (Evans N, 2003). However, once a preterm infant has been diagnosed with hypovolemia, LVEDD is a useful measurement for evaluation.

Thus, echocardiography is the most suitable test for evaluating cardiac activity and systemic perfusion in hypotensive preterm infants. Its drawback is that it does not allow for continuous observation. Additionally, there is no evidence that its use is associated with better outcomes. Alternatively, ultrasound Doppler, which continuously monitors CO, has also been used in neonates (Meyer et al., 2009).

4.3.3 Assessment of systemic and organ blood flow

Near-infrared spectroscopy (NIRS) measures hemoglobin flow and venous saturation in the forearm to calculate oxygen delivery and consumption and fractional oxygen extraction. In a previous study, Nagdyman et al. used NIRS to measure the cerebral tissue oxygenation index (TOI), regional cerebral oxygenation index (rSO2), venous oxygen saturation SjO2, and central SvO2 from the SVC. They found an association between cerebral TOI and SjO2, between cerebral TOI and SvO2, between cerebral rSO2 and SjO2, and between rSO2 and SvO2 (Nagdyman et al., 2008).

Peripheral and mucosal blood flow can be monitored using laser Doppler (Stark et al., 2009; Ishiguro et al., 2011), side-stream dark field imaging (Hiedl et al., 2010), and visible light T-

Sta (Van Bel et al., 2008) technologies. However, these devices have only been used in neonates for research purposes.

4.3.4 Further assessment of hypotension in preterm infants

As previously described, the diagnosis, treatment determination, and outcome evaluation of hypotension must be based on a combination of findings rather than a single marker. If possible, a time-course observation can improve the prognosis of hypotensive neonates.

Soleymani et al. designed a system for hemodynamic monitoring and data collection in neonates (Soleymani et al., 2010; Cavabvab et al., 2009). The system integrated conventional technologies (i.e., continuous monitoring of heart rate, blood pressure, SpO2, and transcutaneous CO2) with novel technologies, including impedance IEC for continuous assessment of CO and stroke volume and NIRS to monitor blood flow distribution to the brain, kidney, intestine, and/or muscle.

5. Treatment/ assessment of neonatal hemodynamics during postnatal transition

The first priority in treating hypotensive preterm infants is to maintain hemodynamics while the primary etiology is identified and its pathogenesis is addressed. Hemodynamic therapy consists of 3 broad categories: fluid resuscitation, vasopressor therapy, and inotropic therapy.

5.1 Fluid bolus

There is no evidence from randomized trials to support the routine use of early volume expansion in very preterm infants with hypotension. Fluid boli are useful in treating hypovolemia caused by twin-to-twin transfusion, third-space losses, or hemorrhage. However, circulating blood volumes are normal in most hypotensive infants, and there is little to no response to volume administration (Bauer et al., 1993). Moreover, preterm infants have immature cardiac contractile systems and vascular regulation; as such, volume management through fluid boli is not always effective.

Goldberg et al. observed an increased incidence of IVH among preterm infants receiving rapid volume expansion (Goldberg et al., 1980). Additionally, adverse neurological outcomes have been reported in preterm infants receiving colloid infusions (Greenough et al., 2002). The use of multiple fluid boli is also associated with an increased mortality in preterm infants (Ewer et al., 2003). Moreover, the administration of fluid boli has been reported be ineffective for cardiopulmonary resuscitation in cases other than at birth (Wyckoff et al., 2005).

There is insufficient evidence to determine the ideal type of volume expansion for preterm infants or for early red cell transfusions. Normal saline is equally effective as albumin in restoring blood pressure in hypotensive preterm infants. Normal saline is efficacious, safe, readily available, and inexpensive; therefore, it has become the fluid of choice for volume expansion (Oca et al., 2003). Furthermore, other crystalloids are costly and increase the risk of infection and neurodevelopmental deficits (Greenough et al., 2002).

5.2 Vasopressors and inotropes

5.2.1 Catecholamines

5.2.1.1 Mechanisms of action of catecholamines

The term "catecholamines" encompasses dopamine (DOA), NE (norepinephrine), and epinephrine (E). Catecholamines are produced by adrenal medullary cells and by neurons, specifically sympathetic postganglionic neurons. Indeed, adrenal medullary cells can be considered a subtype of postganglionic sympathetic neurons. Secretion of catecholamines by the adrenal medulla is regulated mainly by acetylcholine released from sympathetic nerve endings.

5.2.1.2 Biosynthesis of catecholamines (Fig.4)

First, tyrosine is hydroxylated to form dihydroxyphenylalanine (DOPA) in the rate-limiting step. DOPA is then converted into DOA through decarboxylation. DOA is packaged into secretory granules (chromaffin granules). Dopamine-β-hydroxylase inside the granules processes DOA to produce NE. In nerve cells, biosynthesis ends at this stage. In adrenal

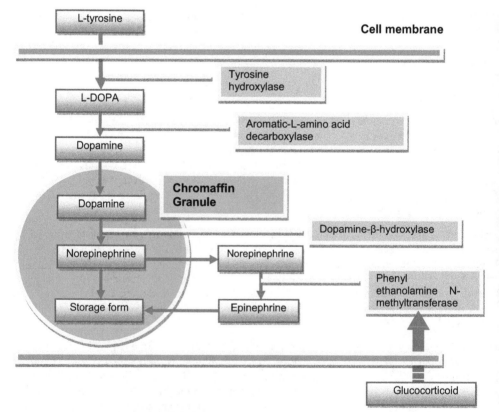

Fig. 4. Catecholamine biosynthesis

medullary cells, NE continues to be processed into E. Once NE is released from the secretory granules into the cytoplasm, it is processed by phenylethanolamine-N-methyltransferase (PNMT) to form E. E binds to a protein known as chromogranin and is recaptured into secretory granules, where it is stored (Goldstein et al., 2003).

The enzyme PNMT, which catalyzes the transformation of NE into E, is induced by glucocorticoids. The direction of blood flow in the adrenal gland travels from the cortex toward the medulla; as a result, medullary cells are in contact with the highest levels of cortisol. Therefore, E production may be regulated by adrenocortical cells.

Acetylcholine is secreted from preganglionic neurons upon stimulation of a sympathetic nerve. Acetylcholine acts at nicotinic receptors to depolarize chromaffin cells. This opens voltage-gated Ca2+ channels, increasing intracellular Ca2+ concentration.This is believed to result in the exocytosis of chromaffin granules.

5.2.1.3 Metabolism of catecholamines

E and NE secreted from the adrenal medulla are incorporated into various tissues and are metabolized by the kidneys. Their half-life in the blood is approximately 2 minutes. They are metabolized by 2 enzymes, catecholamine-O-methyltransferase (COMT) and monoamine oxidase (MAO), which convert them into metanephrine, normetanephrine, and vanillylmandelic acid. In addition to their actions on the heart and blood vessels, catecholamines act on the respiratory tract, gastrointestinal tract, urinary tract, sensory organs, skeletal muscles, adipose tissues, and pancreatic islets. With glucocorticoids, catecholamines also inhibit the proliferation of Th1 cells and promotes their differentiation into Th2 cells.

5.2.1.4 Adrenergic receptors

The physiological effects of catecholamines are elicited through receptors. The basic structure of adrenergic receptors is a seven-transmembrane protein that binds to GTP-binding proteins. There are 2 major types of adrenergic receptors, α and β, which are further classified into subtypes.

There are 2 major α-adrenergic receptor subtypes, α1 and α2, which are subdivided into several pharmacological subtypes. α1 receptors are present at postsynaptic membranes; their activation causes contraction of vascular smooth muscles. α2 receptors are present at presynaptic membranes and inhibit the release of NE caused by sympathetic stimulation. α2 receptors are also present in other various cells, such as blood platelets, pancreatic β-cells, and adipocytes. α1 receptors activate phospholipase C by conjugating with Gq protein. α2 receptors act by inhibiting the production of cAMP through inhibitory GTP-binding proteins (Gi).

β-adrenergic receptors are divided into 3 subtypes: β1, β2, and β3. β1 receptors are mainly distributed in the heart; β2 receptors are mainly distributed in blood vessels, bronchi, and glomerulus, and β3 receptors are mainly distributed in adipocytes. Therefore, β1 receptors promote cardiac stimulation; β2 receptors promote bronchodilation, vasodilation, and glycogenolysis in muscles, and β3 receptors promote lipolysis. β-adrenergic receptors increase the production of cAMP through stimulatory GTP-binding proteins, Gs. This activates cAMP-dependent protein kinase A.

5.2.1.5 Action of catecholamines

Catecholamines act through α and β receptors. The catecholamines differ in their action at α versus β receptors. For instance, while E acts on α and β receptors, NE acts mainly on α receptors (Fig. 5)

5.2.1.6 Cardiovascular effects of catecholamines

Through their actions at β1 receptors, catecholamines increase heart rate and cardiac contractile force. In coronary arteries, when the α-adrenergic effects of catecholamines trigger vasoconstriction, there is a compensatory β2-receptor-mediated vasodilation. In general, the vasodilatory effect predominates. Catecholamines also have vasoconstrictive α-adrenergic effects in arteries of the mucosa, kidney, spleen, and skeletal muscles and in venous vasculature. The β-adrenergic vasodilating effects of catecholamines include arterial vasodilation due to β2-adrenergic receptors in skeletal muscle. Because of their differential effects on adrenergic receptors, each catecholamine differently affects blood pressure and blood flow (Fig.6).

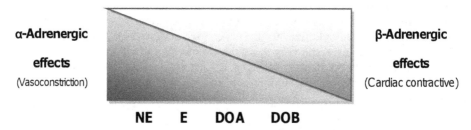

α-Adrenergic		β-Adrenergic
effects		effects
(Vasoconstriction)		(Cardiac contractive)
	NE E DOA DOB	

NE: Nor epinephrine, E: Epinephrine, **DOA** :Dopamine, **DOB**:Dobtamine

Fig. 5. α-and β-Adrenergic receptors effects of vasoactive inotropes

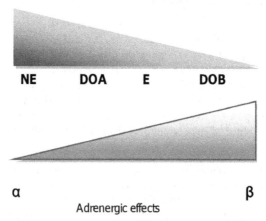

NE   DOA   E   DOB

α   β

Adrenergic effects

NE: Nor epinephrine, E: Epinephrine, **DOA** :Dopamine, **DOB**:Dobutamine

Fig. 6. Effects of catecholamines on blood pressure and blood flow (partly modified from Vincent, 2009)

5.2.1.7 Downregulation of adrenergic receptors

Recently, it has been proposed that exogenous catecholamine administration downregulates adrenergic receptors and their associated second-messenger systems (Hausdorff et al., 1999; Collins et al., 1991). During receptor downregulation, adrenergic receptors undergo lysosomal destruction; therefore, reversal of this process requires new protein synthesis.

5.2.1.8 Levels of catecholamines in hypotensive preterm infants

In extremely low birth-weight infants with hypotension, those in need of high doses of dopamine (DOA>10µg/kg/min) already had high levels of endogenous dopamine compared to those needing low doses of dopamine (DOA ≤10µg/kg/min) (p<0.05) (Ezaki et al., 2009b). The ratio of conversion from NE to E before the use of dopamine and 24 hours after administration were correlated in both infants who needed high doses of dopamine and in those who did not. This suggested that there was successful conversion of NE to E. In infants who did not need high doses of dopamine, there was a similar correlation between conversion of DOA to NE before and 24 hours after administration of dopamine. However, no correlation was found in infants who needed high doses of dopamine, suggesting that the conversion from DOA to NE was limited (Ezaki et al., 2009b) (Fig.7). Therefore, an understanding of the underlying pathological condition is important when administering catecholamines.

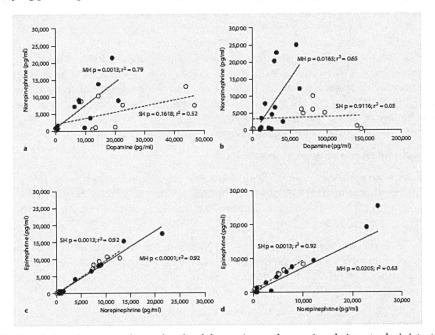

Fig. 7. Correlations between plasma levels of dopamine and norepinephrine at administration (a) and 24 h later (b) and between norepinephrine and epinephrine at administration (c) and 24 h later (d). The severe hypotension (SH, DOA>10µg/kg/min) group (n = 9) is represented by open circles with dotted regression lines, and the mild hypotension (MH, DOA≤10µg/kg/min) group (n = 13) is represented by closed circles with solid regression lines Correlation coefficients and p-values are shown in the respective graphs.

5.2.2 Dopamine

5.2.2.1 Treatment of dopamine in preterm hypotension

Dopamine is the most commonly used vasopressor/inotrope for the treatment of systemic hypotension in preterm infants (Seli,1996). DOA stimulates α-adrenergic receptors, β-adrenergic receptors, and dopaminergic receptors (See 5.2.1.4). DOA stimulates dopamine receptors at low doses (0.5 µg · kg-1 · min-1), mainly triggering effects in renal, mesenteric, and coronary blood vessels. At doses of 2–4 µg · kg-1 · min-1, DOA acts at α-adrenergic receptors, and at doses of 4–8 µg · kg-1 · min-1, DOA acts at β-adrenergic receptors (Seli, 2006).

With the exception of E administration, DOA administration is the most effective treatment for elevating blood pressure in preterm infants. The increase in CBF following DOA administration was found to be greater in hypotensive preterm infants compared to normotensive preterm infants, suggesting the presence of pressure-passive CBF in hypotensive neonates (Sassano et al., 2011). Therefore, we recommend the use of DOA as a first-line inotrope for the treatment of hypotension in preterm infants.

DOA is also an important neurotransmitter that affects both cerebral vasculature and neuronal activity. This is exemplified by pathological conditions caused by dopaminergic dysfunction, including abnormalities in CBF and neuronal metabolism (Edvinsson and Krause, 2002). In the mature brain, CBF is coupled to oxygen consumption (CMRO2). In contrast, CBF coupling to metabolism is strikingly different in the brains of very preterm infants, in which cerebral oxygen extraction, not CBF, sustains CMRO2. However, preterm infants receiving DOA treatment exhibit flow-metabolism coupling similar to that of the mature brain. This suggest a role for DOA in promoting flow-metabolism coupling in the preterm brain (Wong et al., 2009). In addition, we previously reported that high-dose administration of DOA can limit the conversion of NE to DOA (Ezaki et al., 2009b). Therefore, extreme caution must be taken when administering high doses of DOA.

5.2.2.2 Adverse effects of dopamine treatment

α2-adrenergic receptors are important in endocrine regulation; as such, even low doses of systemically administered DOA have profound endocrine effects. For instance, DOA infusion reduces thyroid stimulating hormone and thyroxine levels in very low birth-weight infants (Filippi et al., 2004).

Doses of DOA should rarely exceed 20 µg · kg-1 · min-1, because there is a risk of excessive α-adrenergic-receptor-mediated peripheral vasoconstriction and a subsequent reduction in CO (Rozé et al., 1993). DOA failed to raise blood pressure in more than 30% of preterm infants with systemic hypotension (Pellicer et al., 2005).

5.2.3 Norepinephrine

5.2.3.1 The use of norepinephrine in the treatment of preterm hypotension

NE is a potent vasopressor with α-and, to a lesser extent, β-1 receptor agonist activity (Hollenberg et al., 2004). In the adult, NE is primarily used as a vasopressor in states of hyperdynamic shock, in which SVR is decreased and mean arterial blood pressure is low (Corley, 2004). Experimental studies in fetal lambs have shown that NE may decrease basal pulmonary vascular tone (Houfflin-Debarge et al., 2001) and elevate pulmonary blood flow through activating α2-adrenergic receptors and NO release (Magnenant et al., 2003).

NE can reduce damage incurred by neuroinflammatory and neurodegenerative conditions. It induces the expression of the chemokine CCL2 in astrocytes, which is neuroprotective against excitotoxic damage (Madrigal et al., 2009). Indeed, early associative somatosensory conditioning requires NE (Landers and Sulliyan, 1999).

Thus, NE plays an important role not only in the cardiovascular system, but also in neonatal development. However, there are few studies on the use of NE in the treatment of hypotension in preterm infants. While no studies have compared NE to other drugs, its therapeutic effects in neonates have recently been reported (Paradisis and Osborn, 2004). The use of NE (0.5-0.75 µg · kg-1 · min-1) is effective in the treatment of term and near-term infants with septic shock that are resistant to DOA and dobutamine (Tourneux et al., 2008a). In neonates with persistent pulmonary hypertension-induced cardiac dysfunction, NE can reduce O2 requirements and normalize the systemic artery pressure (Tourneux et al., 2008b).

5.2.3.2 Adverse effects of norepinephrine treatment

In all previous reports describing the use of NE in neonates, NE was administered after other inotropes, making it impossible to describe the side effects solely attributable to NE. In addition, there are no reports on the long-term consequences of the use of NE in preterm infants. In general, excessive peripheral vasoconstriction causes a decrease in the contractile forces of the immature heart. This may result in tachycardia or decreased tissue perfusion. Therefore, capillary refill time, lactate levels, and peripheral and organ blood flow should be monitored.

5.2.4 Epinephrine

5.2.4.1 The use of epinephrine for the treatment of preterm hypotension

Low and moderate doses of E (0.125-0.5 µg · kg-1 · min-1) have found to be as effective as low and moderate doses of DOA (2.5-10 µg · kg-1 · min-1) for the treatment of hypotension in preterm infants (Valverde et al., 2006). In addition, the infusion of E increases mean arterial blood pressure and heart rate without decreasing urine output in very low birth-weight infants with hypotension that do not respond to dopamine infusion up to 15 µg · kg-1 · min-1 (Heckmann et al., 2002).

5.2.4.2 Adverse effects of epinephrine

Compared DOA, E use cases temporary dysfunction of carbohydrate and lactate metabolism (Valverde et al., 2006) and increased metabolic acidosis (Heckmann et al., 2002). E directly affects lactate metabolism by increasing lactate production and decreasing lactate metabolism, thus increasing serum lactate concentrations (Cheung et al., 1997). At very high doses, E induces vasoconstriction sufficient to counteract its inotropic benefits, and CO may fall (Barrington et al., 1995).

Pellicer et al. recently reported that the long-term prognosis of E use was the same as DOA use, and that both were safe (Pellicer et al., 2009). This important study provided an additional treatment option for preterm hypotension.

5.3 Non-catecholamine inotropic/pressor agents

5.3.1 Dobutamine

5.3.1.1 Physiology of dobutamine in preterm hypotension

Dobutamine is a racemic mixture of 2 isomers, the D-isomer with α1- and α2-adrenergic effects and the L-isomer with α1- and α1- adrenergic effects. Dobutamine is predominantly inotropic via stimulation of α1 receptors and has a variable effect on blood pressure (Hollenberg, 2011). Dobutamine administration results in a variable decrease in total SVR. Unlike DOA, dobutamine increases myocardial contractility exclusively through direct stimulation of myocardial adrenergic receptors (Noori et al., 2004).

5.3.1.2 The use of dobutamine for the treatment of preterm hypotension

At a dose of 2–15 µg · kg-1 · min-1, dobutamine increases CO mainly through augmenting stroke volume (Noori et al., 2004; Roze et al., 1993; Bhatt-Mehta and Nahata, 1989).

5.3.1.3 Adverse effects of dobutamine treatment

Adverse effects of dobutamine occur at high doses and include increased heart rate. At very high doses, dobutamine may increase blood pressure and SVR (Cheung et al., 1999), likely due to stimulation of á-receptors (Fig.5 and 6). One study suggested that dobutamine's potential benefit of increased oxygen delivery to the tissues was offset by increased tissue metabolic rate (Penny et al., 2001).

5.3.2 Vasopressin

5.3.2.1 Physiology of vasopressin in preterm infants

Vasopressin induces its physiological responses through 4 receptors, V1, V2, V3, and oxytocin receptors (OTR) (Holmes et al., 2001). When vasopressin binds to V1 receptors in vascular smooth muscle (Va1 receptors), it activates phospholipase C, triggering calcium release from intracellular calcium stores (Fig. 2). This results in vasoconstriction and a subsequent increase in blood pressure. Activation of V2 receptors in the stomach increases intracellular cyclic AMP levels through the mediation of adenylate cyclase and have an anti-diuretic effect. V3 receptors (also known as V1b receptors) are involved in vasopressin's adrenocorticotropic hormone (ACTH)-stimulating effects. Finally, OTR receptors mediate vasopressing's oxytocic effects on uterine contractility.

V2 receptors and OTR receptors also have vasodilating effects that are antagonistic to the effects of V1 receptors. In addition, V1 receptors and OTR receptors have diuretic effects, which are antagonistic to the anti-diuretic effects of V2 receptors. Vasopressin's effects are most adapted to disease-induced changes.

Previous reports have indicated that blood levels of endogenous vasopressin show a two-phased response in adults with shock (Holmes et al., 2001; Landry et al., 1997; Morales et al., 1999). During the initial phase of shock, endogenous vasopressin is released in large amounts and reaches high blood levels in order to maintain tissue perfusion. However, its concentration in the blood decreases over time. As such, vasopressin may be depleted due to its initial release in large amounts. The release of vasopressin from the pituitary gland may also be inhibited by NO produced by the vascular endothelium or due to autonomic nervous system disorders (Holmes et al., 2001; Landry et.al, 1997; Morales et al., 1999).

The effects of the small amounts of exogenous vasopressin may be a result of enhancing the effects of catecholamines, inhibiting inducible NO synthase (iNOS), inhibiting increased cGMP induced by NO and ANP, or inactivating KATP channels in vascular smooth muscles (Fig.2) (Landry et al., 2001; Hamu et al.,1999).

In preterm infants, the levels of vasopressin were high during the first 24 hours following birth (Ezaki et al., 2009b). The effects of these high levels of endogenous vasopressin on the cardiovascular system are not fully understood.

5.3.2.2 The use of vasopressin for the treatment of hypotension in preterm infants

Meyer et al. reported that vasopressin (0.035–0.36 U · kg-1 · hr-1) may be a promising rescue therapy for catecholamine-resistant shock in extremely-low-birth-weight infants with acute renal injury (Meyer et al., 2006). Similarly, Ikegami et al. found that administration of vasopressin (0.001–0.01 U · kg-1 · hr-1) was effective in extremely-low-birth-weight infants resistant to treatment with catecholamines and steroids (Ikegami et al., 2010).

5.3 Adverse effects of vasopressin treatment

The side effects of vasporessin include severe cutaneous ischemia, hepatic necrosis, neurological deficits, and dysmetria (Meyer et al., 2006; Rodríguez-Nunez et al., 2006; Zeballos et al., 2006). Unlike DOA, E, and dobutamine, there are few reports on the side effects of vasopressin. Moreover, it is unclear whether its side effects are dose-dependent and what the long-term prognoses are. However, vasopressin is a pharmacological agent that can be considered for use in patients in whom other drugs are ineffective.

5.4 Lusitropes

5.4.1 Physiology of phosphodiesterase-III inhibitors in preterm hypotension

Phosphodiesterase inhibitors increase intracellular cyclic AMP and thus have inotropic effects independent of α-adrenergic receptors. As such, they result in fewer chronotropic and arrhythmogenic effects than catecholamines. However, increased cyclic AMP in vascular smooth muscle cells can cause vasodilation, thus reducing SVR, which can exacerbate hypotension. In addition, this can reduce pulmonary artery pressure. (Chen et al.,1997,1998; Kato et al.,1998). Milrinone, a cyclic nucleotide phosphodiesterase-III inhibitor, improves contractility and reduces afterload in adults and newborns with cardiac dysfunction.

5.4.2 The use of phosphodiesterase-III inhibitors for the treatment of preterm hypotension

McNamara et al. reported that intravenous Milrinone (0.33–0.99 µg · kg-1 · min-1) administration produced early improvements in oxygenation without compromising systemic blood pressure in patients with severe persistent pulmonary hypertension (McNamara et al., 2006). One randomized clinical trial did not support the use of Milrinone (0.75 µg · kg-1 · min-1 for 3 hrs, then 0.2µ g · kg-1 · min-1 until 18 hours after birth) in the prevention of low SVC in the early transitional circulation of preterm infants (Paradisis et al., 2009).

5.4.3 Adverse effects of Milrinone treatment

Milrinone can cause hypotension and tachycardia (Chang et al., 1995). The long-term effects of Milrinone in preterm infants have not been reported.

5.5 Corticosteroids

5.5.1 Physiology of corticosteroids

The adrenal glands are involved in the growth and maturation of fetal organs during intrauterine life. In most mammals, a cortisol surge occurs as the full gestational term approaches; this triggers increased synthesis of pulmonary surfactant, reduced sensitivity of the arteries to prostaglandins, and increased conversion of pancreatic β-cells from T4 to T3 in the mature liver. These changes allow the fetus to survive in the extrauterine environment. There is also a surge in catecholamines produced by the adrenal medulla during delivery. This surge also allows adaptation to the extrauterine environment by influencing the cardiovascular system, including elevating the blood pressure and increasing the heart function, and by influencing glucose metabolism, fat metabolism, and water absorption in the lungs (Fisher, 2002).

The hypothalamic-pituitary-adrenal system in fetuses and neonates has been implicated in late-onset circulatory collapse (Masumoto et al., 2008) and in the fetal programming of the cardiovascular system. Preterm infants have low adrenal function due to their low levels of 3β-hydroxysteroid dehydrogenase (HSD) (Mesiano and Jaffe, 1997) and weak 11b-HSD2 activity (Donaldson et al.,1991).

Corticosteroids reverse neonatal hypotension by improving capillary-leak syndrome (Briegel et al., 1994), potentiating transmembrane calcium currents, increasing β-receptor sensitivity to catecholamines, reversing the downregulation of β-receptors, increasing the density of β-receptors, and inhibiting NO synthase expression (Prigent et al., 2004).

5.5.2 The use of corticosteroids in the treatment of preterm hypotension

Hydrocortisone administration is effective in the treatment of hypotension and vasopressor dependence in hypotensive preterm infants. Its clinical benefits include increasing blood pressure and decreasing the requirement for vasopressor administration (Higgins et al., 2010). Fernandez et al. have reviewed the use of hydrocortisone in the treatment of premature infants (Fernandez and Watterberg, 2009). Before initiating therapy with hydrocortisone in extremely preterm infants with refractory hypotension, a blood specimen should be analyzed for cortisol concentration. Pending that result, an initial dose of 1 mg/kg can be administered. If the blood pressure improves within 2 to 6 h, 0.5 mg/kg can be administered every 12 h (approximately 8–10 mg/m^2 per day). This long dosing interval is used, because hydrocortisone has a longer half-life in immature infants (Watterberg et al., 2005). This dosing strategy increases serum values by an average of 5 μg/100 ml; higher doses are associated with very high serum concentrations. If the initial cortisol concentration is high (>15–20 μg/100 ml), drug administration may be discontinued, especially in the absence of a clinical response.

5.5.3 Adverse effects of corticosteroid treatment

Although corticosteroid therapy improves blood pressure and circulation, there are many potential complications, including spontaneous gut perforation, hyperglycemia, and hypertension and long-term consequences, including cerebral palsy and intellectual impairment. These complications necessitate the judicious use of corticosteroids to support blood pressure in preterm infants (Yeh et al., 2004).

Hydrocortisone therapy administered simultaneously with indomethacin or ibuprofen has been associated with acute spontaneous gastrointestinal perforation in extremely preterm infants. Therefore, care should be taken to avoid concurrent therapy (Watterberg et al., 2004; Peltoniemi et al., 2005). Infants who develop spontaneous perforation often have high endogenous cortisol concentrations (Watterberg et al., 2004; Peltoniemi et al., 2005).

Watterberg et al. reported that early, low-dose hydrocortisone treatment was not associated with an increased risk of cerebral palsy. In fact, infants treated with hydrocortisone displayed improved developmental outcomes. Together with the short-term benefits, these data support the use of hydrocortisone for the treatment of adrenal insufficiency in extremely premature infants (Watterberg et al., 2007).

6. Conclusion

The major findings of the present chapter summarized in the following figure (Fig.8).

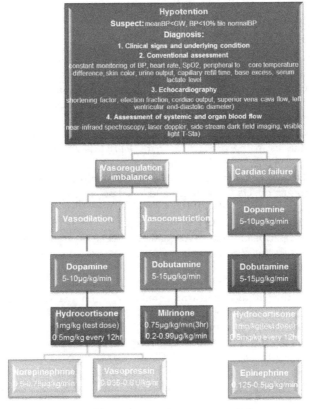

Fig. 8. Evaluation and treatment of hypotension in premature infants

7. Acknowledgment

We express gratitude to the efforts of the authors whose research is cited in this article. First author (FA)'s personal research on vasoactive factors in neonates was inspired by my wife, a physician who introduced me to the use of vasopressin for the management of shock. Therefore, FA offer my wife, Yuko Ezaki, my most sincere gratitude. Finally, FA dedicate this chapter to my famiiy: Munenori, Tomi, Yuko, Yoshiko, Yukiko, and Saeka Ezaki.

FA hope that this work will promote future advances in neonatal care.

8. References

Bauer, K. & Linderkamp, O. & Versmold, HT. (1993). Systolic blood pressure and blood volume in preterm infants. *Archives of disease in childhood*, Vol. 69, 5 Spec No, (Nov), pp. 521-522, ISSN 0003-9888

Barrington, KJ. & Finer, NN. & Chan, WK. (1995). A blind, randomized comparison of the circulatory effects of dopamine and epinephrine infusions in the newborn piglet during normoxia and hypoxia. *Critical Care Medicine*, Vol. 23, No. 4, (Apr). pp. 740-748, ISSN 0090-3493

Belik, J., Light, RB. (1989). Effect of increased afterload on right ventricular function in newborn pigs. *Journal* of *Applied Physiology*, Vol. 66, No. 2, (Feb), pp. 863-869, ISSN 8750-7587

Bhatt-Mehta, V. & Nahata, MC. (1989). Dopamine and dobutamine in pediatric therapy. *Pharmacotherapy*, Vol. 9, No. 5, (May), pp. 304-314, ISSN 0277-0008

Briegel, J. & Kellermann, W. & Forst, H et al. (1994). Low-dose hydrocortisone infusion attenuates the systemic inflammatory response syndrome. The Phospholipase A2 Study Group. *The Clinical investigator*, Vol. 72, No. 10, (Oct), pp. 782-787, ISSN 0941-0198

Cayabyab, R. & McLean, CW. & Seri, I. (2009). Definition of hypotension and assessment of hemodynamics in the preterm neonate. *Journal of Perinatology*, Vol. 29, Suppl. 2, (May), pp. S58-S62, ISSN 0743-8346

Chang, AC. & Atz, AM. & Wernovsky, G et al. (1995). Milrinone: systemic and pulmonary hemodynamic effects in neonates after cardiac surgery. *Critical care medicine*, Vol. 23, No. 11, (Nov), pp. 1907-1914, ISSN 0090-3493

Cheung, PY. & Barrington, KJ. & Pearson, RJ et al. (1997). Systemic, pulmonary and mesenteric perfusion and oxygenation effects of dopamine and epinephrine. *American Journal of Respiratory and Critical Care Medicine*, Vol. 155, No. 1, (Jan), pp. 32-37, ISSN 1073-449X

Cheung, PY. & Barrington, KJ. & Bigam, D. (1999). The hemodynamic effects of dobutamine infusion in the chronically instrumented newborn piglet. *Critical Care Medicine*, Vol. 27, No. 3, (Mar), pp. 558-564, ISSN 0090-3493

Chen, EP. & Bittner, HB. & Davis, RD Jr et al. (1997). Milrinone improves pulmonary hemodynamics and right ventricular function in chronic pulmonary hypertension. *The Annals of Thoracic Surgery*, Vol. 63, No. 3, (Mar), pp. 814-821, ISSN 0003-4975

Chen, EP. & Bittner, HB. & Davis, RD et al. (1998), Hemodynamic and inotropic effects of milrinone after heart transplantation in the setting of recipient pulmonary hypertension. *The Journal of Heart and Lung Transplantation*, Vol. 17, No. 7, (Jul), pp. 669-678, ISSN 1053-2498

Collins, S. & Caron, MG. & Lefkowitz, RJ. (1991). Regulation of adrenergic receptor responsiveness through modulation of receptor gene expression. *Annual Review of Physiology*, Vol. 53, pp. 497-508, ISSN 0066-4278

Corley, KT. (2004). Inotropes and vasopressors in adults and foals. *The Veterinary clinics of North America. Equine practice*, Vol. 20, No. 1, (Apr), pp. 77-106, ISSN 0749-0739

Cunningham, S. & Symon, AG. & Elton, RA et al. (1999). Intraarterial blood pressure reference ranges, death and morbidity in very low birth weight infants during the first seven days of life. *Early Human Development*, Vol. 56, No. 2-3, (Dec), pp. 151-165, ISSN 0378-378256.

Dempsey, EM. & Al Hazzani, F. & Barrington, KJ. (2009). Permissive hypotension in the extremely low birthweight infant with signs of good perfusion. *Archives of Disease in Childhood Fetal & Neonatal Edition*, Vol. 94, No. 4, (Jul), pp. F241-F244, ISSN 1359-2998

Donaldson, A. & Nicolini, U. & Symes, EK et al. (1991). Changes in concentrations of cortisol, dehydroepiandrosterone sulphate and progesterone in fetal and maternal serum during pregnancy. *Clinical endocrinology*, Vol. 35, No. 5,(Nov), pp. 447-451, ISSN 0300-0664

Edvinsson, L. & Krause, D. (2002). Catecholamines, In: *Cerebral blood flow and metabolism*, Edvinsson, L & Krause, D, (Eds.), 191-211, Lippincott Williams & Wilkins, ISBN 978-0781722599, Philadelphia

El-Khuffash, AF. & McNamara, PJ. (2011). Neonatologist-performed functional echocardiography in the neonatal intensive care unit. *Seminars in fetal & neonatal medicine*, Vol. 16, No. 1, (Feb), pp. 50-60, ISSN 1744-165X

Engle, WD. (2001). Blood pressure in the very low birth weight neonates. *Early Human Development*, Vol. 62, No. 2, (May), pp. 97-130, ISSN 0378-3782

Evans, N. (2003). Volume expansion during neonatal intensive care: do we know what we are doing? *Semin Neonatol*, Vol. 8, No. 4, (Aug), pp. 315-323, ISSN1744-165X52.

Evans, N. & Kluckow, M. (1996). Early determinants of right and left ventricular output in ventilated preterm infants. *Archives of disease in childhood. Fetal and neonatal edition*, Vol. 74, No. 2, (Mar), pp. F88-F94, ISSN 1359-2998

Ewer, AK. & Tyler, W. & Francis, A et al. (2003). Excessive volume expansion and neonatal death in preterm infants born at 27-28 weeks gestation. *Paediatric and Perinatal Epidemiology*, Vol. 17, No.2, (Apr), pp. 180-186, ISSN 0269-5022

Ezaki, S. & Suzuki, K. & Kurishima, C et al. (2009a). Resuscitation of preterm infants with reduced oxygen results in less oxidative stress than resuscitation with 100% oxygen. *Journal of clinical biochemistry and nutrition*, Vol. 44, No.1, (Jan), pp. 111-118, ISSN 0912-0009

Ezaki, S. & Suzuki, K. & Kurishima, C et al. (2009b). Levels of catecholamines, arginine vasopressin and atrial natriuretic peptide in hypotensive extremely low birth weight infants in the first 24 hours after birth. *Neonatology*, Vol. 95, No. 3, (Nov 4), pp. 248-255, ISSN 1661-7800

Fernandez, EF. & Watterberg, KL. (2009). Relative adrenal insufficiency in the preterm and term infant. *Journal of Perinatology*, Vol. 29, Suppl 2, (May), pp. S44-S49, ISSN 0743-8346

Fisher, D. (2002). Endocrinology of Fetal Development, In: *Williams Textbook of Endcrinology · 11th*, Kronenberg, HM. & Melmed, S, & Polonsky, KS. & Larsen, (Eds.), pp.756-776, WB Saunders, ISBN 978-1437703245, Phil ad elphia

Filippi, L. & Cecchi, A. & Tronchin, M et al. (2004). Dopamine infusion and hypothyroxinaemia in very low birth weight preterm infants. *Early Human Development*, Vol. 163, No. 1, (Jan), pp. 7-13, ISSN 0378-3782

Goldberg, RN. & Chung, D. & Goldman, SL et al. (1980). The association of rapid volume expansion and intraventricular hemorrhage in the preterm infant. *The Journal of Pediatrics*, Vol. 96, No. 6, (Jun), pp. 1060-1063, ISSN 0022-3476

Goldstein, DS. & Eisenhofer, G. & Kopin IJ. (2003). Sources and significance of plasma levels of catechols and their metabolites in humans. *Journal of Pharmacology and Experimental Therapeutics*, Vol. 305, No. 3, (Jun), PP. 800-811, ISSN 0022-3565

Goldstein, RF. & Thompson, RJ. & Oehler, JM et al. (1995). Influence of acidosis, hypoxemia, and hypotension on neurodevelopmental outcome in very low birth weight infants. *Pediatrics*, Vol. 95, No. 2, (Feb), pp. 238-243, ISSN 0031-4005

Greenough, A. & Cheesemen, P. & Kawadia, V et al. (2002). Colloid infusion in the perinatal period and abnormal neurodevelopmental outcome in very low birth weight infants. *European Journal of Pediatrics*, Vol. 161, No. 6, (Jun), pp. 319-323, ISSN 0340-6199

Greisen G. (2005). Autoregulation of cerebral blood flow in newborn babies. *Early Human Development*, Vol. 81, No. 5, (May), pp. 423-428, ISSN 0378-3782

Hausdorff, WP. & Hnatowich, M. & O'Dowd BF et al. (1990). A mutation of the beta 2-adrenergic receptor impairs agonist activation of adenylyl cyclase without affecting high affinity agonist binding. Distinct molecular determinants of the receptor are involved in physical coupling to and functional activation of Gs. *The Journal of Biological Chemistry*, Vol. 265, No. 3, (Jan), pp.1388-1393, ISSN 0021-9258

Hamu, Y. & Kanmura, Y. & Tsuneyoshi, I et al. (1999). The effects of vasopressin on endotoxin-induced attenuation of contractile responses in human gastroepiploic arteries in vitro. *Anesthesia & Analgesia*, Vol. 88, No. 3, (Mar), pp. 542-548, ISSN 0003-2999

Heckmann, M. & Trotter, A. & Pohlandt, F et al. (2002). Epinephrine treatment of hypotension in very low birthweight infants. *Acta Paediatrica*, Vol. 91. No. 5, (May), pp. 566-570, ISSN 0803-5253

Higgins, S. & Friedlich, P. & Seri, I. (2010). Hydrocortisone for hypotension and vasopressor dependence in preterm neonates: a meta-analysis. *Journal of Perinatology*, Vol. 30, No. 6, (Jun), pp. 373-378, ISSN 0743-8346

Hiedl, S. & Schwepcke, A. & Weber, F et al. (2010). Microcirculation in preterm infants: profound effects of patent ductus arteriosus. *The Journal of Pediatrics*, Vol. 156, No. 2, (Feb), pp. 191-196, ISSN 0022-3476

Hollenberg, SM. & Ahrens, TS. & Annane, D et al. (2004). Practice parameters for hemodynamic support of sepsis in adult patients: 2004 update. *Critical Care Medicine*, Vol. 32, No. 9, (Sep), pp, 1928-1948, ISSN 0090-3493

Hollenberg, SM. (2011). Vasoactive drugs in circulatory shock. *American Journal of Respiratory and Critical Care Medicine*, Vol. 183, No. 7, (Apr 1), pp. 847-855, ISSN 1073-449X

Holmes, CL. & Patel, BM. & Russell, JA et al. (2001). Physiology of vasopressin relevant to management of septic shock. *Chest*, Vol. 120, No. 3, (Sep), pp. 989-1002, ISSN 0012-3692

Ikegami, H. & Funato, M. & Tamai, H et al. (2010). Low-dose vasopressin infusion therapy for refractory hypotension in ELBW infants. *Pediatrics International*, Vol. 52, No. 3, (Jun), pp. 368-373, ISSN 1328-8067

Ishiguro, A. & Sekine, T. & Suzuki, K et al.(2011). Changes in skin and subcutaneous perfusion in very-low-birth-weight infants during the transitional period. *Neonatology*, Vol. 100, No. 2, (Mar), pp. 162-168, ISSN 1661-7800

Jaillard, S. & Houfflin-Debarge, V. & Riou Y et al. (2001). Effects of catecholamines on the pulmonary circulation in the ovine fetus. *American journal of physiology. Regulatory, integrative and comparative physiology*, Vol. 281, No. 2, (Aug), pp. R607-R614, ISSN 0363-6119

Kato, R. & Sato, J. & Nishino, T. (1998). Milrinone decreases both pulmonary arterial and venous resistances in the hypoxic dog. *British Journal of Anaesthesia* , Vol. 81, No. 6, (Dec), pp. 920-924, ISSN 0007-0912

Kluckow, M. & Evans, N. (2000). Superior vena cava flow in newborn infants: a novel marker of systemic blood flow. *Archives of Disease in Childhood Fetal & Neonatal Edition*, Vol. 82, No. 3, (May), pp. F182-F187, ISSN 1359-2998

Kluckow, M. & Seri, I. & Evans, N. (2007). Functional echocardiography: an emerging clinical tool for the neonatologist. *The Journal of Pediatrics*, Vol. 150, No. 2, (Feb), pp. 125-130, ISSN 0022-3476

Kluckow, M. (2005). Low systemic blood flow and pathophysiology of the preterm transitional circulation. *Early Human Development*, Vol. 81, No. 5, (May), pp. 429-437, ISSN: 0378-3782

Landry, DW. & Levin, HR. & Gallant, EM et al. (1997). Vasopressin deficiency contributes to the vasodilation of septic shock. *Circulation*, Vol. 95, No. 5, (Mar 4), pp. 1122-1125, ISSN 0009-7322

McNamara, PJ. & Laique, F. & Muang-In, S et al. (2006). Milrinone improves oxygenation in neonates with severe persistent pulmonary hypertension of the newborn. *Journal of Critical Care*, Vol. 21, No. 2, (Jun), pp. 217-222 ISSN 0883-9441

Landers, MS. & Sullivan, RM. (1999). Norepinephrine and associative conditioning in the neonatal rat somatosensory system. *Brain research. Developmental brain research*, Vol. 114, No.2, (May 14), pp. 261-264, ISSN 0165-3806

Landry, DW. & Oliver, JA. (2001). The pathogenesis of vasodilatory shock. *The New England Journal of Medicine*, Vol. 345, No. 8, (Aug 23), pp. 588-595, ISSN 0028-4793

Liedel, JL. & Meadow, W. & Nachman, J et al. (2002). Use of vasopressin in refractory hypotension in children with vasodilatory shock: five cases and a review of the literature. *Pediatric Critical Care Medicine*, Vol. 3, No. 1, (Jan), pp. 15-18, ISSN 1529-7535

Masumoto, K. & Kusuda, S. & Aoyagi, H et al. (2008). Comparison of serum cortisol concentrations in preterm infants with or without late-onset circulatory collapse due to adrenal insufficiency of prematurity. *Pediatric Research*, Vol. 63, No. 6, (Jun), pp. 686-690, ISSN 0031-3998

Magnenant, E. & Jaillard, S. & Deruelle, P et al. (2003). Role of the alpha2-adrenoceptors on the pulmonary circulation in the ovine fetus. *Pediatric Research*, Vol. 54, No. 1, (Jul), pp. 44-51, ISSN 0031-3998

Madrigal, JL. & Leza, JC. & Polak P et al. (2009). Astrocyte-derived MCP-1 mediates neuroprotective effects of noradrenaline. *Journal of Neuroscience*, Vol. 29, No. 1, (Jan 7), pp. 263-267, ISSN 0270-6474

McLean, CW. & Cayabyab, R. & Noori, S et al. (2008). Cerebral circulation and hypotension in the premature infant- diagnosis and treatment, In: *Neonatology Questions and Controversies: Neurology*, Perlman, JM. (Ed.), pp. 3–26, Saunders/Elsevier, ISBN, 978-1416031574, Philadelphia

Meyer, S. & Gottschling, S. & Baghai, A et al. (2006). Arginine-vasopressin in catecholamine-refractory septic versus non-septic shock in extremely low birth weight infants with acute renal injury. *Critical Care*, Vol. 10, No. 3, (May 5), R71, ISSN 1364-8535

Meyer, S. & Todd, D. & Shadboldt, B. (2009). Assessment of portable continuous wave Doppler ultrasound (ultrasonic cardiac output monitor) for cardiac output measurements in neonates. *Journal of Paediatrics and Child Health*, Vol. 45, No. 7-8, (Jul-Aug), pp. 464-468, ISSN 1034-4810

Mesiano, S. & Jaffe, RB. (1997). Developmental and functional biology of the primate fetal adrenal cortex. *Endocrine* Reviews, Vol. 18, No. 3, (Jun), pp. 378-403, ISSN 0163-769X

Morales, D. & Madigan, J. & Cullinane, S et al. (1999). Reversal by vasopressin of intractable hypotension in the late phase of hemorrhagic shock. *Circulation*, Vol. 100, No. 3, (Jul 20), pp. 226-229, ISSN 0009-7322

Munro, MJ. & Walker, AM. & Barfield, CP. (2004). Hypotensive extremely low birth weight infants have reduced cerebral blood flow. *Pediatrics*, Vol. 114, No. 6, (Dec), pp. 1591-1596, ISSN 0031-4005

Nagdyman, N & Ewert, P. & Peters, B et al. (2008). Comparison of different near-infrared spectroscopic cerebral oxygenation indices with central venous and jugular venous oxygenation saturation in children. *Pediatric Anesthesia*, Vol. 18, No. 2, (Feb), pp. 160-166, ISSN 1155-5645

Ng, PC. & Lam, CW. & Fok, TF et al. (2001) Refractory hypotension in preterm infants with adrenocortical insufficiency. *Archives of Disease in Childhood Fetal & Neonatal Edition*, Vol. 84, No. 2, (Mar), pp. F122-F124, ISSN 1359-2998

Noori, S. & Seri, I. (2005). Pathophysiology of newborn hypotension outside the transitional period. *Early Human Development*, Vol.81, No.5, (May), pp. 399-404, ISSN 0378-3782

Noori, S. & Friedlich, P. & Seri, I. (2004). Pharmacology Review: The Use of Dobutamine in the Treatment of Neonatal Cardiovascular Compromise. *NeoReviews. org*, Vol. 5, No. 1, (Jan 1), pp. e22-e26

Nuntnarumit, P. & Yang, W. & Bada-Ellzey, HS. (1999). Blood pressure measurements in the newborn. *Clinics in Perinatology*, Vol. 26, No. 4, (Dec), pp. 981-996, ISSN 0095-5108

Oca, MJ. & Nelson, M. & Donn, SM. (2003). Randomized trial of normal saline versus 5% albumin for the treatment of neonatal hypotension. *Journal of Perinatology*, Vol. 23, No. 6, (Sep), pp. 473-476, ISSN 0743-8346

Osborn, DA. & Evans, N. & Kluckow, M. (2004). Clinical detection of low upper body blood flow in very premature infants using blood pressure, capillary refill time, and central-peripheral temperature difference. *Archives of Disease in Childhood Fetal & Neonatal Edition*, Vol. 89, No. 2, (Mar), pp. F168-F173, ISSN 1359-2998

Paradisis, M. & Evans, N. & Kluckow, M et al. (2009). Randomized trial of milrinone versus placebo for prevention of low systemic blood flow in very preterm infants. *The Journal* of *Pediatrics*, Vol. 154, No. 2, (Feb), pp. 189-195, ISSN 0022-3476

Paradisis, M. & Osborn, DA. (2004). Adrenaline for prevention of morbidity and mortality in preterm infants with cardiovascular compromise. *Cochrane database of systematic reviews*, No.1, CD003958, ISSN 1469-493X

Pellicer, A. & Valverde, E. & Elorza, MD et al. (2005). Cardiovascular support for low birth weight infants and cerebral hemodynamics: a randomized, blinded, clinical trial. *Pediatrics*, Vol. 115, No. 6, (Jun), pp. 1501-1512, ISSN 0031-400568. Pellicer, A. & Bravo, MC. & Madero, R et al. (2009). Early systemic hypotension and vasopressor support in low birth weight infants: impact on neurodevelopment. *Pediatrics*, Vol. 123, No. 5, (May), pp. 1369-1376, ISSN 0031-4005

Penny, DJ. & Sano, T. & Smolich, JJ. (2001). Increased systemic oxygen consumption offsets improved oxygen delivery during dobutamine infusion in newborn lambs. *Intensive Care Medicine*, Vol. 27, No. 9, (Sep), pp. 1518-1525, ISSN 0342-4642

Peltoniemi, O. & Kari, MA. & Heinonen, K et al. (2005), Pretreatment cortisol values may predict responses to hydrocortisone administration for the prevention of bronchopulmonary dysplasia in high-risk infants. *The Journal of Pediatrics*, Vol. 146, No. 5, (May), pp. 632-637, ISSN 0022-3476

Prigent, H. & Maxime, V. & Annane, D. (2004). Clinical review: corticotherapy in sepsis. *Critical Care*, Vol. 8, No. 2, (Apr), pp.122-129, ISSN 1364-8535

Tourneux, P. & Rakza, T. & Abazine, A et al. (2008a). Noradrenaline for management of septic shock refractory to fluid loading and dopamine or dobutamine in full-term newborn infants. *Acta Paediatrica*, Vol. 97, No. 2, (Feb), pp. 177-180, ISSN 0803-5253

Tourneux, P. & Rakza, T. & Bouissou, A et al. (2008b). Pulmonary circulatory effects of norepinephrine in newborn infants with persistent pulmonary hypertension. *The Journal of Pediatrics*, Vol. 153, No. 3, (Sep), pp. 345-349, ISSN 0022-3476

Rodríguez-Núñez, A. & López-Herce, J. & Gil-Antón, J et al. (2006). Rescue treatment with terlipressin in children with refractory septic shock: a clinical study. *Critical Care*, Vol. 10, No. 1, (Jan 31), R20, ISSN 1364-8535

Rowland, DG. &, Gutgesell, HP. (1995). Noninvasive assessment of myocardial contractility, preload, and afterload in healthy newborn infants. *American Journal of Cardiology*,Vol. 75, No.12, (Apr 15), pp. 813-821, ISSN: 0002-9149

Rozé, JC. & Tohier, C. & Maingueneau C et.al. (1993). Response to dobutamine and dopamine in the hypotensive very preterm infant. *Archives of disease in childhood*, Vol. 69, 1 Spec No, (Jul), pp. 59-63, ISSN 0003-9888

Sassano-Higgins, S. & Friedlich, F. & Seri, I. (2011). A meta-analysis of dopamine use in hypotensive preterm infants: blood pressure and cerebral hemodynamics. *Journal of Perinatology*, Vol. 31, No. 10, (Oct 31), pp. 647-655, ISSN 0743-8346

Seri, I. (1995). Cardiovascular, renal, and endocrine actions of dopamine in neonates and children. *The Journal of Pediatrics*, Vol. 126, No. 3, (Mar), pp.333-344, ISSN 0022-3476

Seri, I. & Evans, J. (2001). Controversies in the diagnosis and management of hypotension in the newborn infant. *Current Opinion in Pediatrics*, Vol.13, No.2, (Apr), pp. 116-123, ISSN 1040-8703

Seri, I. (2006). Management of hypotension and low systemic blood flow in the very low birth weight neonate during the first postnatal week. *Journal of Perinatology*, Vol. 26, Suppl. 1, (May 26), pp. S8-S13, ISSN 0743-8346

Shiao, SY. & Ou, CN. (2007). Validation of oxygen saturation monitoring in neonates. *American Journal of Critical Care*, Vol. 16, No. 2, (Mar), pp. 168-178, ISSN 1062-3264

Skelton, R. & Gill, AB. & Parsons, JM. (1998). Reference ranges for cardiac dimensions and blood flow velocity in preterm infants. *Heart*, Vol. 80, No. 3, (Sep), pp. 281-285, ISSN 1468-201X 124, No. 1, (Jul), pp. 277-284, ISSN 0031-4005

Soleymani, S. & Cayabyab, R. & Borzage, TM et al. (2010). Comparison between charted and continuously recorded vital signs and hemodynamic data. *Annual PAS/SPR Meeting*, Vancouver, Abstract.

Stark, MJ. & Clifton, VL. & Wright, IM. (2009). Carbon monoxide is a significant mediator of cardiovascular status following preterm birth. *Pediatrics*, Vol.

Teitel, DF. & Sidi, D. (1985). Developmental changes in myocardial contractile reserve in the lamb. *Pediatric Research*, Vol. 19, No. 9, (Sep), pp. 948-955, ISSN 0031-3998

Valverde, E. & Pellicer, A. & Madero, R et al. (2006). Dopamine versus epinephrine for cardiovascular support in low birth weight infants: analysis of systemic effects and neonatal clinical outcomes. *Pediatrics*, Vol. 117, No. 6, (Jun), pp. e1213-e1222, 1098-4275

Van Hare, GF., & Hawkins, JA., & Schmidt, KG et al. (1990). The effects of increasing mean arterial pressure on left ventricular output in newborn lambs. *Circulation Research*, Vol. 67, No. 1, (Jul), pp. 78-83, ISSN 0009-7330

Van Bel, F. & Lemmers, P. & Naulaers, G. (2008). Monitoring neonatal regional cerebral oxygen saturation in clinical practice: value and pitfalls. *Neonatology*, Vol. 94, No. 4, (Sep 119), pp. 237-244, ISSN 1661-7800

Vincent, JL. (Ed.). (2009). *Critical care medicine: Churchill's ready reference*, Churchill Livingstone, pp. 12–13, ISBN 978-0080451367, Philadelphia

Watkins, AM. & West, CR. & Cooke, RW. (1989). Blood pressure and cerebral haemorrhage and ischaemia in very low birthweight infants. *Early Human Development*, Vol. 19, No. 2, (May), pp. 103-110, ISSN 0378-3782

Watterberg, KL. & Gerdes, JS. & Cole, CH et al. (2004). Prophylaxis of early adrenal insufficiency to prevent bronchopulmonary dysplasia: a multicenter trial. *Pediatrics*, Vol. 114, No.6, (Dec), pp. 1649-1657, ISSN 0031-4005

Watterberg, KL. & Shaffer, ML. & The PROPHET Study Group. (2005), Cortisol concentrations and apparent serum half-life during hydrocortisone therapy in extremely low birth weightinfants. *Pediatric academic societies annual meeting*, Vol 57, p. 1501

Watterberg, KL. & Shaffer, ML. & Mishefske, MJ et al. (2007).
Growth and neurodevelopmental outcomes after early low-
dose hydrocortisone treatment in extremelylow birth weight infants. *Pediatrics*, Vol. 120, No.1, (Jul), pp. 40-48, ISSN 0031-4005

Wong, FY. & Barfield, CP. & Horne, RS et al. (2009). Dopamine therapy promotes cerebral flow-metabolism coupling in preterm infants. *Intensive Care Medicine*, Vol. 35, No. 10, (Oct), pp. 1777-1782, ISSN 0342-4642

Wyckoff, MH. & Perlman, JM. & Laptook AR. (2005). Use of volume expansion during delivery room resuscitation in near-term and term infants. *Pediatrics*, Vol. 115, No. 4, (Apr), pp. 950-955, ISSN 0031-400

Yeh, TF. & Lin, YJ. & Lin, HC et al. (2004).
Outcomes at school age after postnatal dexamethasone therapy for lung
disease of prematurity. *The New England Journal* of *Medicine*, Vol. 350, No. 13, (Mar 25), pp. 1304-1313. ISSN 0028-4793.

Zeballos, G. & López-Herce, J. & Fernández, C et al. (2006). Rescue therapy with terlipressin by continuous infusion in a child with catecholamine-resistant septic shock. *Resuscitation*, Vol. 68, No. 1, (Jan), pp. 151-153 ISSN 0300-9572

10

Psychophysiological Cardiovascular Functioning in Hostile Defensive Women

Francisco Palmero and Cristina Guerrero

Universitat Jaume I

Spain

1. Introduction

Cardiovascular diseases are the leading causes of death and disability in the world, in both developed and developing countries, and also in both sexes. In fact one third of annual deaths worldwide are due to cardiovascular problems, according to the WHO (World Health Organization) estimated 17.3 million people died from CVDs in 2008, over 80% of CVD deaths take place in low- and middle-income countries, and by 2030, almost 23.6 million people will die from CVDs (in http://www.who.int/cardiovascular_diseases). Therefore, is a serious problem, and not only in industrialized countries, indeed, is an epidemic that not only continues but it is precisely in the developing countries, where it currently is increasing dramatically. On the other hand, prevalence and mortality from these diseases among *women* has increased in an exaggerated way. This for several reasons: first, as mentioned, in women the death rate from CVDs has increased significantly, equaling or exceeding that of the male population, so we think it is of great importance to focus on studies considering this sector only a few risk factors have also increased; second, the sample with which we had consisted mostly of women, given the characteristics of it (psychology undergraduates), which were removed the few men who participated in the study. Thus, from these data and indications, and since most studies have focused on people of both sexes or only male, we considered appropriate to carry out research with a sample of only women.

Moreover the etiology of CVD is multidimensional, that is, factors involving genetic, physiological, chemical, nutritional, environmental and psychosocial, and moreover, is not fully known. It is known that a number of cardiovascular risk factors that may contribute to the development, progression or maintenance of CVD, called "classic risk factors". Among the most important are: age, sex, cholesterol, hypertension, smoking, physical inactivity and obesity. However, surprisingly, these factors fail to explain more than 50% of the variance in predicting cardiovascular risk, whether considered independently or when considered together (Chesney, 1996; Gump & Matthews, 1999). Nevertheless a large proportion of CVDs are preventable, but they continue to increase mainly because preventive measures are inadequate.

Therefore, research about this topic has been long and extensive, especially directed to seek and discover other factors, beyond the "classics", are also contributing to the development

CVD (Brydon et al., 2010; Chida & Steptoe, 2009; Everson-Rose & Lewis, 2005; Jorgensen & Kolodziej, 2007; Vella & Friedman, 2009). We refer to *psychosocial factors*. Thus, the relationship between different psychosocial variables and the risk of CVD has been studied extensively since the mid past century, mainly for these two reasons.

2. Psychosocial risk factors and cardiovascular disease

In the search and exploration for other risk factors that may explain the etiology of CVD, psychosocial factors have gained importance to such an extent that research has been able to explain the mechanisms of action of these variables on CVD. The results obtained in various research studies have confirmed the relationship between psychosocial factors and the atheromatous plaque, which constitutes the basic injury occurring in CVD (Kaplan, et al, 1983; Kaplan, et al, 1987; Manuck, et al, 1983; Manuck, Kaplan & Matthews, 1986; Manuck, et al, 1989; Jennings, et al, 2004; Vale, 2005). The mechanisms involved in its formation, which are mechanical and chemical factors are seriously affected by psychosocial processes, and especially by the stress response. In these processes, emotions cause a faster heart rate and higher blood pressure, leading to increased blood flow and turbulence. In addition, there is a mobilization of lipids which exceeds the body's metabolic requirements, and which facilitates aggregation to artery walls and heart tissue. This relationship between psychosocial factors and CVD has received the generic name of "Hypothesis of the cardiovascular reactivity", and has been supported by various prospective studies (Keys & Taylor, 1971; Schiffer, et al, 1976; Manuck, et al, 1992; Steptoe, et al, 2000).

To date, research has shown that individuals who tend to display strong responses and reactivity are at increased risk of CVD (Manuck et al., 1992; Palmero et al., 2006; Treiber, et al, 2003; Matthews, et al, 2006). The argument that defends this refers to the stereotype response: if the cardiovascular reactivity is a characteristic of an individual and is physiological stable and consistent, then the same response patterns will be seen every time the individual is faced with a situation of stress. Evidently with certain limitations, laboratory situations can be regarded as a procedure that provides information on an individual's physiological functioning in real life (Allen, et al, 1987; Allen & Matthews, 1997; Palmero, et al, 2002; Moseley & Linden, 2006; Palmero, et al, 2007). Thus individuals, whose pattern of cardiovascular functioning is characterized by the expression of exaggerated responses, are those who, with time, are likely to experience some cardiovascular dysfunction (Everson, et al, 1996; Markovitz, et al, 1998; Strike, et al, 2003). Given this relationship between excessive cardiovascular response and CVD, research efforts have focused on finding any variable causing an increase in such responses as this will mean an increase in the likelihood of suffering from one of these diseases.

From the study on the classic Type A behavior pattern through the anger-hostility complex and hostility were conducted, in recent years, research has focused on the *defensive hostility* (high hostility and high defensiveness) as a risk factor in CVD (Guerrero & Palmero, 2010; Helmers & Krantz, 1996; Jamner, et al, 1991; Larson & Langer, 1997; Shapiro, et al, 1995; Palmero, et al, 2007; Vella & Friedman, 2007). The trait of defensive hostility reflects an approach–avoid conflict between the desire for social approval and distrust of those who can provide such support, and currently can be considered as one of the psychosocial factors with more weight and empirical support in its relationship with CVD.

Several studies of CVD patients demonstrate that subjects with high scores in defensive hostility show higher rates of ischemia during a mental stress situation, greater damage by infusion and a longer duration of ischemia during daily activities (Helmers, et al, 1995). As well, a field study conducted with paramedics showed a higher cardiac response by people with a high hostility defensive when they deal with stress situations (Jamner, et al, 1991). These results, usually obtained from real situations, appear to be supported by laboratory studies (Jorgensen, et al, 1995; Shapiro, et al, 1995; Helmers & Krantz, 1996; Larson & Langer, 1997; Palmero et al., 2002; Palmero et al., 2007), which indicates the existence of a subgroup of people who are characterized by high "Defensive Hostility" (DH), as well as a greater cardiovascular response. In general, DH individuals show greater cardiovascular response during the task phase that other groups can be formed when combining hostility and defensiveness variables (Larson & Langer, 1997). And, unlike this group, find another subgroup which is characterized by low hostility and low defensiveness and show a lower cardiovascular response -low risk group-.

However as these studies show, various inconsistencies were also found, which originated, at least in part, from the different tasks used to measure the cardiovascular variables. These results suggest the relevance of broadening the research spectrum whose aim it is to strengthen the association between psychological variables and cardiovascular response from the understanding that the exaggerated response would be the link between these and CVD. In other words, it seems appropriate to establish whether defensive hostility can be seen as the toxic component in relation to CVD.

Therefore, the *general objective* pursued with this study refers to the delimitation of the effects of defensive hostility on cardiovascular response in women, in a real stress situation. Specifically, exploring the relationship between defensive hostility, which is a better predictor than hostility alone, and cardiovascular responses (HR, SBP and DBP) in this tonic dimension. That is, considering all three phases of the experiment (adaptation: A, task: T and recovery: R) to establish the significance of the functional psychophysiological profiles in the four experimental groups (DH: high hostility-high defensiveness, HH: high hostility-low defensiveness, Def: low hostility-high defensiveness, LH: low hostility-low defensiveness).

From these premises and the proposed main objective has been carried out this research with the ultimate aim to contribute both to the development of the theoretical basis on psychosocial variables that can be considered as cardiovascular risk factors and its subsequent application in clinical practice as well as contribute to methodological development in the field of psychophysiological research.

The *general hypothesis* suggests that individuals with high scores in defensive hostility display the highest values with the psychophysiological variables. Specifically, we expect that these individuals show the greatest average values recorded in the variables (HR, SBP and DBP), and in all the phases of the experiment (A, T and R), compared to those shown by the individuals of the other three groups. In addition, DH group will be characterized by less adaptive psychophysiological profile.

3. Empirical study

3.1 Study design

In this section we show data from a recent study published by the authors (Guerrero and Palmero, 2010). One hundred and thirty female students from a *Universitat Jaume I* participated in this research. The mean age of the participants was 20.34 years (*SD*=2.06). The criteria to form the groups were the scores obtained with both the Ho Inventory (Cook & Medley, 1954) and the Social Desirability Questionnaire (Crowne & Marlowe, 1960). We used the median as the cut-off point to classify participants as "high" or "low" in each variable, thus the sample was composed as follows: 30 Defensive Hostility (DH), 40 High Hostility (HH), 42 Defensive (Def), and 18 Low Hostility (LH).

3.2 Instrumentation

Cardiovascular responses were measured with the registration system Biopac MP150 with NIBP module 100A, both were connected to a personal computer to monitor and store all the responses. Specifically, this registration system was used to measure the physiological responses: heart rate, systolic blood pressure and diastolic blood pressure. Also, this system recorded these cardiovascular parameters continuously and noninvasively.

Hostility was measured with the Hostility Inventory of Cook and Medley (1954), specifically the Composite Hostility Score (Chost) consisting in three subscales: cynicism, hostile feelings and aggressive responses. In previous studies, this information led to a scale being provided with a greater ability to predict the response and cardiovascular reactivity in comparison with the Ho scale provided as a whole (Barefoot et al., 1989; Christensen & Smith, 1993; Guerrero, 2008).

Defensiveness was measured with the Spanish version (Ávila & Tomé, 1989) of the Social Desirability Questionnaire of Crowne and Marlowe (1960). It consists of 33 items of choice alternatives (true or false) that reflect socially desirable behaviors and cognitions.

Also, reports and self-reports were also used to collect some data on behavioral habits related to health issues, and various personal and socio-demographic data.

3.3 Study procedure

A real academic exam was used as a situation of stress. More specifically, we used an exam of the degree of Psychology; this situation represents a real mental stress task for students.

Data were collected individually in one session. Following informed consent, each subject completed a questionnaire of demographics, previous medical history and noted any medication. Then, they went into the experimental cabin where they were asked to sit comfortably in an armchair and a sensor was connected to their non dominant wrist. From this time onward, both instructions and exam questions were submitted through the projector.

Following this registration session, it was necessary to remove the sensors and to go to another room to complete the corresponding scales. Finally, they were thanked for their collaboration and left.

The recording session consisted in three phases: adaptation (A), task (T) and recovery (R), with duration of 10, 20 and 10 minutes, respectively.

a. *Adaptation phase* (10 min): there was no stimulus. The purpose of this period was for participants to become familiar with the environment. The psychophysiological variables were recorded in their tonic dimension to establish baseline levels with the aim of obtaining the participants' usual levels under rest conditions.

b. *Task phase* (20 min): the 20 stimuli that formed the experimental task were presented: an objective test of 20 questions with four alternative answers. The stimuli were separated by a one-minute period, and the duration of this phase was therefore 20 minutes. This phase was considered an overall stressful period, and its variables were recorded in their phasic dimension.

c. *Recovery phase* (10 min): no stimulus was presented. The variables were considered in their tonic dimension to see how these variables recovered their usual levels after the stress situation. These data allow us to ascertain how long the organism needs to achieve its usual values following a situation of stress. This is extremely relevant when considering the consequences caused by the stress situation from a neuroendocrinological viewpoint because the greater the time needed by the organism to recover its baseline levels, the greater the exposure to the effects of substances released by the organism because of this situation of stress (catecolamnines and cortisol).

3.4 Statistical analysis

The first approaches were the descriptive analysis and correlations, and an analysis of variance (ANOVA) was carried out for a more detailed analysis of the results. Then, according to the main objective, that of analyzing the relationship between defensive hostility and the cardiovascular responses to study the functional significance of each group's profiles during all three phases, namely in their tonic dimension, an ANOVA was carried out whose design was 4 groups (DH, HH, LH and Def) x 3 phases (adaptation, task and recovery) with repeated measures for the phase variable. Subsequently, a univariate analysis of variance has been conducted for each phase to obtain a more accurate description of the potential differences encountered should such differences be given from the post hoc Tukey test with which the groups involved in them will be determined.

3.5 Study results

Data will be presented in the following figures, which reflect the psychophysiological profiles obtained from analysis of data for each physiological variable separately.

Although, before that, we like to refer to the profiles described by Kelsey (1993) on which we relied. There are different ways to respond physiologically to stressful events, which depends on external factors (situational) and internal factors (personality variables). In this regard, and from the classic proposal Kelsey, we noted three response patterns, which reflect corresponding profiles associated with different forms of reaction to stressful events: *habituation, sensitization* and support or *constant*.

-   Habituation.

When you perceive a situation as potentially threatening or novel, occurs an increase in cardiovascular reactivity. After an exposure time in such a situation, and after that initial increase, there is a phenomenon of habituation, during which we see a progressive decrease of the initial values. This phenomenon is considered essential in the process of adaptation and regulation of humans and lower animals, demonstrating the ability to self-regulatory organism, that is, it can be activate to deal with a potentially dangerous or threatening situation and, in turn, is able to return to baseline (BL) once the situation has gone or is under control.

- Sensitization.

In this case, the individual responds to an agent or stressor stimulus with a high cardiovascular reactivity (the phenomenon of sensitization), similar to the previous pattern but without habituation occur. Instead, it produces a progressive increase in reactivity over the situation. It shows a organism's inability to return to baseline, which is highly detrimental to the heart muscle and overall health.

- Constant.

In this third pattern occurs an initial increase, similar to that of the other two patterns, but no habituation or sensitization occurs. This increase remains constant throughout the stress. Thus, this pattern is also maladaptive; since there is no preparation behavior is essential in the adaptation to the environment (Cannon, 1932) or has the ability to return to baseline levels.

From these profiles is observed that only the first is adaptive, decreasing when the individual cardiovascular reactivity to stressful events faced long periods of time. On the one hand, the initial increase in activation allows for better coping with the situation and the subsequent decline after a period of time, it is necessary to avoid damaging the body and maintain homeostasis (Palmero, Breva, et al., 1994; Palmero, Espinosa et al., 1995).

Concerning *heart rate* in Figure 1 shows the obtained profiles by different groups.

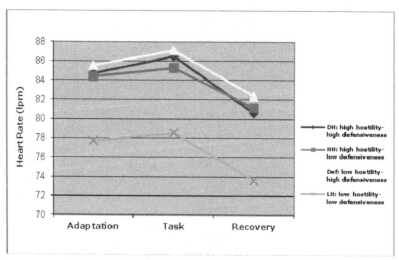

Fig. 1. Heart rate and defensive hostility during three phases.

As for the functional significance of the various profiles, as seen in Figure 1, all groups show the habituation trend, so profiles are adaptive. Although, LH group shows the more adaptive pattern, as it presents a greater and faster recovery to their baseline levels.

Concerning to *systolic blood pressure* as seen in Figure 2, all groups show the habituation trend. Again, LH group presents a more adaptive pattern, with lower values in the recovery phase.

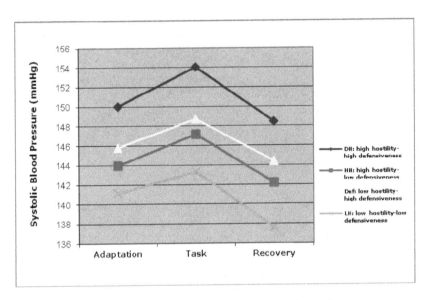

Fig. 2. Systolic blood pressure and defensive hostility during three phases.

Here we also find that DH is the group that obtained the greatest values in systolic pressure in all three phases.

An additional interesting fact is the effect of variable defensiveness, although the difference was not statistically significant, we see that the two groups with high defensiveness, DH and Def, presented the higher SBP values in all three phases (A, T and R)

Concerning *diastolic blood* pressure as seen in Figure 3, all groups show the habituation trend, and again LH group presents a more adaptive pattern.

Again, we see that DH is the group that shows the highest values in all three phases. In this case also notes the effect of variable defensiveness, although neither are statistically significant differences. Two groups with high defensiveness, DH and Def, presented the higher DBP values, but only in adaptation and task phases.

Figure 2 and 3 demonstrate clear differences between SBP and DBP between the psychophysiological patters of extreme groups: DH presents higher values than LH group. And the other two groups are in an intermediate position, with values very similar among them and throughout the three phases.

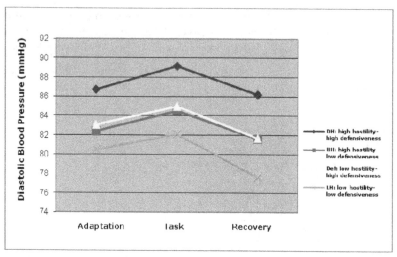

Fig. 3. Diastolic blood pressure and defensive hostility during three phases.

4. Conclusion

In general, the DH group presented higher values for the cardiovascular variables during the three phases, as well as a slow recovery. Thus, we believe that *defensive hostility* has proved to be a more appropriate criterion than hostility alone when determining the possible risk of cardiovascular dysfunction.

So, consistent with our main objective, and in relation to establishing the functional significance of the general profiles in the four groups through considering the three experiment phases, our results are in the expected direction. Specifically, the DH group obtains the highest values in the three phases and variables, particularly in the blood pressure index. Additionally, extending the findings available to therefore include the recovery phase, we have found that this group of individuals takes longer to recover after a stress situation, that is, they score the highest values encountered during the recovery phase.

About the *cardiovascular parameters*, the three most commonly used in these studies were HR, SBP and DBP (Swain & Suls, 1996), to combine the criteria and to enhance the comparison between different results from various research studies. All the parameters have been captured, recorded, stored and analyzed in a highly reliable, non invasive and continuous manner, which is especially relevant in the case of blood pressure. They are easily accessible and provide us with highly reliable information on cardiac and vascular functioning over different time periods, that is, to reflect the changing psychophysiology profile of individuals at all times.

Among these parameters, we note blood pressure reflects the greatest differences between the two extreme groups (DH and LH): introducing a greater response, activation and recovery for the DH group. On the other hand, HR reveals a clear difference in the lowest values submitted by the low-risk group (LH) compared to a more homogeneous response from the other three groups in all the phases. So, we suggest that the cardiovascular functioning of hostile defensive individuals in such situations is best reflected through blood pressure, specifically through diastolic pressure, an index which seems to appear truer for the recovery phase, as reflected by the significant differences found between the two extreme groups.

More specifically, showing each cardiovascular physiological variable separately, the following was observed.

Regarding the *HR*, although there is no effect of interaction between hostility and defensiveness, since the group HD presents values very similar to those groups HH and Def, HR shows how the low-risk group, LH , presents the lowest values along the three phases compared to the other groups.

We must also emphasize for the three groups with higher levels in HR, which is the group Def -although differences are not statistically significant- which presents the highest levels in all three phases, reflecting a major effect of the variable defensiveness, specifically in the adaptation and task phases where groups with high defensiveness (DH and Def) show the highest levels.

Our data also specifies that it is in the recovery phase where there are statistically significant differences between the Def group and the LH group.

Regarding the *SBP*, beside show the effect of interaction between hostility and defensiveness, a fact that reflects the important values of the DH group, the main effect of the defensiveness variable also exist in three phases, which means that subjects with high scores in defensiveness obtain higher values than subjects with low scores in defensiveness.

In addition, our data indicate that statistically significant differences that exist between DH and LH groups are specifically at the task and the recovery phases, in turn, indicates that there are no differences between groups with respect to their baseline levels.

The fact that the DH group presents higher scores for these values, leads us to suggest that defensive hostility rather than hostility alone better predicts the cardiovascular function in situations of stress.

Regarding the *DBP*, it seems that the real meaning of this variable can be seen only with the consideration of defensive hostility, such as denoting the effects of interaction in all three phases. Like the previous case, our data indicate that statistically significant differences also exist between DH and Def groups, but in this case appear in the recovery phase. There was also a main effect of the defensiveness variable, but is almost imperceptible.

Regarding the *functionality of the profiles* all four groups in three variables were adaptive. But in blood pressure case, it seems interesting to note that while the four groups that tend to indicate profiles of habituation, the fact that the individuals' defensive hostile obtains these statistically significant values during the recovery phase means that this group of individuals takes significantly longer to return to the baseline values of situations without stress. Thus, the profile of hostile defensive subjects would be less adaptive, because in this group the recovery is more slow and gradual. The profiles of the three remaining groups are adaptive, with a faster recovery.

Specifically, in our view, while DBP continues the pattern of other variables during the task, and displays an interaction effect between hostility and defensiveness, it is the most important variable to detect the cardiovascular functioning of hostile defensive individuals in the recovery phase. Once again, these arguments lead us to suggest that it is desirable to consider this variable, along with the inclusion of the recovery phase.

In short, along with the results corresponding to the tonic dimension of the cardiovascular variables being studied, it appears that *defensive hostility* is more appropriate than hostility alone to understand cardiovascular functioning in stressful situations. So, defensive hostility identifies a dimension of personality that, ultimately, would be a better predictor of the cardiovascular response in particular and of cardiovascular disease in general. It would be more fitting than hostility alone to explain and understand cardiovascular functioning in stressful situations.

The DH group, which shows that those individuals with high scores in hostility and high scores in defensiveness, are those who reflect the highest values in activation and cardiovascular response, but only when faced with the demands of a challenging task. For this reason, and as we have pointed out, it seems appropriate to use a real situation of stress as an experimental task because this specific environment is the best scenario to see the psychophysiological response style that characterizes the individuals being studied. In addition, if the situation of stress is sufficiently long, there is also the possibility of locating the adjustment mechanism of individuals to the sustained demands of this stressful activity. Those hostile individuals seeking to perform an action that is not disagreeable to others display the greatest difficulty in controlling their hostile experiences. The result of this inability to properly monitor hostility experiences produces a sustained increase in the activation of the sympathetic system which, in turn, gives rise to significant increases in the cardiovascular variables studied: HR, SBP and DBP. One particular sensitivity of the SBP is to capture this sympathetic activation which suggests its suitability differential in such studies.

Thus, these findings show the relationship between defensive hostility and cardiovascular functioning in situations of stress by the various cardiovascular register indexes (HR, SBP and DBP) and by considering the various parameters analyzed, namely response, activation and cardiovascular recovery, have been demonstrated. As mentioned above, we believe that defensive hostility has proved to be a more appropriate criterion than hostility alone when determining the possible risk of cardiovascular dysfunction.

Regarding the three *experimental phases*, we can state the following. About the *recovery phase*, we think that its inclusion in the experimental research laboratory is especially important since it provides vital information on restoring physiological parameters. This phase is a basic and essential element in the detection of the possible risks of future dysfunctions (Guerrero & Palmero, 2006). As seen, the recovery phase profile in the DH group has shown a slower recovery, especially in terms of blood pressure, and more specifically in DBP. Thus, the inclusion of the recovery phase in this type of experimental laboratory, it constitutes a basic and essential element in the detection of possible risks of future dysfunctions. From a neuroendocrinological viewpoint, it is important to consider the consequences caused by the situation since the more time the organism needs to recover the baseline levels, the greater the exposure to the effects of the substances released (catecholamines and cortisol).

About the *task phase*, by considering the *duration* parameter, which is scarcely taken into account in such research, we believe it appropriate to propose an experimental task that is long enough to establish a genuine cardiovascular functioning, that is more likely to be correct, by appreciating how the adjustment to a stressful situation is produced, or not. The fact that short or moderately long tasks have been systematically used may have masked the dysfunctional connotations of the response profiles in the different groups.

Regarding the *tasks* used as a stressful situation in the laboratory, the importance of creating and using a type of task that involves a real stress situation must be highlighted, that is, one as close as possible to everyday situations. Thus, one can understand some of the inconsistencies found which, in turn, provide the ecological laboratory experiments in this field with more validity. In this respect, we believe that the task used in this research, a real exam, is a task with connotations of personal and social threats, which also requires investing considerable effort to be able to deal with it actively and successfully, and this has been reflected by the significant differences obtained in the three experiment phases.

Concluding, in our modest opinion, with this and other research we have conducted we provide more empirical support about the great relevance within the theoretical framework on DH as a possible psychosocial cardiovascular risk factor also in women. However, as a future research direction, probable variability among females as compared to males necessitates concentrated research in this area, and we recognize the need for separate data analysis for males. Also, the study should be replicate with other samples to see if there are similar results and generalize these obtained data.

5. References

Allen, M.T. & Matthews, K.A. (1997). Hemodynamic responses to laboratory stressors in children and adolescents: The influences of age, race, and gender. *Psychophysiology*, 34, 329-339.

Allen, M.T., Sherwood, A., Obrist, P.A., Crowell, M.D., & Grange, L.A. (1987). Stability of cardiovascular reactivity to laboratory stressors: A 2 ½ year follow-up. *Journal of Psychosomatic Research*, 31, 639-645.

Brydon L., Strike P.C., Bhattacharyya M.R., Whitehead D.L., McEwan J., Zachary I., and Steptoe A. (2010). Hostility and physiological responses to laboratory stress in acute coronary syndrome patients. *J Psychosom Res*, 68 (2), 109-116.

Cannon, W.B. (1932). *The wisdom of the body.* New York: Norton.

Chida Y. and Steptoe A. (2009). The Association of Anger and Hostility with Future Coronary Heart Disease. A Meta-Analytic Review of Prospective Evidence. *J Am Coll Cardiol*, 53 (11), 936-946.

Cook, W.W. & Medley, D.M. (1954). Proposed hostility and pharisaic-virtue scales for the MMPI. *Journal of Applied Psychology*, 38, 414-418.

Crowne, D. P. & Marlowe, D. (1960). A new scale of social desirability independent of psychopathology. *Journal of Consulting Psychology*, 24 (4), 349-354.

Chesney, M.A. (1996). New behavioral risk factors for coronary heart disease: Implications for intervention. In K. Orth-Gomer y N. Schneiderman (eds.): *Behavioral Medicine Approaches to Cardiovascular Disease Prevention* (pp. 169-182). Mahwah, NJ: Erlbaum.

Everson, S.A., Kaplan, G.A., Goldberg, D.E., & Salonen, J.T. (1996). Anticipatory blood pressure response to exercise predicts future high blood pressure in middle-aged men. *Hypertension, 27,* 1059-1064.

Everson-Rose, S.A.; Lewis, T.T. (2005). Psychosocial factors and cardiovascular diseases. *Annual Review of Public Health, 26,* 469-500.

Guerrero, C., and Palmero, F. (2006). Percepción de control y respuestas cardiovasculares. *International Journal of Cliniccal and Health Psychology, 6* (1), 145-168.

Guerrero, C. (2008). Metodología en psicofisiología cardiovascular: procedimiento alternativo para la medición de la reactividad y su relación con la hostilidad defensiva. Tesis doctoral publicada. Universitat Jaume I, Castellón. En http://www.tesisenxarxa.net/TDX- 0206108-131614/index.html.

Guerrero, C., and Palmero, F. (2010). Impact of defensive hostility in cardiovascular disease. *Behavioral Medicine, 36* (3), 77-84.

Gump, B.B. &Matthews, K.A. (1999). Do background stressors influence reactivity to and recovery from acute stressors? *Journal of Applied Social Psychology, 29,* 469-494.

Helmers, K. F., Krantz, D. S., Merz, C. N. B., Klein, J., Kop, W. J., Gottdiener, J.S., & Rozanzki, A. (1995). Defensive hostility: Relationship to multiple markers of cardiac ischemia in patients with coronary disease. *Health Psychology, 14,* 202-209.

Helmers, K.F. & Krantz, D.S. (1996). Defensive hostility, gender and cardiovascular levels and responses to stress. *Annals of Behavioral Medicine, 18,* 246-254.

Jamner, L.D., Shapiro, D. Goldstein, I.B., & Hug, R. (1991). Ambulatory blood pressure and heart rate in paramedics: Effects of cynical hostility and defensiveness. *Psychosomatic Medicine, 51,* 285-289.

Jennings, J.R., Kamarck, T.W., Everson-Rose, S.A., Kaplan, G.A., Manuck, S.B., & Salonen, J.T. (2004). Exaggerated blood pressure responses during mental stress are prospectively related to enhanced carotid atherosclerosis in middle-aged Finnish men. *Circulation, 110*: 2198–2203.

Jorgensen, R.S.; Abdul-Karim, K.; Kahan, T.A., & Frankowsi, J.J. (1995). Defensiveness, cynical hostility and cardiovascular reactivity: A moderator analysis. *Psychotherapy and Psychosomatics, 64(3-4),* 156-161.

Jorgensen, R.S., and Kolodziej, M.E. (2007). Suppressed anger, evaluative threat, and cardiovascular reactivity: a tripartite profile approach. *International Journal of Psychophysiology, 66(2),* 102-8.

Kaplan, J.R., Manuck, S.B., Adams, M.R., Weingand, K.W., & Clarkson, T. B. (1987). Inhibition of coronary atherosclerosis by propanolol in behaviorally predisposed monkeys fed an atherogenic diet. *Circulation, 76,* 1364-1372.

Kaplan, J.R., Manuck, S.B., Clarkson, T.B., Lusso, F.M., Taub, D.M., & Miller, E.W. (1983). Social stress and atherosclerosis in normocholesterolemic monkeys. *Science, 220,* 733-735.

Keys, A. & Taylor, H.L. (1971). Mortality and coronary heart disease among men studied for 23 years. *Archives of Internal Medicine, 128,* 201-214.

Larson, MR. & Langer, AW. (1997). Defensive hostility and anger expression: relationship to additional heart rate reactivity during active coping. *Psychophysiology, 34,* 177-184.

Manuck, S.B., Kaplan, J.R., & Clarkson, T.B. (1983). Behaviorally induced heart rate reactivity and atherosclerosis in cynomolgus monkeys. *Psychosomatic Medicine, 45,* 95-108.

Manuck, S.B., Kaplan, J.R., & Matthews, K.A. (1986). Behavioral antecedents of coronary heart disease and atherosclerosis. *Arteriosclerosis, 7,* 485-491.

Manuck, S.B., Kaplan, J.R., Adams, M.R., & Clarkson, T.B. (1989). Behavioral elicited heart rate reactivity and atherosclerosis in female cynomolgus monkeys. *Psychosomatic Medicine, 51,* 306-318.

Manuck, S.B., Olsson, G., Hjemdahl, P., & Rehnqvist, N. (1992). Does cardiovascular reactivity to mental stress have prognostic value in postinfarction patients? A pilot study. *Psychosomatic Medicine, 54,* 102-108.

Markovitz, J.H., Raczynski, J.M., Wallace, D., Chettur, V., & Chesney, M.A. (1998). Cardiovascular reactivity to video game predicts subsequent blood pressure increases in young men: The CARDIA study. *Psychosomatic Medicine, 60,* 186-191.

Matthews, K.A., Zhu, S., Tucker, D.C, & Whooley, M.A. (2006). Blood pressure reactivity to psychological stress and coronary calcification in the coronary artery risk development in young adults study. *Hypertension, 47*(3): 391-395.

Mente, A. & Helmers, K.F. (1999). Defensive hostility and cardiovascular response to stress in young men. *Personality and Individual Differences, 27*(4), 683-694.

Moseley, J.V. & Linden, W. (2006). Predicting blood pressure and heart rate change with cardiovascular reactivity and recovery: results from 3-year and 10-year follow up. *Psychosomatic Medicine, 68:* 833-843.

Palmero, F., Guerrero, C., Gómez, C. y Carpi, A. (2006). Certezas y controversias en el estudio de la emoción. *Revista Electrónica de Motivación y Emoción, 9,* 23-24. *Psychosomatic Medicine, 68:* 833-843.

Palmero, F., Breva, A. & Landeta, O. (2002). Hostilidad defensiva y reactividad cardiovascular en una situación de estrés real. *Ansiedad y Estrés, 8*(2-3), 115-142.

Palmero, F., Iñiguez, C., Guerrero, C., Carpi, A., Díez, J.L. & Diago, J.L. (2007). Hostilidad, psicofisiología y salud cardiovascular. *Avances de Psicología Latinoamérica. Colombia,* 25 (1), 22-43.

Schiffer, F., Hartley, L.H., Schulman, C.L., & Abelmann, W.H. (1976). The quiz electrocardiogram: A new diagnostic and research technique for evaluating the relation between emotional stress and ischemic heart disease. *American Journal of Cardiology, 37,* 41-47.

Shapiro, D., Goldstein, I.B., & Jamner, L.D. (1995). Effects of anger/hostility, defensiveness, gender, and family history of hypertension on cardiovascular reactivity. *Psychophysiology, 32,* 425-435.

Steptoe, A., Cropley, M., & Joekes, K. (2000). Task demands and the pressures of everyday life: Associations between cardiovascular reactivity and work blood pressure and heart rate. *Health Psychology, 19,* 46-54.

Strike, P.C., Magid, K., Brydon L., Edwards, S., McEwan, J.R., & Steptoe, A. (2003). Exaggerated platelet and hemodynamic reactivity to mental stress in men with coronary artery disease. *Psychosomatic Medicine, 66:* 492–500.

Swain, A., & Suls, J. (1996). Reproducibility of blood pressure and heart rate reactivity: A meta-analysis. *Psychophysiology, 33,* 162-174.

Treiber, F.A., Kamarck, T., Schneiderman, N., Sheffield, D., Kapuku, G, & Taylor, T. (2003). Cardiovascular Reactivity and Development of Preclinical and Clinical Disease States. *Psychosomatic Medicine, 65,* 46-62.

Vale, S. (2005). Psychosocial stress and cardiovascular diseases. *Postgraduate Medical Journal, 81,* 429-435.

Vella, E.J. (2003). *Autonomic Characteristics of Defensive Hostility: Reactivity and Recovery to Active and Passive Stressors.* Published thesis. Blacksburg, Virginia.

Vella, E.J. y Friedman, B.H. (2007). Autonomic characteristics of defensive hostility: Reactivity and recovery to active and passive stressors. *International Journal of Psychophysiology, 66,* 95-101.

Vella, E.J., and Friedman, B.H. (2009). Hostility and anger-in: Cardiovascular reactivity and recovery to mental arithmetic stress. *Int J Psychophysiol, 72,* 253-259.

Permissions

The contributors of this book come from diverse backgrounds, making this book a truly international effort. This book will bring forth new frontiers with its revolutionizing research information and detailed analysis of the nascent developments around the world.

We would like to thank David C. Gaze, for lending his expertise to make the book truly unique. He has played a crucial role in the development of this book. Without his invaluable contribution this book wouldn't have been possible. He has made vital efforts to compile up to date information on the varied aspects of this subject to make this book a valuable addition to the collection of many professionals and students.

This book was conceptualized with the vision of imparting up-to-date information and advanced data in this field. To ensure the same, a matchless editorial board was set up. Every individual on the board went through rigorous rounds of assessment to prove their worth. After which they invested a large part of their time researching and compiling the most relevant data for our readers. Conferences and sessions were held from time to time between the editorial board and the contributing authors to present the data in the most comprehensible form. The editorial team has worked tirelessly to provide valuable and valid information to help people across the globe.

Every chapter published in this book has been scrutinized by our experts. Their significance has been extensively debated. The topics covered herein carry significant findings which will fuel the growth of the discipline. They may even be implemented as practical applications or may be referred to as a beginning point for another development. Chapters in this book were first published by InTech; hereby published with permission under the Creative Commons Attribution License or equivalent.

The editorial board has been involved in producing this book since its inception. They have spent rigorous hours researching and exploring the diverse topics which have resulted in the successful publishing of this book. They have passed on their knowledge of decades through this book. To expedite this challenging task, the publisher supported the team at every step. A small team of assistant editors was also appointed to further simplify the editing procedure and attain best results for the readers.

Our editorial team has been hand-picked from every corner of the world. Their multi-ethnicity adds dynamic inputs to the discussions which result in innovative outcomes. These outcomes are then further discussed with the researchers and contributors who give their valuable feedback and opinion regarding the same. The feedback is then collaborated with the researches and they are edited in a comprehensive manner to aid the understanding of the subject.

Apart from the editorial board, the designing team has also invested a significant amount of their time in understanding the subject and creating the most relevant covers. They scrutinized every image to scout for the most suitable representation of the subject and create an appropriate cover for the book.

The publishing team has been involved in this book since its early stages. They were actively engaged in every process, be it collecting the data, connecting with the contributors or procuring relevant information. The team has been an ardent support to the editorial, designing and production team. Their endless efforts to recruit the best for this project, has resulted in the accomplishment of this book. They are a veteran in the field of academics and their pool of knowledge is as vast as their experience in printing. Their expertise and guidance has proved useful at every step. Their uncompromising quality standards have made this book an exceptional effort. Their encouragement from time to time has been an inspiration for everyone.

The publisher and the editorial board hope that this book will prove to be a valuable piece of knowledge for researchers, students, practitioners and scholars across the globe.

List of Contributors

Raul A. Martins
University of Coimbra, Faculty of Sport Science and Physical Education, Portugal

Michihiro Suwa
Department of Cardiology, Hokusetsu General Hospital, Takatsuki, Osaka, Japan

Reza Amani and Nasrin Sharifi
Ahvaz Jondishapour University of Medical Sciences, Iran

Tassadit Benaissa and Angela Tesse
INSERM, UMR 915, Institut de recherche thérapeutique (IRT), Nantes, France

Thierry Ragot
CNRS, UMR 8203, Institut de Cancérologie Gustave Roussy, Villejuif, France

Servy Amandine, Jones Meriem and Valeyrie-Allanore Laurence
Department of Dermatology, Hôpital Henri Mondor, Créteil, France

Steve Ogbonnia
Department of Pharmacognosy, University of Lagos, Lagos, Nigeria

G.P. Arutyunov and N.A. Bylova
The Russian State Medical University (RSMU), Russia

Ana Olga Mocumbi
National Health Institute & University Eduardo Mondlane, Mozambique

Shoichi Ezaki and Masanori Tamura
Division of Neonatal Medicine, Center for Maternal, Fetal and Neonatal Medicine, Saitama Medical Center, Saitama Medical University, Japan

Francisco Palmero and Cristina Guerrero
Universitat Jaume I, Spain

Printed in the USA
CPSIA information can be obtained
at www.ICGtesting.com
JSHW011420221024
72173JS00004B/613